Handbook of Clinical Chiropractic Care

Second Editio

Lawrence H. Wyatt, DC, DACBR, FICC

Professor
Division of Clinical Sciences
Texas Chiropractic College
Pasadena, Texas

JONES AND BARTLETT PUBLISHERS
Sudbury, Massachusetts
BOSTON TORONTO LONDON SINGAPORE

World Headquarters
Jones and Bartlett Publishers
40 Tall Pine Drive
Sudbury, MA 01776
978-443-5000
info@jbpub.com
www.jbpub.com

Jones and Bartlett Publishers
Canada
6339 Ormindale Way
Mississauga, ON L5V 1J2
CANADA

Jones and Bartlett Publishers
International
Barb House, Barb Mews
London W6 7PA
UK

Library of Congress Cataloging-in-Publication Data
Wyatt, Lawrence H.
Handbook of clinical chiropractic care / Lawrence H. Wyatt.
p. ; cm.
Includes bibliographical references and index.
ISBN 0-7637-3249-4 (pbk.)
1. Chiropractic—Handbooks, manuals, etc.
[DNLM: 1. Manipulation, Chiropractic—Handbooks. 2. Chiropractic—Handbooks. WB 39 W975h 2004] I. Title.
RZ242.9.W93 2004
615.5'34—dc22
6048 2004006402

ISBN-13: 978-0-7637-3249-3
ISBN-10: 0-7637-3249-4

Production Credits
Executive Editor: Jack Bruggeman
Production Manager: Amy Rose
Associate Production Editor: Tracey Chapman
Editorial Assistant: Kylah McNeill
Marketing Manager: Ed McKenna
V.P., Manufacturing and Inventory Control: Therese Connell
Composition: ATLIS Graphics
Cover Design: Diana Coe
Printing and Binding: Malloy, Inc.
Cover Printing: Malloy, Inc.

Printed in the United States of America
10 09 08 07 06 10 9 8 7 6 5 4 3 2

Dedication

To my son, Cole Kenneth Wyatt
You are my rainbow and I love you

My Rainbow

In every life, a miracle arrives
A gift sent from heaven above.
Mine is a rainbow, a brand new life
Graced by unconditional love.

A million adventures for you await
But none as important as these.
Learn how to give and to create
Of comfort, a provider be.

I pray the Lord will keep you safe
And ever questioning why.
Marveling at the beauty of life
And why stars fill an evening sky.

Do not regret your choices, my son
Be they good or bad, you'll see.
Lessons taught are not undone
If we learn, we'll better be.

I wish you peace in every way
That indifference may pass you by.
Fear not the future and live for the day
When you are a better man than I.

Someday I will leave and forever be gone
To be in heaven with a watchful eye.
But never forget that my love lives on
Until we're together again on high.

LHW (Dad)
December 2002

Contributors

Connie D'Astolfo, DC
Staff Chiropractor and Co-Director of Pain Management
Tendercare Living Centre
Toronto, Ontario, Canada

Randy J. Ferrance, DC, MD
Hospitalist: Internal Medicine and Pediatrics
Riverside Tappahannock Hospital
Tappahannock, VA

Timothy A. Mirtz, DC, MSE, CHES
Graduate Student
Department of Health, Sport, and Exercise Science
University of Kansas
Lawrence, KS

Stephen M. Perle, DC, MS
Associate Professor of Clinical Services—College of Chiropractic
Adjunct Professor of Mechanical Engineering—School of Engineering
University of Bridgeport
Bridgeport, CT

Table of Contents

Foreword *xix*
Acknowledgments *xxi*
Preface to the Second Edition *xxiii*

PART I—Professional Protocols and Specialized Patient Populations 1

Chapter 1—Health Promotion in Clinical Practice 3
TIMOTHY A. MIRTZ, DC, MSE, CHES
Introduction 3
Understanding Community Health 4
Delivering Individual Health Promotion with Evidence-Based Medicine 4
EBM Principles in Clinical Health Promotion 5
Appropriate Versus Effective Health Promotion 7
Individual Health Behaviors 8
Conclusion 9

Chapter 2—Medical Recordkeeping 11
LAWRENCE H. WYATT, DC, DACBR, FICC
Introduction 11
Problem-Oriented Medical Record System 12
Comprehensive Database 13
Problem List 14
Initial Plans 14
Progress Notes 15
Specialized Notes 16
Writing Orders 16
Types of Orders 17
Prescription Writing 18
Patient Confidentiality 19

Chapter 3—Geriatrics 21
CONNIE D'ASTOLFO, DC AND LAWRENCE H. WYATT, DC, DACBR
Introduction 21
Theories on Aging 21
Geriatric Clinical Assessment 23
Geriatric Vital Signs 25
Chiropractic Treatment of the Geriatric Patient 26

Chapter 4—Pediatrics 31
R.J. Ferrance, DC, MD
The Pediatric History and Physical Examination 31
Growth and Development 34
Pre-participation Physical Examination of the Adolescent Athlete 34
The Pediatric Cervical Spine 36
Pediatric Orthopedic and Sports Injuries 38
Common Pediatric Conditions 42

Chapter 5—Hospital and Long-Term Care 47
Connie D'Astolfo, DC
Introduction 47
General Institutional Protocols 47
Case Presentations 48
Charting Procedures 48
Clinics and Ward Rounds 48
Institutional Committees 48
Surgery 49
Roles for the Chiropractor in the Institutional Setting 50

PART II—Clinical Investigations 53

Chapter 6—History, Physical Examination, and Differential Diagnosis 55
Lawrence H. Wyatt, DC, DACBR, FICC
History 55
Physical Examination 62
General Signs (Table 6.4) 62
Vital Signs 63
Skin 68
Head/Face 68
Eyes (Figure 6.2) 69
Ears 73
Nose 74
Throat 74
Thorax/Lungs 75
Heart and Great Vessels 77
Abdomen 79
Extremities 84
Special Tests/Signs in Physical Examination 84
Differential Diagnosis of Common Signs and Symptoms 86
Abdominal Pain 86
Ascites 86

Chest Pain 86
Constipation 86
Cough 86
Diarrhea 86
Dysphagia 86
Dyspnea 86
Dysuria 86
Edema, Peripheral 88
Fever of Unknown Origin 88
Heartburn (Pyrosis) 88
Hematemesis 88
Hematuria 88
Hemoptysis 88
Hepatomegaly/Splenomegaly 88
Jaundice 88
Lymphadenopathy 89
Melena 89
Oliguria/Anuria 89
Weight Loss, Unexplained 89
Wheezing 89

Chapter 7—Orthopedics 93
LAWRENCE H. WYATT, DC, DACBR, FICC
Introduction 93
Useful Orthopedic Tests/Signs 93
General Spine Tests 94
Malingering Tests 95
Cervical Spine Tests 97
Thoracic Spine Tests 102
Lumbar Spine Tests 102
Thoracic Outlet Tests 112
Shoulder Tests 114
Elbow Tests 122
Wrist/Hand Tests 124
Hand Tests 126
Hip Tests 126
Knee Tests 129
Ankle/Foot Tests 133
Range of Motion 135
Scoliosis Evaluation 135
Spondylolisthesis 143

Screening Orthopedic Examinations 146
Upper Body Screening Examination (with patient sitting) 146
Lower Body Screening Examination 147
Deformities of the Skeleton 150

Chapter 8—Neurology 153
LAWRENCE H. WYATT, DC, DACBR, FICC
Introduction 153
Location of the Lesion 153
Deep Tendon Reflexes 154
Paralysis/Paresis/Muscle Tone 154
Fasciculations or Fibrillations 155
Pathologic Reflexes 155
Spinal Cord Lesions 157
Brain Lesions 159
Radiculopathy 162
Peripheral Neuropathy 162
Etiology of the Lesion 162
Peripheral Lesions 162
Nerve Root Lesions 162
Spinal Cord Lesions 163
Brain Stem Lesions 165
Cerebral Lesions 166
Treatment of the Lesion and Contraindications to Treatment 166
The Neurologic Examination 167
Peripheral Neuropathy 169
Abnormal Gait 169
Abnormal Involuntary Movements 171
Differential Diagnosis of Common Signs and Symptoms 172
Anisocoria 172
Bitemporal Hemianopsia 172
Dementia 172
Diplopia 172
Dizziness 173
Headache 173
Hyperreflexia 174
Hyporeflexia 174
Ophthalmoplegia 174
Polyneuropathy 174
Syncope 174
Tremors 175
Vertigo 175
Weakness (Muscular) 175

Specialized Neurologic Testing 176
Evoked Responses 176
Motor Evoked Potentials (MEP) 177
Electromyography (EMG) 177
Nerve Conduction Velocity (NCV) 178
Electroencephalogram (EEG) 179
Lumbar Puncture (LP) 179
Glossary of Neurologic Signs, Symptoms, and Diseases 180

Chapter 9—Clinical Laboratory Diagnosis 187
LAWRENCE H. WYATT, DC, DACBR, FICC
Introduction 187
Complete Blood Count (CBC) 187
Interpreting the CBC (common reference ranges in parentheses) 188
Red Blood Cell Morphology 188
Poikilocytosis: Irregular shape of red blood cells 188
Cellular Inclusions 189
Mean Corpuscular Hemoglobin 189
White Blood Cell Count 189
White Blood Cell Differential 190
Hemoglobin 190
Hematocrit 190
Platelets 190
Urinalysis 190
Specific Gravity 191
Ph 191
Glucose (negative) 191
Ketones (negative) 192
Blood (negative) 192
Nitrites (negative) 192
Bilirubin (negative) 192
Urobilinogen 193
Serum Chemistries 193
Acid Phosphatase 193
Alanine Aminotransaminase (ALT) 193
Albumin 193
Albumin/Globulin Ratio (A/G Ratio) 195
Alkaline Phosphatase 195
Alpha fetoprotein (AFP) 196
Amylase 196
Anti-double stranded DNA Antibody (Anti-dsDNA) (negative) 196
Antinuclear Antibody (ANA) (negative) 196

Antistreptolysin-O Titre (ASO) 196
Aspartate Aminotransferase (AST) 197
Bicarbonate 197
Bilirubin 197
Blood Urea Nitrogen (BUN) 197
Calcium 197
Chloride 198
Cholesterol 198
Creatine Phosphokinase (CPK) 198
Creatinine 198
Fluorescent Treponemal Antibody Absorbed (FTA-ABS) (nonreactive) 198
Gamma-glutamyl Transpeptidase (GGT) 198
Globulin 198
Glucose 198
Glycosylated Hemoglobin 199
Hemoglobin A1C (Glycosylated Hemoglobin) 199
High-density lipoprotein (HDL) cholesterol 199
Human Chorionic Gonadotropin (HCG) 199
Human Immunodeficiency Virus (HIV) 199
Human T-Lymphocyte Virus (HTLV) (negative) 199
Iron 199
Iron Binding Capacity (Total) (TIBC) 199
Lactate Dehydrogenase (LDH) 200
Lipase 200
Low-density lipoprotein (LDL) Cholesterol 200
Lupus Erythematosus Cell Preparation (LE Prep) (none seen) 200
Monospot (negative) 200
Parathyroid Hormone (PTH) 200
Phosphorus 200
Potassium 201
Protein Electrophoresis (Serum) (SPE) (variable) 201
Protein, Serum 202
Rheumatoid Factor (RA Latex) 202
Schilling's Test 202
Serum Glutamic-oxaloacetic Transaminase (SGOT) 202
Serum Glutamic-pyruvic Transaminase (SGPT) 202
Sodium 202
Thyroid Stimulating Hormone (TSH) 202
Thyroxine (14 Total) 203
Triglycerides 203
Triiodothyronine (T3 RIA) 203
Troponin I 203

Uric Acid 203
Venereal Disease Research Laboratory (VDRL) (nonreactive) 203
Special Studies 203
Specific Laboratory Panels 204

Chapter 10—Diagnostic Imaging 205
Lawrence H. Wyatt, DC, DACBR, FICC
Introduction 205
Ten Rules of Radiology 205
Basic Rules of Radiographic Interpretation 207
General Bone Radiology 208
Bone Tumors 208
Arthritides 209
Trauma 209
Infection 210
Congenital Lesions 210
Soft Tissues 210
Differential Diagnosis and Follow-Up Imaging 211
Common Causes of Common Lesions 211
Radiographic Evaluation in the Abdomen and Chest 211
Abdomen 216
Adrenal Calcification 216
Dysphagia 218
Hematemesis 222
Hematochezia 222
Hepatomegaly 222
Abdominal Mass (Adult) 222
Melena 222
Pancreatic Calcification 222
Pneumoperitoneum 223
Renal Calcification 223
Splenic Calcification 223
Splenomegaly 223
Vas Deferens Calcification 223
Chest 223
Consolidation 223
Effusion (Pleural) 224
Extrapleural Sign 224
Hilar Enlargement (Bilateral) 224
Hilar Enlargement (Unilateral) 224
Mediastinal Mass (Anterior) 224
Mediastinal Mass (Middle) 224

Mediastinal Mass (Posterior) 225
Multiple Pulmonary Nodules 225
Unresolving Pneumonia 225
Solitary Pulmonary Nodule 225
Radiation Physics Made Easy 225
Basic Rules 225
Radiography Procedure 226
Standard Radiographic Views 229
Radiology Reports 229
Advanced Diagnostic Imaging 233
Computerized Tomography (CT) 233
Magnetic Resonance Imaging (MRI) 234
Radionuclide Bone Scanning 236
Diagnostic Ultrasound (US) 236
Plain Film Interpretation 237
Chest Radiographs 237
Abdomen Radiographs 237
Spine Radiographs 238
Extremity Radiographs 238
Skull Radiographs 238

Chapter 11—Specialized Procedures 245
LAWRENCE H. WYATT, DC, DACBR, FICC
Introduction 245
Venipuncture (Phlebotomy) 245
Urine Specimen Collection 245
Electrocardiogram (ECG) 249
Digital Rectal Examination 250
Cardiopulmonary Resuscitation (CPR) 252

PART III—Differential Diagnosis 255

Chapter 12—Rheumatology 257
LAWRENCE H. WYATT, DC, DACBR, FICC
Introduction 257
Classification of Rheumatologic Diseases 257
History 257
Physical Examination 259
Laboratory Investigation 260
Radiographic Investigation 261
Rheumatologic Diseases 261
Rheumatoid Arthritis 261
Ankylosing Spondylitis 262

Arthritis Associated with Psoriasis 263
Reiter's Syndrome 263
Arthritis Associated with Enteropathy 264
Gouty Arthritis 264
Calcium Pyrophosphate Crystal Deposition Disease 264
Hydroxyapatite Deposition Disease 265
Degenerative Joint Disease 265
Diffuse Idiopathic Skeletal Hyperostosis (DISH) 266
Fibromyalgia Syndrome 266

Chapter 13—Clinical Oncology 269
LAWRENCE H. WYATT, DC, DACBR, FICC
Introduction 269
Screening Methods 269
Lung Cancer 269
Colon Cancer 270
Breast Cancer 270
Female Genital Cancer 271
Prostate 271
Clinical Examination 271
Bladder 271
Brain 271
Spinal Cord 271
Bone 272
Breast 272
Lung 272
Genital (Female) 272
Genital (Male) 272
Colon 272
Liver 272
Pancreas 273
Kidney 273
Stomach 273
Leukemia 273
Lymphoma 273
Laboratory Investigation of Cancer 273
Diagnostic Imaging of Cancer 275
Malignant Bone Tumors 276
Multiple Myeloma 276
Chordoma 278
Osteosarcoma 278
Chondrosarcoma 278
Fibrosarcoma 279

Ewing's Sarcoma 279
Giant Cell Tumor of Bone 279
Lymphoma of Bone 280
Benign Bone Tumors 280
Hemangioma 280
Enostoma (Bone Island) 280
Osteochondroma (Exostosis) 280
Enchondroma 281
Chondroblastoma 281
Chondromyxoid Fibroma 281
Osteoma 282
Osteoblastoma 282
Osteoid Osteoma 282
Simple Bone Cyst (Unicameral Bone Cyst) 283
Aneurysmal Bone Cyst 283
Fibroxanthoma (Fibrous Cortical Defect, Nonossifying Fibroma) 283
Fibrous Dysplasia 283
Glossary of Oncology Terms 284

Chapter 14—Spine Pain 287
Lawrence H. Wyatt, DC, DACBR, FICC
Introduction 287
Structural Spinal Landmarks 287
Spinal Biomechanics 288
Facet Planar Motions 288
Coupled Motions 288
Vertebrogenic Spine Pain 288
Arthritides 288
Biomechanical 290
Developmental 290
Infectious 291
Metabolic 291
Miscellaneous 292
Trauma 292
Tumors 292
Referred Spine Pain 293
Cervical Spine 293
Thoracic Spine 293
Lumbar Spine 294
Mimicry Syndromes 295
Chronic Pelvic Pain Syndrome (CPPS) 295
Cervical Spine Dysfunction 296

Thoracic Spine Dysfunction 296
Lumbar Spine Dysfunction 297
SI Joint Dysfunction 297
Trigger Points (with Muscle Generators) 297

Chapter 15—Clinical Conditions 301
LAWRENCE H. WYATT, DC, DACBR, FICC
Introduction 301
Abdominal Aortic Aneurysm 301
Achilles Tendinopathy 302
Acromioclavicular (AC) Joint Separation 302
Angina Pectoris 302
Ankle Sprain 303
Appendicitis 303
Baker's Cyst 304
Bankart Lesion 304
Bell's Palsy 304
Benign Essential Tremor 305
Benign Prostatic Hyperplasia 305
Berry Aneurysm 305
Bicipital Tendinitis 306
Bursitis 306
Carpal Tunnel Syndrome 306
Cerebrovascular Accident 307
Cholecystitis/Cholelithiasis 307
Chronic Obstructive Pulmonary Disease 307
Cruciate Ligament Tears 308
De Quervain's Disease (Stenosing Tenosynovitis) 308
Disc Protrusion/Extrusion/Sequestration 308
Diverticulitis 309
Facet Syndrome 309
Fever 309
Gastroesophageal Reflux Disease 310
Guillain-Barre Syndrome (Ascending Paralysis) 310
Headache 311
Headache, Cervicogenic 311
Headache, Cluster 311
Headache, Migraine (without Aura) 313
Headache, Migraine (with Aura) 313
Headache, Migraine-Basilar Artery 313
Headache, Nervous System Etiology 314
Herpes Zoster (Shingles) 314

Hodgkin's Lymphoma 314
Hypertension 315
Lateral Epicondylitis 315
Leukemia 316
Lyme Disease 316
Meniscus Tears, Knee 316
Multiple Sclerosis 317
Myasthenia Gravis 317
Osteochondritis Dissecans 317
Osteoporosis 318
Pancoast Tumor 318
Peptic Ulcer Disease 318
Phlebitis/Thrombophlebitis 319
Prirformis Syndrome 319
Plantar Fascitis 320
Pronator Teres Syndrome 320
Raynaud's Disease 321
Rotator Cuff Disease 321
Sacroiliac Joint Dysfunction 321
Spinal Canal Stenosis (Neurogenic Claudication) 322
Thoracic Outlet Syndrome 322
Transient Ischemic Attack 323
Transitional Segment, Lumbosacral 323
Trigeminal Neuralgia (Tic Douloureux) 323
Vascular Claudication 324
Vertebral Artery Dissection 324
Vertigo, Benigh Paroxysmal Positional (BPPV) 325
Vertigo, Cervicogenic 325
Vitamin B-12 Deficiency (Sub-Acute Combined Degeneration) 325

PART IV—Clinical Practice Protocols **327**

Chapter 16—Ethics in Chiropractic Clinical Practice 329
Stephen M. Perle, DC, MS
Introduction 329
Caveat Emptor vs. Credat Emptor 329
Duties 330
Rights 331
Self-regulation 332
Informed Consent 332
Research Subjects 333
Boundaries between Practice and Research 333

Institutional Review Boards 334
Abandonment 334
Boundary Issues 335
"Gaming the System" or Fraud 335
Advertising 336
Conclusion 336

Chapter 17—Sprain/Strain Management 339
Lawrence H. Wyatt, DC, DACBR, FICC
Introduction 339
Management of Sprains and Strains 340
Sprain Management 342
Strain Management 343
Prognosis 344

Chapter 18—Cervical Spine Trauma Management 347
Lawrence H. Wyatt, DC, DACBR, FICC
Introduction 347
Examination 348
Radiography 350
Ancillary Diagnostic Testing 352
Treatment 352
Prognosis 353
Ancillary Therapies 353
Conclusion 355

Chapter 19—Low Back Pain Management 359
Lawrence H. Wyatt, DC, DACBR, FICC
Introduction 359
Diagnostic Evaluation 360
Treatment 361
Acute Low Back Pain 362
Chronic Low Back Pain 364
Prognosis for Manipulative Therapy Success 365

Chapter 20—Joint Manipulation and Mobilization 371
Lawrence H. Wyatt, DC, DACBR, FICC
Introduction 371
Rationale for Spinal Manipulation 372
Indications for Joint Manipulation 373
Contraindications to Joint Manipulation 374
Absolute Contraindications 375
Relative Contraindications 376
Adverse Reactions to Manipulation 377
Manipulation Under Anesthesia/Conscious Sedation 380

Joint Mobilization 380
Principles of Mobilization 381
Mobilization Grades 381
Types of Mobilization 381
Clinical Examples of Mobilization 383

Chapter 21—Physical Medicine and Rehabilitation 391
LAWRENCE H. WYATT, DC, DACBR, FICC
Introduction 391
Effects of Physical Medicine Modalities 391
Specific Physical Medicine Modalities 391
Cryotherapy 392
Spray and Stretch Technique 393
Heat Therapy 394
Contrast Bath 395
Ultrasound 396
Galvanic Current 398
Sinusoidal Current 398
Interferential Current (IFC) 399
Microcurrent Therapy (MCT) 400
Traction 401
Massage 401
Muscle Energy Techniques 402
Trigger Point (TrP)/Tender Point Therapy 404
Spinal Stabilization Exercises 405
Orthoses and Mechanical Supports 407
Joint Mobilization 407
Neural Mobilization 414

Appendix A—Abbreviations 417
Index 431

Foreword

I was pleased to provide a foreword for the first edition of "The Handbook of Clinical Chiropractic Care" and am equally honored to provide this foreword for the second edition. This handbook now offers ninety photographs, which demonstrate technique. There has been a significant improvement in the tables, algorithms, and clinical charts. The comprehensive nature of this publication, to include physical examination, neurology, orthopedics, laboratory investigation, diagnostic imaging, manipulation, and physical therapy procedures is very thorough and elevates this book to represent the "Merck Manual" of chiropractic.

The clinical application and easy access to all of the material in this text makes this a "must-have" reference source for practicing doctors of chiropractic and chiropractic students.

Dr. Wyatt is to be commended for his outstanding effort in upgrading an already excellent first edition. His second edition of "The Handbook of Clinical Chiropractic Care" is a publication that he can be proud of and will be embraced by the profession as an excellent contribution to the published literature of chiropractic.

Terry R. Yochum, DC, DACBR, Fellow, ACCR
Adjunct Professor of Radiology
Southern California University of Health Sciences
Los Angeles, CA

Director, Rocky Mountain Chiropractic Radiological Center
Denver, CO

Clinical Instructor of Skeletal Radiology
Department of Radiology
University of Colorado School of Medicine
Denver, CO

Acknowledgments

It is not without perseverance and hard work that any manuscript is completed. Importantly, it must be acknowledged that many people, other than the author, yield their time and energy toward completion of such a project.

I would like to extend my heartfelt thanks and profound respect to a number of people who were instrumental in the completion of this book. I would especially like to thank God and Harvey Slusky, MD, for giving me a second chance at life. To my wife Cheryl: thank you, once again, for your love and patience and for looking after our son during this time. You are still my best friend. To my son Cole: sorry I've not been able to spend as much time with you as I wanted over the last few months, but look out boy, because Daddy's back and it's our turn to have some fun. To my co-authors Stephen Perle, DC; Connie D'Astolfo, DC; Tim Mirtz, DC; and Randy Ferrance, MD, DC: I thank you and respect you all for taking the time to contribute such important facets of this book. Your work is sincerely appreciated. To Rosemary Calio, RN, DC, and Jimmy Jackson: thank you for your invaluable editorial assistance. To Jack Bruggeman: thank you, kind sir, for your encouragement, patience, and editorial assistance. To Joseph W. Howe, DC, and Kenneth Linder, PhD: you are gentlemen, scholars, and my mentors, and you will never be able to appreciate how much you both mean to me.

To my students, who are one of the important audiences for this text: thank you for being my inspiration and for making me one of the lucky people in this world who enjoy going to work every day. I pray you will become involved and make a difference in the future of the chiropractic profession.

Preface to the Second Edition

The chiropractic profession is a dynamic, eclectic, and ever-expanding part of the healthcare delivery team. Multi-disciplinary practices, integrated chiropractic and medical practices, and chiropractic care integration into hospital and long-term care facilities are an important part of the evolution of this profession.

The demands of evidence-based health care are also now applied to the chiropractic profession. Manipulation has received much attention in the last 20 years in the scientific arena as a safe and effective tool for the management of many neuromusculoskeletal conditions and for the management of the neuromusculoskeletal comorbidities of organic disease.

The second edition of the *Handbook of Clinical Chiropractic Care* addresses these challenges by presenting an expanded, but still concise, quick-access handbook that covers the more common conditions seen in a chiropractic practice. Where possible, an evidence-based approach is presented, but it must be understood that a purely evidence-based practice is impossible to achieve in any form of health care. Instead the clinician must use the best available evidence, clinical experience, and a "pinch" of intuition to manage his or her patients.

This book is filled with quick-reference tables, algorithms, and lists that are designed to assist the busy clinician in daily practice. Emphasis is on the conditions that are seen in a chiropractic practice, both organic and biomechanical.

It is hoped that the use of this manual will help the chiropractic physician assume a more integral role in the delivery of health care to the patients in need of our care.

PART I

Professional Protocols and Specialized Patient Populations

Chapter 1

Health Promotion in Clinical Practice

Using evidence-based medicine and understanding the basics of health behaviors

Timothy A. Mirtz, DC, MSE, CHES

Introduction

Chiropractic practice has been traditionally identified as a neuro-musculo-skeletal-based type of practice. There has been a recent push by chiropractors to consider themselves as health promotion and disease prevention practitioners. Yet there are few data on how this is accomplished and whether or not the concept is practical. Moreover, there are few data on what encompasses health promotion as it applies to chiropractic practice. Does it mean answering individual questions from a patient? Does it entail giving a handout on various disease states that can easily be avoided by the patient? Does it take into consideration the health behavior possessed by the patient? Is the patient already in a wellness behavior or in another health behavior realm? Such questions provide more clues to what is known about how to deliver appropriate and effective health promotion in clinical practice.

The purpose of this chapter is to provide the practitioner with the basic concepts of health promotion and how clinical health promotion can be delivered. This chapter aims to provide the clinician with tools to deliver individual health promotion, understand the difference between community needs versus that of individual needs, and to understand the various health behaviors that need to be identified in order to deliver the appropriate information. This chapter will attempt to provide to the reader essential tools for effectively delivering pertinent health care advice/health promotion using evidence-based medicine (EBM) principles.

Understanding Community Health

Community health is defined as both private and public (government) efforts of individuals, groups, and organizations to promote, protect, and preserve the health of those in the community. (1) This differs from personal health in that community health seeks to protect or improve the health of the population or community. (1)

Differences with Personal and Community Health

Personal	*Community*
a. individual actions and decision making b. preventive or curative in nature c. seldom directed to affect behaviors of others	a. improving and protecting population

Due to the very nature of clinical practice, the emphasis will likely be on personal health promotion per individual and not at the community level. The community, however, will benefit more from a knowledgeable person than from an uninformed or misinformed person.

Delivering Individual Health Promotion with Evidence-Based Medicine

Clinical health promotion is defined as the application of health promotion principles in the clinical setting. (2) Clinical health promotion assumes that the application of psychological and behavioral principles to change health behaviors will result in improved health and well-being for patients. (2) Patient education and self-care education (where people are motivated to cure or control a disease) offer the best evidence for health education practice. (3) Health promotion in chiropractic clinical practice should go beyond the concept of delivery of manipulation as the health promoting aspect. It (health promotion) must go beyond the concept of giving a handout or brochure that may be outdated or not answer the patient's most pressing need. One should be wary of undue enthusiasm and carefully evaluate the interventions before they are offered. (2)

The method by which one can confine claims to those that are clearly supported through the research record is through EBM. EBM is a lifelong learning model for physicians that takes into account three aspects: the *best available evidence* along with *individual clinical experience* taking into consideration a *patient's value system.* (4) This model can easily be placed in the confines of individual health promotion at the health-care setting.

EBM Principles in Clinical Health Promotion

The first step in delivering health promotion to individuals can be appreciated in "asking an answerable question." An example of asking an answerable question is if, in the patient encounter, the patient asks about vitamin C intake with his or her diabetic condition. Construction of an answerable question would possibly be "How much vitamin C can a diabetic ingest? Is there any potential harm with vitamin C intake and diabetes? What are the short-term and/or long-term benefits of vitamin C with diabetes?" Questions need to be constructed to allow the physician to effectively answer a clinical concern.

Once the answerable question has been constructed, the next task is to find an adequate resource. Internet access to the National Library of Medicine's MEDLINE should be within one's grasp. This database system is considered by many experts to be the most up-to-date data source on medically related topics. (4) The next step is to determine keywords to place in the search engine. From your answerable question(s) it can be appreciated that the initial keywords will be "vitamin C" and "diabetes." If further literature is needed that should be more specific, the inclusion of "harms" or "adverse effects" and/or "dose" can be added to the search. This search would constitute the third step. In initiating the search, one should look for the search engine's "limits" area. In this area one can designate an age group (ex: 45 to 60), literature years (ex: 1998 to 2003), and to find either English language or worldwide articles.

Once the search has been completed, the articles that may answer your question are isolated and can be read. Step four involves isolating your evidence to answer your answerable question. In this search you may find answers that you did not know existed and information that may challenge an already preconceived answer. As per the example of "how much vitamin C can a diabetic ingest and is it beneficial?", the evidence summary need only list the data that apply to the question. An evidence summary does not need to go into any lengthy detail. The evidence summary should also list the main author and year in order to retrieve data if the patient wishes to examine the source and to help the clinician find the data without having to perform the search all over again. An example of an evidence summary for this question would be:

Author (Year)	*Data*
Brown (1998)	Persons with diabetes may benefit from supplemental vitamin C. (5)
Hasanain (2002)	*Lack* of data to substantiate benefit of anti-oxidant vitamins *in excess* of dietary allowance. (6)
Mullan (2002)	500 mg daily for one month lowered arterial blood pressure and improved arterial stiffness in patients with type II diabetes. (7)
Peponis (2002)	50 non-insulin dependent patients given 1000 mg/day of vitamin C for 10 days; reduces oxidative damage and improves ocular surface. (8)
Kulbertus (2002)	250 mg/day of vitamin C; all comparisons between vitamin supplementation and placebo failed to reveal any difference in favor or against supplementation. (9)
Darko (2002)	1.5 grams daily for three weeks did not significantly improve oxidative stress, blood pressure, or endothelial function in type II diabetes. (10)
Yu (2002)	200 mg of vitamin C daily for four weeks; can inhibit LDL oxidation and protect against vascular disease in type II diabetes. (11)
Gaede (2001)	Short-term treatment with vitamin C in pharmacologic dosages lowers albumin excretion rate (a predictor of end stage renal disease); 1250 mg/day for four weeks with a three-week washout reduces albumin excretion rate by 19%. (12)
Price (2001)	Vitamin C is recommended during periods of both acute and chronic hyperglycemia to preserve endothelial function. (13)
Will (1999)	Diabetes lowers vitamin C concentrations. (14)

It is at this time that the clinician is ready for the final step of applying the evidence. The above evidence summary indicates several things. First, a basic science review is given. Secondly, a clinical primer is given to review the clinician. Thirdly, clinical data from the experimental literature indicate that there is a benefit to short-term vitamin C ingestion given a dose amount that will match your patient's clinical needs. The clinician is in the position to initiate a short-term trial of vitamin C ingestion with a dose not exceeding the recommended daily allowance.

One of the criticisms leveled against EBM is that it is "cookbook" medicine. Nonetheless, the above evidence summary indicates that such is hardly the case in the example given. It is now up to the clinician to weigh the evidence and make recommendations as per the patient specifics. EBM has thus made the clinical decision much more difficult and does not provide easy answers. However, it does give the patient more information than that of a brief brochure and is up-to-date. The clinician, along with the patient, can now formulate a treatment plan together knowing that there are no exact answers taking into consideration the patient's particular wants, needs, and desires.

Steps to delivering individual health promotion using EBM

Step 1: Asking an answerable question
Step 2: Selecting an evidence resource
Step 3: Executing the search strategy
Step 4: Examining the evidence summary
Step 5: Applying of the evidence

From utilizing this process the individual clinician has now completed the evidence-based triad of best available evidence and improved individual clinical experience taking into consideration the patient's value system. This can be appreciated in that the clinician has now added to the process of lifelong learning by finding new clinical evidence in answering a patient's concern. Furthermore, the clinician has gained valuable clinical experience and has armed the patient with data to help make an informed decision. The concept of informed consent has been accomplished by giving the patient as much pertinent data as seen from the evidence summary.

Appropriate versus Effective Health Promotion

In health promotion there is a wide gap of difference between appropriate health promotion and effective health promotion. Appropriate health promotion can be defined as the delivery of appropriate and timely information in an effort to inform the patient on who, what, when, where, and how of a particular health issue or disease state. Effective health promotion, on the other hand, can be defined as that aspect of health promotion delivered that created a change in the state of the patient's behavior to effectively make a change for the better. An example of this can be seen in alcoholism. The following table shows the difference between the concepts of appropriate health promotion versus effective health promotion.

Health behavior/disease state

Alcoholism

Appropriate promotion

Assuring patient of confidentiality; concern; empathy
Giving patient addiction information
Offering resources such as Alcoholics Anonymous (AA)
Giving information on short-term and long-term effects of alcoholism as per patient history, patient individual concern, and family history

Effective promotion

Patient elects to read information; patient couples this with other people he/she has sought out on this question
Patient self-examines his/her situation
Patient makes decision to initiate action
Patient enters himself/herself into AA, attends meetings, gets a sponsor, thus attempting to gain sobriety

It should be pointed out that if effective promotion is not achieved, this does not imply that an inappropriate promotion occurred. Motivation is a term that is loosely defined and not completely understood by many physicians. Motivation is something that happens within a person, not something done *to* a person by others. (3) It (motivation) refers to the internal dynamics of behavior, not to the external stimuli use of motive-arousing appeals. (3) In other words, we can appeal to people's motives, but we cannot "motivate" them. (3) Thus physicians need not become concerned that their efforts were in vain.

Individual Health Behaviors

Effective health promotion is hindered by what is least understood in chiropractic circles, and this is in the concept of wellness. Nelson (15) suggested that the concept of wellness was largely unexamined. However, what remains unknown about wellness in chiropractic circles is that wellness is a behavior and not really a state of being. If we know now that one cannot motivate someone and that lifestyle behaviors play a large role in many of today's disease states, it stands to reason that wellness is a behavior that is individual and not delivered to someone.

If effective health promotion is based upon the person's willingness to change for something better and wellness is a behavior, then what causes effective promotion to fall short? The answer is quite simple once the concept of multiple health behaviors is realized and appreciated. Green and Kreuter (3) provide the following definitions that may be encountered in the clinical setting.

Behavior	*Definition*
Wellness	Activity undertaken by a person, who believes himself to be healthy, for the purpose of attaining a greater level of health.
Preventive health	Activity undertaken by a person, who perceives himself to be healthy, for the purpose of preventing illness or detecting it in an asymptomatic state.

At-risk	Activity undertaken by a person, who believes himself to be healthy, but at greater risk of developing a specific health condition, for the purpose of preventing that condition or detecting it in an asymptomatic state.
Illness	Activity undertaken by a person, who perceives himself to be ill, to define the state of his health and discover a suitable remedy.
Sick role	Activity undertaken by a person, who considers himself to be ill, for the purpose of getting well. It includes receiving treatments, involves few dependent behaviors, and leads to some degree of neglect of one's usual duties.
Self care	Activity undertaken by a person, who considers himself to be ill, for the purpose of getting well. It includes minimal reliance on therapists, involves a few dependent behaviors, and leads to little neglect of one's usual duties.

The above table indicates that patients are more than likely presenting more than a desire to achieve a wellness behavior. By acknowledging that patients may present such behaviors, the clinical encounter will become more exacting as well as educational. The knowledge of such behaviors will aid in identifying patients to help meet their unique individual needs.

Conclusion

This chapter attempts to introduce the physician to individual health promotion using EBM principles. Using the steps outlined in this chapter, the answering of a patient's question and helping promote his or her individual health can be utilized. Once these steps are learned, they can be easily repeated, thus making more efficient use of the clinician's time and efforts.

Included in this chapter was a brief introduction between individual health promotion and community health promotion. Along with the understanding of individual behaviors as it applies to health, the clinician should feel more confident in understanding the patient's present behavior, thus making the delivery of individual health promotion more efficient.

References

1. McKenzie, J.F., Pinger, R.R., & Kotecki, J.E. *An Introduction to Community Health.* 3rd edition. Jones and Bartlett Publishers. Boston. 1999.
2. Bishop, G.D. *Health Psychology.* Allyn & Bacon. Boston. 1994.

3. Green, L.W., & Kreuter, M.W. *Health Promotion Planning.* Mayfield Publishing Company. Mountain View, CA. 1999.
4. Sackett, D.L., Straus, S.E., Richardson, W.S., Rosenberg, W., & Haynes, R.B. *Evidence-based Medicine.* Churchill-Livingstone. London. 2000.
5. Brown, D.J., & Goodman, J. A review of vitamins A, C, and E and their relationship to cardiovascular disease. *Clinical Excellence for the Nurse Practitioner.* 1998. Jan;2(1):10–22.
6. Hasanain, B., & Mooradian, A.D. Antioxidant vitamins and their influence in diabetes mellitus. *Current Diabetes Report.* 2002. Oct;2(5):448–456.
7. Mullan, B.A., Young, I.S., Fee, H., & McCance, D.R. Ascorbic acid reduces blood pressure and arterial stiffness in type II diabetes. *Hypertension.* 2002. Dec;40(6):804–809.
8. Peponis, V., Papathanasious, M., Kapranou, A., Magkou, C., Tyligada, A., Melidonis, A., Drosos, T., & Sitaras, N.M. Protective role of oral antioxidant supplementation in ocular surface of diabetic patients. *British Journal of Ophthalmology.* 2002. Dec;86(12):1369–1373.
9. Kulbertus, H., & Scheen, A.J. Clinical study of the month: the MRC/BHF Heart Protection Study. *Review Medical Liege.* 2002. Sep;57(9):613–616.
10. Darko, D., Dornhorst, A., Kelly, F.J., Ritter, J.M., & Chowienczyk, P.J. Lack of effect of oral vitamin C on blood pressure, oxidative stress and endothelial function in type II diabetes. *Clinical Science* (London). 2002. Oct;103(4):339–344.
11. Yu, Y.M., Chang, W.C., Chang, C.T., Hsieh, C.L., & Tsai, C.E. Effects of young barley leaf extract and antioxidative vitamins on LDL oxidation and free radical scavenging activities in type II diabetes. *Diabetes Metabolism.* 2002. Apr;28(2):107–114.
12. Gaede, P., Poulsen, H.E., Parving, H.H., & Pedersen, O. Double-blind, randomized study on the effect of combined treatment with vitamins C and E on albuminuria in type II diabetic patients. *Diabetes Medicine.* 2001. Sep;18(9):756–760.
13. Price, K.D., Price, C.S., & Reynolds, R.D. Hyperglycemia-induced ascorbic acid deficiency promotes endothelial dysfunction and the development of atherosclerosis. *Atherosclerosis.* 2001. Sep;158(1):1–12.
14. Will, J.C., Ford, E.S., & Bowman, B.A. Serum vitamin C concentrations and diabetes; findings from the Third National Health and Nutrition Examination Survey, 1988–1994. *American Journal of Clinical Nutrition.* 1999. July;70(1):49–52.
15. Nelson, C.F. Chiropractic and wellness care. *Journal of Chiropractic Humanities.* 1994. 4(1):3–17.

Chapter 2

Medical Recordkeeping

Lawrence H. Wyatt, DC, DACBR, FICC

Introduction

The "chart" is a written record of the patient's health while under a physician's care. It serves as a database of important clinical, social, and demographic information on each and every patient. While the requirements for each state differ, statutes require that these records, including radiographs and special studies, be maintained by the physician for a number of years. Many times special requirements concerning the length of time records must be kept on file are made for persons under legal age. The statutes require that medical records on children be kept until they at least reach the age of majority or until a specific time period elapses, whichever is longer. All physicians should become familiar with the relevant state statutes where they practice.

Many jurisdictions also require that physicians report special or unusual circumstances about a patient's health to local, county, or state authorities. The more commonly required reportable circumstances are outlined in Table 2.1.

Accurate recordkeeping is essential for chiropractors. Not only will immaculate records assist the physician in collating information concerning the patient, but they will assist the physician if he or she is called to a court of law. The patient chart is also helpful when it becomes necessary to produce records for third-party payers. Communication among physicians concerning a patient's status or progress is also notably enhanced with meticulously kept records. It must be understood, however, that the chart is not a magic document that, by itself, prevents liability or even responsibility. It is such an important document that it should not be altered, nor is it the place to attempt to improve your

Table 2.1 Common Reportable Patient Care Circumstances

Non-accidental injury caused by a weapon
Birth
Stillborn birth
Death
Cancer cases
Certain communicable diseases (e.g., HIV, tuberculosis)
Sexually transmitted diseases
Suspected abuse (child, spouse, parent)

position in the face of the possibility of a liability claim. The patient chart may actually create liability if the records are not accurate and correct. When one undertakes the responsibility for patient care, one also carries the obligation to chart all interactions with patients.

The patient's chart should be organized so that pertinent information is easily accessible. A common problem in charting is the misconception that a blank space beside a question or a test is the equivalent of a negative response. A blank space provides the reader with no information whatsoever. All queries and spaces on forms should be answered/filled in, thereby leaving no question as to the status of that finding. Illegible records are also troublesome. Should the patient see another physician, by choice or necessity, legible notes allow the new physician to interpret the patient's previous health care accurately.

There are a number of useful hints to be used when writing in a patient's chart. Each note should be titled and dated, including the time that the patient was seen. The source of the information, especially with pediatric, geriatric, and mentally impaired patients, should be recorded. A signature and title should follow any entry into the records. All charting should be performed on official institutional forms.

Problem-Oriented Medical Record System

There are many different forms of charting, the most popular of which is probably the problem-oriented medical record (POMR) system developed by Dr. Larry

Weed. This system permits a standardized analysis of each of the patient's problems with good cross-referencing. The major disadvantage of this system is that it is somewhat more cumbersome than many others.

The POMR system is divided into a number of component parts including the comprehensive database, problem list, initial plans, and progress notes. Outlines of the components of each part can be found in Tables 2.2A, 2.2B, and 2.2C.

Comprehensive Database

Creation of a POMR begins with the collection of all historical and physical examination data, supplemented by data from any diagnostic tests that are

Table 2.2A Complete Problem List Components

Patient identification
Each problem entered separately
Date/time problem entered into chart
Active problems (chief complaint should be highlighted)
Inactive problems
Physician signature

Table 2.2B Initial Plans Components

Patient identification
Date/time
Initial plans for each problem (listed separately)
Diagnostic plans
Therapeutic plans
Physician signature

Table 2.2C Progress Notes Components

Patient identification
Date
Time
Subjective complaints
Objective tests
Assessment
Plans
Diagnostic plans
Therapeutic plans
Physician signature

appropriate for the patient's age, sex, and physical status. Copies of reports of any examinations should become a permanent part of the patient's chart.

Problem List

The problem list is a compilation of the patient's problems, both past and present, most often collected from the comprehensive database. Each problem is recorded and dated in descending order of severity on a problem list sheet and assigned a number for future reference. Patient problems can be a symptom, sign, abnormal laboratory finding, abnormal diagnostic study, or abnormal special study. The problem that has brought the patient to the physician's attention is marked with an asterisk to identify it as the chief complaint. Each problem is also listed as active (still causing the patient distress) or inactive (no longer a problem for the patient). Inactive problems are listed with the date they became inactive. As the signs, symptoms, and other problems are collated to form a specific diagnosis, the problem list should be updated accordingly by deleting the compilation of problems previously noted and noting a diagnosis as a new active problem.

Initial Plans

The initial plans formally list the diagnostic and therapeutic procedures to be performed on the patient, along with their rationale, as well as patient education plans. Initial plans should be formulated for any active problem on the problem list. This rule applies even if the problem is not treatable with chiropractic health care, in which case a note stating that the problem is being handled by another physician will suffice. If the problem is to be co-managed, that fact should also be noted.

Listing the rationale for procedures is also important. Any diagnostic test required should contribute significant data to the treatment or prognosis for the patient. There are also admission protocols, which vary with each institution, that are many times performed. For example, any patient with an acute cervical acceleration-deceleration injury (whiplash) may be required to have a Davis series of radiographs performed while in a cervical collar. Complete blood count and urinalysis are often part of an admission protocol as well.

Progress Notes

Progress notes are a short notation of the progress or regress in the patient's status. Each active problem being treated by the physician, with its appropriate number from the problem list, should be recorded. There are four divisions of the progress notes, which form the mnemonic SOAP.

- *Subjective*—New symptoms or a change in symptoms since the last note are recorded here. These are expressed in the patient's words, surrounded by quotation marks, if that format is appropriate. Have the patient quantify the symptoms, if at all possible. For example, if the patient had one dollar's worth of pain on the first visit, have him or her quantify how much pain is still being experienced—e.g., 50 cents worth of pain.
- *Objective*—Record new or changed examination, laboratory, or imaging findings since the last note. Again, quantify the changes if possible. For example, a straight leg test that was initially positive at 45 degrees and now is not positive until 75 degrees helps quantify the amount of patient progress.
- *Assessment*—Diagnoses, whether working or final, along with any concomitant and complicating factors, are noted here. These should be as specific as possible and include any complicating co-morbidities, as they may affect the patient's prognosis.
- *Plans*—Include new or continuing diagnostic, therapeutic, or patient education plans in this section. For example, if it is important that the patient remain in bed with only bathroom privileges until the results of a magnetic resonance imaging scan are known, this should be noted. Specific types of manipulation, physical therapy, or any other therapeutic

procedures; their location; and the patient's tolerance of any procedures performed should also be charted here.

Specialized Notes

Many facilities will add an admission note and a discharge note to the medical record. These notes summarize the patient's status at admission to the facility and at the time of discharge from care, including the patient's complaint, status, and progress. For discharge notes, the reason for discharge should also be noted. If the patient is discharged after not following a diagnostic or treatment plan, then a "discharged against medical advice" form should be signed by the patient. It is important for medicolegal reasons to inform the patient of the reason for the discharge. In cases of discharge against medical advice, it is vital to suggest another physician and to emphasize the importance of the patient seeking further care, both verbally and in writing.

Written and verbal informed consent should be obtained from patients undergoing diagnostic and therapeutic procedures. A witness should also sign the informed consent form. In the case of a minor, parental or guardian consent is also necessary.

Operative notes may be used in some instances, as with those patients undergoing manipulation under anesthesia or conscious sedation.

Writing Orders

Orders are instructions to patients, assistants, interns, clerks, and consultants concerning the management of a case. They can be general or specific depending upon what is required. For example, an order for "vitamin C as needed (p.r.n.) for acute coryza" is obviously inadequate because no dosage or route of administration is noted. A complete order should state the order, date, and time; what is to be administered; to whom, how, and when it is to be given; and where it is to be administered.

There are many templates for writing orders. *Standing orders* (SOs) are instructions that are to be performed on specific types of patients under specific circumstances without the need for consultation with the clinician. For example, if a patient has been involved in a motor vehicle accident, the SO might be for a seven-view cervical spine (Davis) series, the lateral being performed while the patient is in a cervical collar.

Orders that vary and require discussion with the attending clinician before being performed may be given by the clinician as *written orders, verbal orders,* or *telephone orders.* The type of orders given should be placed in the patient's chart next to the orders.

If the words *STAT* or *ASAP* appear next to a set of orders, the orders should be performed immediately and supersede any routine investigations being performed.

Of course, all chart entries require the signature of a licensed physician.

Orders are the backbone of chiropractic diagnosis and therapy. The more concise and easily understood the orders, the better those interacting on a particular case, including the patient, can effectively carry out those orders.

Types of Orders

The orders described in this section can be easily remembered by the mnemonic LATER DUDES (representing laboratory, activity, treatment, extras, radiology and diagnosis, updates, disability, exercises, and supplements). Each element is briefly described below.

- *Laboratory*—Many facilities have admission protocols concerning laboratory studies. Other studies specific to the case at hand should also be noted. All laboratory orders should include when the studies are to be performed and who the ordering physician is.
- *Activity*—Due to the unique nature of patients seen by chiropractic physicians, all patients should be required to adhere to the level of activity (both work and leisure) prescribed for them. Terms such as light and regular work duty can be used but should be modified by noting both included and excluded activities (e.g., no lifting involving any low back torque). If the patient's activity is unrestricted, the phrase "activities of daily living as much as wanted" (ADL ad lib) can be used.
- *Treatment*—The type of treatment, including adjustment and manipulation, physical therapy, medication, rehabilitation, and patient therapy, medication, rehabilitation, and patient instructions should be outlined. Be as specific as possible, including frequency, duration, and dosage where applicable. Manipulation should be ordered p.r.n. (*pro re nata,* or "as needed"). The type and location of the manipulation should be charted as specifically as possible in the progress notes. Contraindications for any type of procedure should be listed here as well.
- *Extras*—This is where orders for any special diagnostic studies, such as an electromyogram, or special treatment or consultations, such as "neurosurgical consultation to rule out (R/O) cord tumor," should be made. Any special requirements for preparation for these tests should be given to the patient and duly noted. Any orders that do not fit into any of the other categories should be included here.

- *Radiology*—Any requisitions for diagnostic radiography should be included here. Be as specific as possible concerning which views are to be performed and any special preparatory procedures (e.g., cleansing enema) of which the patient should be aware.
- *Diagnosis*—The working clinical diagnosis, including pertinent rule outs, should be included here.
- *Updates*—Reexamination dates and dates for follow-up x-ray, laboratory, and special studies are explained here. The specific examinations and tests to be performed should be listed.
- *Disability*—The amount of disability suffered by the patient should be noted here. The percentage of disability according to standard disability evaluation procedures should be recorded also, if applicable. Any home care instructions for the patient, either by the patient or patient's family, are noted.
- *Exercises*—The type and frequency of exercises to be performed by the patient and the instructions given to the patient should be charted. Specific weights to be used during exercises must be noted.
- *Supplements/Nutraceuticals*—Any nutritional supplementation, including dosage, route of administration, and frequency, should be noted. If written instructions for the patient were given, they should be recorded in the chart.

Using this form of order writing will assure the doctor of excellent patient care and compliance, as the orders can be understood and carried out precisely.

Prescription Writing

Although prescription writing for medications does not occur often in the chiropractic profession, there are states that do allow such prescribing privileges. The following is a format for proper prescription writing. This format may be used for medications, physical therapy, supplements, orthopedic supports, and other such necessities.

Essential components of a prescription include:

- *Name, age, and address.*
- *Date*—State regulations vary, but most states require that a prescription be filled within six months. Check with your state for specific requirements.
- *Rx*—Rx is from the Latin for "recipe." The product or therapy being prescribed and its strength and type (generic or brand name) should be

noted. The form of the product (e.g., tablets, capsules) should also be included.

- *Dispense* ("disp")—The amount (e.g., number of tablets) or the time period (e.g., six weeks) for the treatment is noted here.
- *Sig.*—Sig. is from the Latin "signa," which means "mark through." This is where the patient instructions are noted. This portion of the prescription is typically written in shorthand. (Abbreviations are listed in Appendix A.)
- *Refills*—This lists the number of times the prescription can be filled.

Prescriptions should be written on a prescription pad containing the physician's name, address, and license number. There should also be a place for the physician's signature. All notations should be printed and clearly legible.

If instructions to patients are given, they should not be abbreviated or written in shorthand. Instead, they should be written out and easily understood.

Patient Confidentiality

Since the time of Hippocrates, it has been important to ensure the confidentiality of patients. Over time, this health information has come to be used by many non-medical individuals and organizations, including employers, insurers, and attorneys. These entities are not subject to health care ethics codes. With this increase in the use of this information have come more regulations. The first comprehensive set of federal regulations of health information, the Privacy Rule under the Health Insurance Portability and Accountability Act of 1996 (HIPAA), came into effect in April 2003. The Security Rule, also required under HIPAA, was issued in final form on February 20, 2003, and will become effective in 2005.

The regulations for protecting privacy are complicated. The Privacy Rule establishes a federal mandate for individual rights in health information, imposes restrictions on uses and disclosures of individually identifiable health information, and provides for civil and criminal penalties for violations. The complementary Security Rule includes standards for protection of health information in electronic form. Under these statutes protected health information is defined very broadly. Protected health information includes: individually identifiable health information related to the past, present, or future physical or mental health or condition, the provision of health care to an individual, or the past, present, or future payment for the provision of health care to an individual. Even the fact that an individual received medical care is protected information under the regulation.

For additional information about the specifics of the HIPAA and related regulations, you are advised to consult *http://www.hhs.gov/ocr/hipaa/finalreg.html.*

Chapter 3

Geriatrics

Connie D'Astolfo, DC
Lawrence H. Wyatt, DC, DACBR

Introduction

Geriatrics is defined as "the branch of medicine concerned with the problems of aging." (1) The World Health Organization classifies the geriatric population in three groups. It defines the elderly as individuals ages 65 to 75, the old as ages 76 to 90, and the very old as those over the age of 90. (2,3) Normal consequences of aging include decreased organ function, decreased stress tolerance, increased psychological stress (personal loss, death of friends, loss of independence), increased susceptibility to disease and infection, atypical presentation to disease, adverse drug reactions, and decreased physical conditioning. (4,5,6) Geriatric patients, as other groups, are commonly afflicted by specific conditions. For the geriatric population, these can be grouped using the mnemonic "the Five I's" that include intellectual impairment, immobility, instability, incontinence, and iatrogenic drug reactions. (4,5) The "Five I's" are associated with single, or most often, multiple clinical diagnoses. (Table 3.1)

Theories on Aging

No one really knows how and why people change as they get older. Some theories claim that aging is caused by accumulated injuries from ultraviolet light, "wear and tear" on the body, byproducts of metabolism, and others. Other theories view aging as a predetermined, genetically controlled process. No theory, however, sufficiently explains all the changes of the aging process. Aging is a

Table 3.1 The Five I's

Intellectual Impairment	Decreased attention span, memory loss, personality change, disorientation, social withdrawal 60% associated with Alzheimers DDX: Iatrogenic drug reactions, depression, sensory loss, metabolic disturbances, endocrine abnormalities, trauma (subdural hematoma), nutritional deficiencies, brain tumor, infections, cardiovascular accidents
Immobility	DDX: Weakness: muscle disuse, malnutrition, electrolyte imbalance, anemia, neurological disorders, myopathies Stiffness: osteoarthritis, rheumatoid arthritis, polymyalgia rheumatica Pain: osteoporosis, osteomalacia, Paget's disease, metastatic bone CA, trauma, osteoarthritis polymyalgia rheumatica, intermittent claudication, stenosis Imbalance: general debility, neurologic disorders (stroke, loss of postural reflexes, peripheral neuropathy d/t diabetes, alcohol, malnutrition, vestibulo-cerebellar dysfunction, anxiety, drugs, prolonged bed rest * Complications of immobility: bedsores (decubitus ulcers), muscle weakness and wasting, osteoporosis, venous thrombosis, incontinence
Instability	DDX: Drop attacks (loss of control of antigravity muscles), syncope, vertigo, spasticity, rigidity (pyramidal and extrapyramidal disease), medications causing postural hypotension (antidepressants, neuroleptics, antihypertensives), arrhythmias (antidepressants), dizziness, vertigo, confusion and genitourinary causes (urgency)
Incontinence	DDX: Functional incontinence (inability to get to the toilet), detrusor instability, overflow incontinence, stress incontinence, fecal impaction
Iatrogenic Drug Reactions	Caused by changes in intestinal absorption and renal clearance Chronic multiple conditions equate to multiple drug use in the geriatric population

complex and varied process that varies in how it affects different people and organs. Most gerontologists believe that aging is the cumulative effect of the interaction of many lifelong influences including heredity, environment, cultural influences, diet, exercise and leisure, past illnesses, and many other factors.

Unlike the changes seen during adolescence, which are predictable to within a few years, each person ages at a unique rate. Some systems begin aging as early as 30 years old while other aging processes are not common until much later. Although there are predictable changes that typically occur with aging, they occur at different rates and to different extents. There is no reliable way, including age in years or chronological age, to predict specifically how a patient will age. In fact, even in one person, different organ systems "age" at a different rate.

Geriatric Clinical Assessment

The geriatric assessment needs to include a comprehensive history and physical exam. The clinician must be able to distinguish abnormal signs and symptoms from normal aging (Table 3.2), identify drug toxicity, rule out conditions that require prompt intervention, and be aware of challenges such as underreporting of illnesses, overestimation of cognitive abilities, atypical presentations, and overlapping of symptoms from multiple conditions. (3,19,20) The assessment should include several screening measures including cardiovascular and cerebrovascular risk factors amenable to preventative treatment, co-morbidities (e.g., diabetes mellitus), secondary and reversible causes of dementia, impaired vision, hearing, dehydration, and malnutrition. (16,17) The clinician should assess functional capacity (independence with activities of daily living), assess gait and mobility, and identify patients at risk for falls or in need of walking aids. (16,17) The chiropractor should also have adequate resources to provide referrals to appropriate consultants and community services when required.

Pain should be a special consideration in the assessment of the geriatric patient. (6–15) Pain is not a normal part of aging, and both clinicians and patients need to understand this. Geriatric patients sometimes believe that pain cannot be relieved and are stoic in reporting their pain. The frail and old (>85 years) are at particular risk for undertreatment of pain. (13) Aging does not alter pain thresholds or tolerance. (13) Cognitive impairment, delirium, and dementia are serious barriers to assessing pain in the older person. Sensory problems such as visual and hearing changes may also interfere with the use of some pain assessment scales. When a verbal report from a patient is not possible, clinicians should observe for behavioral cues to pain such as restlessness or agitation. (11–13) The absence of pain behaviors does not negate the presence of pain. Consider pain

Table 3.2 Characteristic Neuromusculoskeletal Changes with Advancing Age (16, 17, 30)

General Neurological Function	- changes in cerebral blood flow - decrease in neuro-endocrine function - decreased olfaction, taste - decreased visual acuity, pupil size and reactivity - limitation of conjugate vertical gaze and convergence - smooth ocular pursuit becomes saccadic - hearing loss - decreased muscle bulk without fasciculations - mild increase in muscle tone and decreased muscle strength (but not generally apparent on examination) - decreased speed and coordination of movement - decreased muscle stretch reflexes (loss of ankle jerks) - increased prevalence and number of primitive reflexes - decreased vibration sensation in distal LE
Postural Changes	- flexed posture - forward head posture - thoracic kyphosis - flexion of elbows, knees, hips, wrists due to ankylosis of joints and ligaments - postural instability
Gait and Extra-pyramidal Conditions	- reduction in stride length and velocity, toe off, toe clearance, arm swing, hip and knee rotation -wide-based gait typically in men -narrow-based waddling gait typically in women * Altered gait due to pathological causes include myelopathy, multiple cerebral infarcts, Parkinson's, hydrocephalus, cerebellar disease, brain tumors, Binswanger's and/or Alzheimer's disease
Spinal Changes	- loss of bone mass - shortening of ligaments or tendons - loss of muscle bulk - decrease in tensile strength of trabecular bone - dry/brittle intervertebral discs

Table 3.2 Characteristic Neuromusculoskeletal Changes with Advancing Age (16, 17, 30) *(continued)*

	- flat uncinate processes (may project laterally and posteriolaterally where they may impinge neural structures) - dural root sleeves may become fibrotic and rigid - ligamentum flavuum may become hypertrophied and may compress spinal canal space
Cortical and Psychological Function	- decrease in brain size - change in sleep patterns, mood, appetite - decline in an ability to memorize a large body of knowledge - reduced semantic skills, name objects quickly - diminished visual spatial ability

predictors such as frailty, history of back and/or leg pain, arthritides, neuropathy, malignancies, increasing age, prolonged sitting, bedridden status, and others. (14,22–29) Nonsteroidal anti-inflammatory drugs can be used safely in the geriatric patient, but their use requires vigilance for side effects, especially gastric and renal toxicity. Opioids are safe and effective when used appropriately in elderly patients. Elderly people are more sensitive to analgesic effects of opiate drugs. They experience higher peak effect and longer duration of pain relief. (8,10,21)

Geriatric Vital Signs

There are normal physiologic changes associated with aging. Normal body temperature does not change significantly with aging, but adequate temperature regulation is more difficult in the aged. Loss of subcutaneous fat makes it harder to maintain body heat, and many older patients find that they must wear extra layers of clothing in order to feel warm. Keeping cool is also more difficult. Skin changes include reduced ability to sweat and elderly people, therefore, become overheated more quickly. The ability to perceive temperature diminishes, and they find it more difficult to tell when they are becoming chilled or overheated.

These changes lead to more susceptibility to heat-related illness such as hypothermia and hyperthermia.

Fever is an important sign of illness in the elderly. Many times, fever is the only symptom of some illnesses for several days. Any fever that is not explained by a known illness should be investigated. Often, older people are unable to create a higher temperature with infection, so very low temperatures and checking the other vital signs play an important role in following these people for signs of infection.

Because of age-related changes in the heart, the resting heart rate may become slightly slower in older patients. In addition, exercise-induced heart rate increases are slower to appear, and the pulse takes longer to slow back down to normal after exercise. In addition, the maximum heart rate reached with exercise is less than in an active younger adult. Bradycardia and atrial fibrillation are relatively common in the elderly.

Blood vessels become less elastic, and the "average" blood pressure increases from 120/80 to 150/90 and may remain persistently high, even with treatment. The blood vessels respond slower to a change in body position, so orthostatic hypotension is more common.

Although lung function decreases slightly in this patient population, the changes are usually only in reserve function and the respiratory rate changes little in the elderly. There is decreased tolerance to exercise in some elderly people as they have a reduced response to decreased oxygen or increased carbon dioxide levels, where the rate and depth of breathing does not increase as it should.

The medications that are used to treat common disorders in the elderly may also have a profound effect on the vital signs. For example, digitalis, which is an inotropic/chronotropic agent used for congestive heart failure, and certain blood pressure medications (e.g., beta blockers) will cause the pulse rate to decrease. Pain medications can affect breathing. Diuretics can cause low blood pressure and aggravate orthostatic hypotension. These changes secondary to medication usage, in addition to interactions between medications, should be remembered when considering an elderly patient's symptom complex.

Chiropractic Treatment of the Geriatric Patient

In the geriatric patient, the restitution of normal neuromusculoskeletal structure is likely not a typical goal due to bone, soft tissue, and nervous system remodeling. However, improving joint mobility, soft tissue elasticity, nervous system functioning, and vascular supply are realistic goals. The emphasis of chiropractic care should be multi-modal, with a focus on addressing the kinetic chain to improve global range of motion, gait and body posture/mechanics, reducing pain as well as providing lifestyle and nutritional counseling. For example, regional considerations can include the neck-shoulder-scapula complex, thoracolumbar junction, wrist-fingers, and foot-knee-hip-pelvis chain. (5) High-velocity low-amplitude spinal and nonspinal manipulation can be a vital component of care; however, the clinician may need to modify his or her technique based on the presenting clinical conditions, relative and absolute contraindications (e.g., compression fractures, anti-coagulant therapy, osteopenia (31), and functional limitation of the patient such as maintaining a broader contact, less torque, and avoiding the thoracic spine during side posture rotational adjustment of lumbar spine.) (5) Soft tissue manipulation, physical modalities, traction, blocking techniques, low force joint mobilization, proprioceptive training, exercise and rehabilitation, and acupuncture can also be components of the treatment plan.

Exercise is a vital component of chiropractic care of the geriatric patient. Patient compliance is not always easily accomplished; however, there are several recommendations to increase patient participation with exercise. Exercise needs to be fun, and adding music and movement to the exercise environment can be helpful. It should also be social (group participation), sustainable (affordable and for brief periods), and a priority (validate exercise as a prescribed health intervention and enlist reinforcement from other health care providers and from family or caregivers). (18) The elderly, especially frail elders, require special precautions and exercise modifications based on functional limitations. (18) For example, patients should always be encouraged to wear supportive foot wear and loose, comfortable clothing while exercising. Patients who require the use of a walker or wheelchair should be seated in a supportive chair, with arms, while exercising. For those who are immobile, there should be a focus on truncal and upper body motion and resistance training and the use of pre-exercise local heat and active stretching for restricted joint movement (e.g., shoulder, knee, neck). Patients should also be encouraged to do pelvic floor strengthening exercises (e.g., Kegel's exercises). (18)

Generally, exercises should be focused on increasing circulation (decreasing symptoms of congestive heart failure and venous insufficiency), strengthening, improving balance and coordination (decreasing risk of falls), and overall improvement in mobility and independence.

The presence of an enlarging aged population is necessitating a shift in the focus of patient needs from healthcare providers. Understanding the normal physiological changes that occur with aging will help the clinician to identify significant pathology, recognize urgent needs, and focus on earlier detection and prevention. Chiropractors can play a significant role in the care of the geriatric patient. This includes neuromusculoskeletal pain management and functional restoration and health promotion through the use of exercise, lifestyle changes, and nutritional counseling.

References

1. *Taber's Cyclopedic Medical Dictionary.* F.A. Davis Co. USA, 1997.
2. Ferri, F., et al. *Practical Guide to the Care of the Elderly Patient.* 2nd ed. St Louis. Mosby Year Book, 1997.
3. World Health Organization. *Implementation of the global strategy for health for all by the year 2000: first evaluation: eighth report on the world health situation.* Geneva. The Organization, 1991.
4. Lonergan, E. Geriatrics. *A Lange Clinical Manual.* 1st ed. Stamford, CT. Appleton and Lange, 1996.
5. Gleberzon, B. *Chiropractic Care of the Older Patient.* Butterworth-Heinemann, MA, 2001.
6. AGS Panel on Chronic Pain in Older Persons (1998) Guidelines. The management of chronic pain in older persons. [Published erratum appears in 46(7):913.] *J Am Geriatr Soc* 46(5):635–651.
7. King, S. Shattering Myths about Geriatric Pain. *Geriatric Times.* May/June 2000:1 (1).
8. AGS Panel. The Management of Persistent Pain in Older Adults. The American Geriatrics Society 2002 Annual Scientific Persons Meeting "Shaping the Future for Older Adults," 2002.
9. ASCP. Improving outcomes of pain management in long term care patients. American Society of Consultant Pharmacists' Annual Meeting, Nov. 13, 1998.
10. AGS Panel. The American Geriatrics Society Guidelines for the Management of Pain: Implications in the LTC Setting. 29th Annual Meeting of the AGS, 1998.
11. Ferrell, B.A. The assessment and control of pain in the nursing home. In: Rubenstein, L.Z., & Wieland, D., editors. *Improving Care in the Nursing Home—Comprehensive Reviews of Clinical Research.* Sage Publication. Newbury Park, CA, 1993.
12. Ferrell, B.A. Pain evaluation and management in the nursing home. *Ann Intern Med.* 1995;123(9):681–687.
13. Ferrell, B.A., Ferrell, B.R., & Rivera, L. Pain in cognitively impaired nursing home patients. *J Pain Symptom Manage.* 1995;10(8):591–598.
14. Thomas, E., et al. Predicting who develops chronic low back pain in primary care: a prospective study. *BMJ.* June 19, 1999:318.
15. Lavsky-Shulan, M., Wallace, R.B., Kohout, F.J., et al. Prevalence and functional correlates of low back pain in the elderly: The Iowa 65+ Rural Health Study. *J Am Geriatr Soc.* 1985; 33:23–28.

16. David J. Gladstone, BSc, MD, et al.. The Neurological Examination in Aging, Dementia and Cerebrovascular Disease Part 1: Introduction, Head and Neck, and Cranial Nerves. *Geriatrics and Aging.* Volume 5, Number 7, September 2002, Pages 36–43.
17. David J. Gladstone, BSc, MD, et al. The Neurological Examination in Aging, Dementia and Cerebrovascular Disease. Part 4: Reflexes and Sensory Examination. Geriatrics and Aging. Volume 5, Number 10, December 2002, Pages 51–57.
18. Heath, J., MD, & Stuart, M., PhD. Prescribing Exercise for Frail Elders. J *Am Board Fam Pract.* 15(3):218–228, 2002.
19. Bowers, L. Clinical assessment of geriatric patients: unique challenges. *Top Clin Chiropractic.* 1996:3(2):10–21.
20. McCarthy, K.A. Management consideration in the geriatric patient. *Top Clin Chiropractic.* 1996;3(2):66–75.
21. American Pain Society (1999). *Principles of Analgesic Use in the Treatment of Acute Pain and Cancer Pain.* 4th ed. Glenview, IL. American Pain Society.
22. Clinical Standards Advisory Group 1994. Back Pain. Report of a CSAG committee on back pain. London. HMSO.
23. Papageorgiou, A.C., Croft, P.R., Ferry, S., Jayson, M.I.V., & Silman, A.J. Estimating the prevalence of low back pain in the general population. Evidence from the South Manchester Back Pain Survey. *Spine.* 1995;20:1889–1894.
24. Croft, P.R., Papageorgiou, A.C., Ferry, S., Thomas, E., Jayson, M., & Silman, A. Psychological distress and low back pain. Evidence from a prospective study in the general population. *Spine.* 1995;20:2731–2737.
25. Thomas, E., Silman, A.J., Croft, P.R., Papageorgiou, A.C., Jayson, M.I., & Macfarlane, G.J. Predicting who develops chronic low back pain in primary care: a prospective study. *Br Med J.* 1999;318:1662.
26. Acello, Barbara. Pain Control. *Nursing.* March 2000.
27. Starck, P., et al. Pain Management Outcomes: Issues for Advanced Practice Nurses. *The Internet Journal of Advanced Nursing Practice.* 2000;4(1).
28. Fox, P., et al. Prevalence and Treatment of Pain in Older Adults in Nursing Homes and LTC Institutions: A Systematic Review. *CMAJ* February 9, 1999:160(3).
29. Thomas, E., et al. Predicting who develops chronic low back pain in primary care: a prospective study. *BMJ.* June 19, 1999:318.
30. Souza, T., et al. Normal Aging. *Top Clin Chiropractic.* 1996;3(2):1–9.
31. Winterstein, J. Perspectives on clinical practice: practical management of the geriatric patient. *J. Aust Chiropractors Assoc.* 1990;20(2):62–65.

Chapter 4

Pediatrics

R.J. Ferrance, DC, MD

Children are not simply small adults. While it would take an entire textbook to delineate and expound on the many differences one must keep in mind when treating children, we will restrict ourselves in this chapter to only those most often encountered by the chiropractor.

The Pediatric History and Physical Examination

While the pediatric history and physical (H&P) examination does not differ vastly from an H&P on an adult, there are some subtle differences that are best kept in mind. The first is, until proven otherwise, mom is always correct. Listen closely to mom's concerns. No one knows the child as well as mom, and no one is better at picking up subtle changes than she is. Remember to add to the past medical history questions about the pregnancy and delivery, noting any complications with either and the impact they had on the child's growth and development. The usual decorum of an H&P can often be disrupted by the presence of the child, so the examiner's attention to detail will often be taxed. Anyone working with children needs a near limitless supply of patience, and a sense of humor.

Pearls to help with the pediatric history:

- The examination room might not be the ideal setting to meet the child.
- Introduce yourself to the caregiver and to the child, and get down on his or her level first.

- Sit opposite the historian and maintain eye contact.
- Social amenities are different with children than with adults. Do not be afraid to play.
- Remember that the child's last name might not be the same as the caregiver's.
- Ask the child what he or she prefers to be called.
- Note the reason for the visit in both the caregiver's and the child's own words.
- Remember to ask about maternal age at birth, health of the mom, medications, drugs, tobacco, alcohol during pregnancy, infections, length of gestation, labor and delivery, complications, birth weight, Apgar scores, jaundice, feeding, and whether the baby left the hospital with mom.
- What has the child's growth and development been up until now? Look especially for delays in major milestones.
- Remember to touch on safety issues: car seats, smoke exposure, smoke alarms, bike helmets.
- In the review of systems, remember to ask about bowel and bladder functions, feeding, sleeping, and overall behavior.
- For adolescents, remember the mnemonic HEADSS (home, education, alcohol, drugs, sexual activity, sexual orientation).

Pearls to help with the pediatric physical examination:

- Be friendly and have a sense of humor (buy one if you have to).
- Have your equipment handy and ready, but not prominent.
- Size up the child's likely reaction.
- Do not expect problems.
- Use games, allow the child to handle the instruments. This takes a lot of the mystique and resulting fear out of the examination.
- Keep up a conversation.
- Warm your hands.
- Be gentle.
- Tell the child what you are going to do and offer the child choices so that he or she has a feeling of some control.
- Remember that vital sign normals for children are different than for adults.
- Pediatric blood pressure normal ranges can be found in Table 4.1. Pediatric pulse normal ranges can be found in Table 4.2.

Table 4.1 Normal Pediatric Blood Pressure

95th Percentile of Blood Pressure in Boys and Girls 3 to 16 Years of Age, According to Height.*

Blood Pressure	Age	Height Percentile for Boys				Height Percentile for Girls			
		5th	25th	75th	95th	5th	25th	75th	95th
	yr	mm Hg				mm Hg			
Systolic	3	104	107	111	113	104	105	108	110
	6	109	112	115	117	108	110	112	114
	10	114	117	121	123	116	117	120	122
	13	121	124	128	130	121	123	126	128
	16	129	132	136	138	125	127	130	132
Diastolic	3	63	64	66	67	65	65	67	68
	6	72	73	75	76	71	72	73	75
	10	77	79	80	82	77	77	79	80
	13	79	81	83	84	80	81	82	84
	16	83	84	86	87	83	83	85	86

*The height percentiles were determined with standard growth curves. Data are adapted from those of the Task Force on High Blood Pressure in Children and Adolescents.[3]

Table 4.2 Normal Range and Mean Pulse for Children

Age	Heart Rate (BPM) Range	Mean
0–7 days	95–160	125
1–3 weeks	105–180	145
1–6 months	110–180	145
6–12 months	110–170	135
1–3 years	90–150	120
4–5 years	65–135	110
6–8 years	60–130	100
9–11 years	60–110	85
12–16 years	60–100	85
>16 years	60–100	80

Source: Adapted from Park, M.K. *Pediatric Cardiology for Practitioners,* 3rd ed. St Louis. Mosby. 1996.

- Watch, be observant, and take the opportunities the child gives you. Not every examination flows in an orderly pattern.
- Positioning: Until six months, on a familiar blanket on the exam table is best; from six months to two years, mom's lap is often best. From three on up, the child will typically enjoy getting up on the exam table "like a big kid."
- Remember to be sensitive not only to what you say, but to what the child and the caregivers hear.
- If you note abnormal findings, pass them along to other care providers. Be a member of the team, and remember that our primary concern should always be the child.

Growth and Development

Children grow and mature constantly and, as a result, what is considered "normal" activity and behavior for them changes nearly continuously. A thorough developmental evaluation is best left to a developmentalist, but a list of common red flags is included in Table 4.3.

Pre-participation Physical Examination of the Adolescent Athlete

The required sports physical examination is the most common reason healthy adolescents visit a physician. While only 2% of potential athletes are disqualified from competition, the pre-participation physical examination (PPE) does give the physician an opportunity for interventions and dialogue. Twelve percent of potential athletes are found to require some type of follow-up (be it strength training, rehabilitation, nutritional counseling, or some undiagnosed medical condition) and, occasionally, previously ignored injuries are discovered. (1)

The optimal timing for the PPE is usually 4–6 weeks prior to the beginning of the season. This should allow time to make any needed changes to the athlete's preparations for the sport. Specifically, one should look for any medical or musculoskeletal conditions that would make a particular sport unsafe, screen for underlying illness through history, review systems and physical examination, recognize any pre-existing injury patterns from previous participation, and then devise a rehabilitation or strength and condition program to help prevent future injuries and/or recurrences of injury.

Table 4.3 Developmental Red Flags Suggesting the Need for Further Work-up and/or Referral

Birth to Three Months	4–6 Months	6–12 Months	12–24 Months
Rolling prior to 3 months	Poor head control	Persistence of primitive reflexes beyond 6 months	Lack of consonant production by 14 months
Persistent fisting at 3 months	Failure to reach for objects by 5 months	Absent babbling by 6 months	Lack of imitation by 16 months
Failure to alert to environmental stimuli	Absent smile	Absent stranger anxiety by 7 months	Lack of protodeclarative pointing by 18 months
		W-sitting and bunny hopping at 7 months	Hand dominance prior to 18 months
		Inability to localize sound by 10 months	Inability to walk up and down stairs at 24 months
		Persistent mouthing of objects at 12 months	Persistent poor transitions 21–24 months
			Advanced non-communicative speech

Specific Issues:

- Subjective weakness, faintness, or syncope during exercise: This is a red flag for cardiac abnormalities. Sudden cardiac death makes up the majority of sports fatalities, occurring in 5–15 out of every 1 million athletes. Keep in mind that asthma, hypoglycemia, and seizures can lead to very similar symptoms.
- Wheezing during sports: 85% of children with asthma have exercise-induced bronchospasm (EIB). It is estimated that 10–35% of student athletes have some form of EIB.
- Recurrent mononucleosis: Splenomegaly can predispose to rupture in high-moderate contact. The swelling of the spleen tends to peak 3–4 weeks after the onset of symptoms.

- Unilateral organ: Any child with a unilateral organ needs to have mandatory protective wear. A unilateral kidney is a contraindication to high contact sports.
- Menstrual Hx: Note, if a female athlete is experiencing either primary or secondary amenorrhea, watch for the "female athlete triad" of anorexia, amenorrhea, and osteoporosis.
- Seizure Disorder: This is of special concern in aquatic sports. Most authorities feel that if the athlete has been seizure free for greater than six months, the risk is negligible.
- Past history of injury: Help design a specific program to limit or prevent such future injuries.
- Ergogenic aids: Be sure to ask about supplements. Many athletes take huge doses of vitamins and other supplements. Nearly 9% of high school athletes and 3% of junior high school athletes admit to taking anabolic steroids. (2) The student athletes taking these drugs rarely know anything more about them than that Arnold Schwarzenegger took them, they are available at health food stores, and one is not supposed to tell the coach they are taking them. Many student athletes do not know that anabolic steroids can increase aggression, decrease HDL (good cholesterol), increase LDL (bad cholesterol), cause atrophy of the testicles, prematurely halt growth through premature skeletal maturation and accelerated puberty changes, and can possibly lead to liver problems and high blood pressure. Counsel them to stop. Some patients do become physically dependent upon the drugs and will have withdrawal symptoms that seem to consist mostly of mood swings, fatigue, restlessness, loss of appetite, insomnia, reduced sexual drive, and a drive to take more steroids. The most dangerous of the withdrawal symptoms is depression, which can persist for over a year or more.
- Family History: Ask especially about cardiac-related death, congenital heart disease, long QT syndrome, hypertrophic cardiomyopathy, or Marfan's syndrome.

Remember that the PPE can serve as one of the few teachable moments that adolescents are likely to give us. Encourage them to think about safety in sports, safety in the choices, safety in life, and help them to realize the power they have and can use to be effective role models to other children.

The Pediatric Cervical Spine

As if to prove the maxim that children are not simply small adults, we have the pediatric cervical spine. It is important to remember that the fulcrum of movement is higher in children, owing in large part to the fact that the pediatric head is disproportionately larger and holds more mass. In children under the age of eight years, the fulcrum typically rests in the C2 region, falling to the C3–C4 interspace between the ages of 8 and 12, and then falling to the more familiar adult level of C5 after the child has reached his or her 12th birthday. Remember also that the pediatric vertebrae might not be fully ossified, that the ligamentous attachments may be stronger than the bone, and that the articular surfaces tend to be more horizontal. All these factors collude to affect the types of neck injuries we might see in children.

Developmentally, it is important to keep in mind that while the neural tube is undergoing segmentation (6–8 weeks of gestation), the branchial arches and urogenital tube are developing as well. These structures have both a close temporal and geographical orientation to the neural tube, so when congenital defects are seen in one system, be on the alert for problems in another.

Atlantoaxial Instability (AAI): AAI is defined as an atlanto-dental interval of greater than 5mm. It is commonly seen in patients with Down Syndrome (15% of children with Downs have AAI), as well as in children with odontoid aplasia or hypoplasia, or in os odontoideum. AAI rarely leads to neurological compromise and when it does, there typically are warning signs weeks to months prior to the C1 dislocation. Those warning signs include ataxia, neck pain, limited cervical spine range of motion, torticollis, sensory deficits, excessive fatigue, and upper motor neuron lesions. The International Special Olympics Committee requires pre-participation flexion/extension films on all children with Downs prior to competition. Eighty-five percent of children with Down Syndrome who have an atlanto-dental interval >5mm will remain asymptomatic throughout their entire lives.

Grisel's syndrome is an acquired form of AAI that is seen after pharyngeal infections such as streptococcal pharyngitis. It is thought that the local infection and inflammation lead to a hyperemia that then leads to a demineralization of the bone and some ligamentous instability. With time, however, re-mineralization occurs and the AAI resolves.

Klippel-Feil Syndrome (KFS): Klippel-Feil Syndrome is a congenital deformity of the cervical spine classically defined as a triad of short neck, low posterior hairline, and limitations in cervical spine range of motion secondary to congenital fusions. The classic triad is actually seen in less than 50% of children with definable KFS, however. Classification of the high-risk variants of KFS include:

Type I: C2–C3 fusion with occipitalization of C1

Type II: Long cervical fusion with an abnormal occipitocervical junction

Type III: Two blocked vertebral segments with a single open interspace.

Associated findings can include congenital heart disease, scoliosis, Sprengel's deformity, hearing impairments, renal abnormalities, facial asymmetry, and upper extremity anomalies, so any child presenting symptoms of KFS should be examined and, if appropriate, have other additional tests ordered to evaluate the possibility of other problems.

Little research has been done into the safety of spinal manipulation in children with KFS.

If neurological compromise is present, then a neurosurgical consult should be considered for possible surgical stabilization.

Congenital Muscular Torticollis (CMT): Congenital muscular torticollis is a condition with several proposed etiologies, the most popular of which is thought to be ischemic muscular injury in a sternocleidomastoid muscle (SCM) causing unilateral SCM fibrosis with failure of elongation of the muscle. The torticollis is progressive over the first several months of life, and in some cases a pseudotumor can be felt in the affected SCM. The deformity has head tilt to the ipsilateral side with rotation to the contralateral side. Plagiocephaly is common from a uniform head position when sleeping and may persist even after the CMT is corrected. Treatment is conservative, with active positioning at home, manual stretching exercises, and gentle spinal manipulation when appropriate. Rarely, surgical intervention is necessary. Positive prognostic indicators include a minimal initial deficit in cervical spine rotation and an early age at presentation. (3)

Kinematic Imbalances Caused by Suboccipital Strain (KISS): Described by Dr. Heider Biedermann, KISS syndrome is defined as two groups: KISS-1, where the lead symptom is lateral fixation of the head and trunk, and KISS-2, where the lead symptom is fixed retroflexion of the head and trunk. These children tend to adopt fairly uniform sleeping postures with difficult sleeping, and they go on to develop asymmetric motor patterns and postures of the trunk and extremities. The arm on the concave side seems to be used less, and develops more slowly. Children with KISS tend to have extreme sensitivity to neck palpation and respond well to gentle mobilization of the upper cervical vertebrae. (4)

Pediatric Orthopedic and Sports Injuries

Children, it seems, are particularly vulnerable to sports injuries. Multiple sources lay the blame for this on:

- Lack of coaching education at the youth level
- Inadequate preparticipation physical examinations for the athletes
- Hazardous playing fields
- Conditioning and training errors
- Lack of improper, poorly fitting, or inadequate safety equipment

- Encouraging children to play while injured or tired
- Grouping teams by age rather than by size
- Poor nutrition
- Incomplete recovery time after stress injuries
- Varying stages of physical maturation

Apophyseal injuries tend to be much more prevalent in children than in adults. This is due in part to the significant loading and tensile stresses on the apophyses and the fact that they are structurally weak when compared to adjacent tissues. They can be more common in juvenile athletes than tendon injuries and may, at times, be associated with avulsions. In general, treatment for apophyseal injuries consists of rest, ice, immobilization, conservative anti-inflammatory measures, and then controlled stretching and strengthening of the affected area.

Proximal Humeral Epiphysitis (Little League Shoulder): Swelling and tenderness anterior and lateral to the humeral head, exacerbated by repetitive and forceful overhand motions. Plain films may show a subtle widening of the physis, but no fracture.

Medial Epicondylar Apophysitis (Little League Elbow): Fragmentation and/or avulsion of the medial epicondyle, oftentimes with osteochondritis/chondrosis of the capitellum. This can lead to abnormalities of apophyseal growth of the medial epicondyle and delayed closure or nonunion of the medial humeral growth plate. Hypertrophy of the ulna can also result, with apophysitis of the olecranon with or without delayed closure. The pain is typically provoked by resisted wrist flexion and pronation, and by valgus stress at a slightly flexed elbow. If ulnar nerve paresthesias are present, this implies more extensive involvement of the ulnar collateral ligaments and/or the flexor carpi ulnaris tendon. X-rays should be performed to rule out avulsions or degenerative changes.

Juvenile Kyphosis (Scheuermann's Disease): An anterior wedging of three or more adjacent vertebrae leading to an increase in kyphosis or decrease in lumbar lordosis. Repetitive trauma or excessive axial loading injures the ring apophyses of the vertebrae and can subsequently lead to end-plate abnormalities and narrowed disk spaces. Most cases are asymptomatic. Bracing is typically only needed if the thoracic kyphosis exceeds 50 degrees. Most care is supportive, with moderate activity restriction and spinal manipulation if indicated to relieve any associated pain.

Legg-Calve-Perthes Disease (LCP): LCP is typically seen in the 4–8 year age range, and then again in the teenaged years. It is an avascular necrosis of the femoral head with resultant collapse and resorption of sequestered bone. Osteochondral new bone formation will continue for one to three years, but with relatively weak subchondral support. The condition is characterized by chronic hip and groin pain, with occasional radiation to the thigh or knee. Early in the course, X-rays may appear normal. In the acute period, rest and anti-inflammatory measures are the mainstay of treatment. Abduction stretching exercises should be implemented, and close follow-up is needed to determine the extent of the necrosis. Surgical correction of gross deformities of the femoral head may be necessary.

Slipped Capital Femoral Epiphysis (SCFE): SCFE is the most common disorder of the hips in adolescents. It is typically seen in overweight teenaged boys and is characterized by hip pain that is most severe in the groin, and often referred to the knee or the anteromedial thigh. The symptoms are minimized with the hip in external rotation and flexion, and most affected boys will assume this as their natural position of comfort. If suspected, both hips should be X-rayed since 25% of patients will have bilateral involvement.

Grade I: <⅓ displacement of the femoral head relative to the femoral neck

Grade II: ⅓–½ displacement

Grade III: >½ displacement

Treatment consists of traction and immobilization. Oftentimes surgery is needed to pin the femoral head in place.

Tibial Tubercle Apophysitis (Osgood Schlatter's Disease): Characterized by pain in the anterior shin just below the knee but without limitation in range of motion except during forced flexion or flexion followed by forced extension (jumping, stairclimbing, rising from a squatting position). Typically results from repetitive traction injury of the tibial tuberosity and physis. Usually is self-limiting, and rarely leads to a nonunion of the tubercle.

Sinding Larsen-Johansson Disease (Jumper's Knee): Characterized by anterior knee pain caused by persistent traction on the immature inferior pole of the patella. Typically seen in children ages 10–13, it can lead to abnormal calcification of the inferior aspect of the patella. Pain is typically isolated to the patella and exacerbated by jumping, climbing, kneeling, and direct trauma. Treatment is conservative in all but the worst cases with rest, anti-inflammatory measures, stretching, and strengthening exercises.

Kohler's Disease: Characterized by pain in the midfoot with localized tenderness over the navicular bone. It tends to affect younger children (ages 5–9) and is exacerbated by weight bearing and exercise. X-rays may show increased density with a narrowing of the tarsal navicular bone.

Calcaneal Apophysitis (Sever's Disease): Characterized by unilateral or bilateral heel pain that increases with activity and decreases with rest. Tenderness is usually noted with lateral and medical compression of the calcaneus, but not on the plantar surface of the heel. Heel cord contraction or weakness of the dorsiflexors tend to contribute to the problem. It tends to affect 8–12 year olds. X-rays are indicated to rule out fragmentation or sclerosis of the calcaneal apophysis. Treatment consists of rest, anti-inflammatory measures, and flexibility exercises to slowly and gently stretch the legs to reduce muscular tension and contraction. Shoe inserts can help, and in rare, severe cases, splinting or casting may be necessary.

Plantar Fascitis: Severe pain with initiating exercise and with first walking in the morning improves with movement and as the day progresses. Microtears of the fascia are to blame, and the exacerbation of symptoms in the morning comes from the shortening of the fibers as they heal overnight. Children with pes planus or cavus, inadequate dorsiflexion, weakness of the plantar flexor muscles, or limited mobility of the subtalar joint are particularly vulnerable. Stretching along with nighttime splinting is, by far, the most effective therapy.

Low Back Pain: In recent years, more attention has been paid to back pain in children, partly because it has lately been found to be more prevalent than previously thought. Recent studies suggest that 10–30% of healthy children experience back pain, especially low back pain, by their teenage years. (5,6) One common suspect for back pain in children is the school backpack, which has also received a great deal of attention in the past few years. A study in Italy found that the average load of a backpack was 22% of the child's weight and that ⅓ of the children surveyed carried in excess of 30% of their body weight at least one time per week. Their point prevalence for reporting back pain was nearly 16%, with a lifetime prevalence of nearly 48%. (7) According to some studies, compensatory forward head posture occurs with backpack loads of only 10–15% of body weight. (8) Therefore, teaching children how to handle the load better would certainly help them with their posture, if not prevent back pain itself.

Choosing the right backpack is important. A good backpack would have two wide, padded shoulder straps, a padded back, and a waist strap, be lightweight in and of itself, and would end above the child's waist.

Tips for using the backpack include always using both straps, tightening the straps, packing as light as possible (using the locker and, if necessary, asking for a second set of textbooks to keep at home to avoid carrying them back and forth each day), organizing, bending with both knees with the arms in flexion, and performing back strengthening exercises.

While there are few good studies on the effects of spinal manipulation in children, studies are now being performed and are promising. (9) More research needs to be directed toward manipulative treatment of the pediatric population.

A few words about injury prevention. It is important, especially with adolescent athletes who often consider themselves invincible, to emphasize the importance of preventing rather than simply treating injuries. Emphasize overall fitness rather than sports-specific skills. Talk about careful introduction of training focused upon development of specific skill sets only when it is age, fitness, and developmentally appropriate to do so. Conditioning should begin a good six to eight weeks before the beginning of the athletic season, and we need to help younger athletes especially control the intensity of their play. All injuries need to be examined early and often and changes made to the training regimen as needed to compensate for and heal the injury. No athlete, but especially no child athlete, should be allowed to "play through" an injury.

Common Pediatric Conditions

Otitis Media (OM): The treatment of otitis media by chiropractors has gained some popularity as of late with many practitioners claiming great response to chiropractic care. Many different possible explanations as to why this has been forwarded exist, but to date, no good studies have validated the anecdotal reports. There are three types of otitis media: Acute OM—defined as a suppurative infection with both systemic and local signs and rapid onset; OM with effusion, a.k.a. "glue ear," which is defined as a persistence of nonsuppurative effusion beyond three months; and chronic suppurative, which is continuing inflammation with otorrhea through a perforated tympanic membrane. Risk factors for OM include young age, attendance at day care, white race, male sex, a history of enlarged adenoids or tonsils, asthma, previous episodes of OM, exposure to tobacco smoke, use of a pacifier, and bottle feeding. The natural course of acute OM is that approximately 80% will resolve in about three days with or without antibiotics. (10) While serious complications, including hearing loss, mastoiditis, meningitis, or recurrent OM are rare, we should keep in mind that the condition itself is far from benign. Approximately 51,000 children die each year in developing countries from complications from OM. (11) Many medical physicians now recommend that a "wait and see" attitude be employed, with antibiotics delayed until after the first 72 hours, and then used only in cases that are not resolving. OM can be very painful, however, and a recent study suggested that although a 2–3 day waiting period is usually fine, analgesia with a naturopathic herbal extract solution may be beneficial to the child. (12) For prevention, there is no evidence that spinal manipulation is helpful, only equivocal evidence that prophylactic antibiotics are helpful, but good evidence that xylitol (sugarless) gum chewing can have a positive effect.

Asthma: Asthma is defined as a reversible airway obstruction caused by airway inflammation, increased mucous production, and bronchial smooth muscle contraction. Attacks or flares of asthma can be triggered by a number of different irritants, including upper respiratory infections, allergens, tobacco smoke, and even emotional stress. Studies to date have found no appreciable improvement in lung function with spinal manipulation, but one study did find a positive impact on quality of life measurements. (13) Traditional medical treatment runs the range from as-needed bronchodilator treatments for occasional bronchospasm up to daily disease modifying agents such as inhaled corticosteroids or leukotriene blockers for more persistent and severe disease. First line therapy should always be environmental modification, including removing common triggers such as dust mites through the use of bed and pillow covers, removing stuffed animals from the bed and/or room, sweeping and dusting daily, and considering removing carpets in favor of hardwood floors. There has been some recent controversy over the efficacy of control of house dust mites, and the issue does not seem to have been fully settled yet. While some reviews suggest no benefit (14), many have shown great benefit. (15) It is probably worth at least a trial. Animals need only be removed from the child if there is a demonstrated allergy to the animal in question.

Atopic Dermatitis (AD): Described as a pruritic, eczematous skin rash, the incidence of AD is increasing with time, now affecting some 12–15% of the pediatric population. AD tends to begin in infancy (50% within the first year of life, 80% by five years) and is characterized by extremely dry and scaly patches of skin that are extremely pruritic and follow a distinctive distribution. Eighty percent of children with AD will go on to develop either asthma or allergic rhinitis, and many will lose the AD component after the onset of respiratory symptoms. Most have elevated serum IgE and nearly all have a family history positive for atopic disease. Food allergies have been found to play a role, and some strategies that have proved helpful in decreasing the severity of AD include withholding peanuts, nuts, fish, shellfish, and soybeans for the first two years of life; breastfeeding as long as possible, mom taking care to avoid eggs, milk, and peanuts while pregnant and breastfeeding; and delaying solid food introduction to the infant until six months of age. (16,17) If a particular food is suspected of causing a food allergy, with or without atopic symptoms, a trial of food withdrawal followed by food challenge can often give the answer. The child should not receive a food challenge at home, however, if anaphylaxis is suspected.

Colic: Colic has received a great deal of attention lately, both because of articles that seem to suggest spinal manipulation can be beneficial, and because of articles that seem to suggest spinal manipulation is not beneficial. Classically, colic is felt to be some sort of infantile gastrointestinal distress, whether from abdominal cramping or from excessive gas. A number of therapies have been tried, few successfully. While it is typically benign and self-limiting, the parental distress it can lead to can be quite disruptive and is a significant risk factor for abuse of the child. Children with colic tend to be between three weeks and three months of age, crying for more than three hours a day, usually at the end of the day, for more than three days a week, for longer than three weeks. Babies otherwise are healthy, growing and thriving. While well controlled studies seem to suggest that spinal manipulation is no more effective than placebo, there are some suggestions that some cases of colic do respond to spinal manipulation. Dr. Joyce Miller at the Anglo-European College of Chiropractic has postulated that some cases of colic might, instead, be what she has termed Irritable Infant Syndrome of Musculoskeletal Origin (IISMO).

She defines IISMO as a child with hypertonia, arching extensor position, limb hyperactivity, restless sleep, general unrest, and unusual posture. She's found that many of these children present sleeping problems, unconsolable crying, appetite or eating problems, a retarded affective development, and postural problems. There is some suggestion that gentle spinal manipulation may lead to some benefit in these children.

Attention Deficit Hyperactivity Disorder (ADHD): An oft-maligned diagnosis, ADHD is not at all a new disorder. It was actually described by Hippocrates, who wrote of "quickened responses to sensory experience, but also less tenaciousness because the soul moves on quickly to the next impression." Formal criteria for diagnosis can be found in the DSM-IV, but it is important to remind the examiner that confounding diagnoses, including many physical ailments, need to be ruled out first. Questionnaires should be gained from teachers, parents, and others who work directly with the child. One such rating questionnaire is the "Connors" rating instrument, which helps toward a more objective diagnosis. While theories about nutritional deficiencies, poor parenting, a chaotic home environment, and just plain laziness abound in the ADHD arena, no clear etiology has come to the forefront. Some children do have improvement with a trial of dietary management, consisting mostly of removal of the more allergenic foods such as milk, soy, wheat, corn, citrus, peanuts, and artificial additives. For most children, however, dietary changes have little effect. Many different nutraceuticals have been employed, also with little effect. The gold standard of treatment remains behavioral modification followed, if necessary, by stimulant medication.

Neonatal Fever: In a recent article on pediatrics and chiropractic, 62% of chiropractors who were "peer-recommended" for the treatment of children said they would manage an infant with fever without referral to a medical physician. (18) While the majority of fevers in a neonate are the result of benign processes, most caused by self-limited viral infections, a small number of infants with fever do have bloodstream or central nervous system infections. Within the medical community, neonatal fever is a cause for alarm because, although morbidity and mortality are rare, those cases that are serious infections often result in death or

Table 4.4 **Benign Laboratory Findings and Risk Factor Delineation in the Work Up of a Neonate with Fever >100.5F.**

Benign Laboratory Findings
- Normal urinalysis
- WBC 5,000–15,000
- If diarrhea is present, no heme or WBCs in stool
- CSF of <10 wbc/hpf (If LP performed)
- CSF of <8 wbc/hpf if bloodless
- Negative CSF gram stain
- Band:Neutrophil ratio of <0.2
- No infiltrate on chest x-ray

Risk Factors:
- High Risk
  - Premature infant, NICU graduates, congenital heart or lung disease
- Low Risk
  - Do not appear toxic, have no obvious source of fever
  - Reliable caregiver and transportation

permanent disability. Studies show that 4–6% of babies with fever greater than 100.5°F rectally will suffer debilitating injury or death if untreated. Current recommendations hold that infants under the age of 30 days with a fever should all be admitted to the hospital for IV antibiotics. If blood, urine, and CSF cultures remain negative at 72 hours, the IV antibiotics can be discontinued and the child discharged home. Infants 1–2 months of age can avoid hospital admission if they have an otherwise benign physical examination, benign laboratory findings, and no significant risk factors for bacteremia (table 4.4). (19,20)

References

1. Smith, J., & Labowski, E.R. The preparticipation physical examination: Mayo clinic experience with 2,729 examinations. *Mayo Clin Proc.* 1998;73:419–429.
2. Metzl, J.D. Strength training and nutritional supplement use in adolescent athletes. *Current Opin Pediatr.* 1999;11:292–296.
3. Cheng, J.C., et al. *J Bone Joint Surg Am.* 2001;83-A(5):679–687.
4. Biedermann, H. Das KISS-syndrom der Neugeborenen und Kleinkinder. *Manuelle Medizine.* 1993;31:97–107.

5. Richards, B.S., McCarthy, R.E., & Akbarnia, B.A. Back pain in childhood and adolescence. AAOS Instructional Course Lectures. 1999;48:525–542.
6. King, H. Disorders of the pediatric and adolescent spine. *Orthop Clin North Am.* 1999;30:467–474.
7. Negrini, S., & Carabalona, R. Backpacks on! Schoolchildren's perceptions of load, associations with back pain and factors determining the load. *Spine.* 2002;27:187–195.
8. Grimmer, K., Williams, M., & Gill, T. The associations between adolescent head-on-neck posture, backpack weight and anthropometric features. *Spine.* 1999;24: 2262–2267.
9. Hayden, J.A., Mior, S.A., & Verhoef, M.J. Evaluation of chiropractic management of pediatric patients with low back pain: A prospective cohort study. *J Manipulative Physiol. Ther.* 2003;26:1–8.
10. Froom, J., Culpepper, L., Jacobs, M., et al. Antimicrobials for acute otitis media? A review from the International Primary Care Network. *BMJ.* 1997;315:98–102.
11. World Health Organization. World development report 1993: investing in health. Oxford. Oxford University Press. 1993:215–222.
12. Sarrell, E.M., Cohen, H.A., & Kahan, E. Naturopathic treatment for ear pain in children. *Pediatrics.* 2003;111:e574–579.
13. Bronfort, G., Evans, R.L., Kubic, P., & Filkin, P. Chronic pediatric asthma and chiropractic spinal manipulation: a prospective clinical series and randomized clinical pilot study. J *Manipulative Physiol. Ther.* 2001 July–Aug;24(6):369–377.
14. Gotzsche, P.C., Johansen, H.K., Burr, M.L., & Hammarquist, C. House dust mite control measures for asthma (Cochrane Review). *Cochrane Database Syst. Rev.* 2002;3:CD001187.
15. Halken, S., et al. Effect of mattress and pillow encasings on children with asthma and house dust mite allergy. *J Allergy Clin. Immunol.* 2003;111:169–176.
16. Sampson, H.A. Role of immediate food hypersensitivity in the pathogenesis of atopic dermatitis. *J Allergy Clin. Immunol.* 1988;71:473.
17. Sampson, H.A., & Sicherer, S.H. Food Allergy: Current knowledge and future directions. *Immunology Clinics of NA.* 1999;19:495–517.
18. Lee, A.C., Li, D.H., & Kemper, K.J. Chiropractic care for children. *Arch Pediatr. Adolesc. Med.* 2000;154:401–407.
19. Baraff, L.J. Management of fever without source in infants and children. *Ann Emerg. Med.* 2000 Dec;36(6):602–614.
20. Jaskiewicz, J.A., McCarthy, C.A., Richardson, A.C., et al. Febrile infants at low risk for serious bacterial infections—an appraisal of the Rochester criteria and implications for management. Febrile Infant Collaborative Study Group. *Pediatrics.* 1994 Sep;94(3): 390–396.

Chapter 5

Hospital and Long-Term Care

Connie D'Astolfo, DC

Introduction

With the advent of medical and surgical rotations for interns and hospital/long-term care (LTC) privileges for chiropractic physicians, it has become necessary for clinicians to become familiar with institutional protocols. Knowledge of the proper procedures used in mainstream institutional settings will allow for rapid integration into the hospital and LTC system. It is also crucial that the chiropractor adopt a clinical role, pertinent to conditions prevalent in the institutional setting or department, which is evidence based, synergistic, and valuable to the healthcare team.

General Institutional Protocols

As a general rule, the expectations of an intern on rotation will be explained at the outset. It is imperative that one understand these responsibilities and protocols and become familiar with schedules for operating suites, rounds, clinics, and conferences. Punctuality is essential since hospitals and most LTC institutions generally operate on a very tight schedule.

In order to save time, one should be aware of the location of each of the various departments in the hospital/LTC facility. Introducing oneself to clerks, receptionists, social workers, nursing staff, physiotherapists, and other registered staff is crucial, as is carrying a small book with room locations, telephone numbers, names, and keeping a daily schedule.

Case Presentations

There are generally two types of case presentations: formal and informal. Keeping notes on an index card on the patient being presented is very useful. Informal presentations are usually given to small groups and consist of a pertinent and concise report of history, examination findings, and treatments administered to patients since their admission. These are typically from one to five minutes in length. Formal presentations, on the other hand, are usually presented to larger groups, typically referred to as "grand rounds" or "in-services," in a conference setting. These presentations may cover a patient's entire medical history and treatment plan or may be focused on a medical issue or new intervention pertinent to the patients in that department. They are usually from 10 to 20 minutes in length. Interns/clinicians should check with the chief of staff/medical director or director of care for exact instructions regarding presentations.

Charting Procedures

Although the problem-oriented medical recordkeeping system is outlined in this text and is commonly used, it is not the system used in all institutions. The chiropractic physician should become familiar with whatever system is used in the hospital or LTC facility and integrate recordkeeping accordingly.

Clinics and Ward Rounds

It is necessary that physicians become familiar with history, physical examination, and infection control procedures commonly used in the institution. Imaging studies and protocols also vary between institutions. Finally, it is expected that interns on rotation and clinicians, especially in internal, family medicine services, and in all LTC facilities, will become somewhat knowledgeable regarding drugs of choice for the diseases most commonly seen in each respective patient population. Services can be provided either as inpatient or outpatient, depending on the department. In the case of LTC, all healthcare is provided as an inpatient service, in the patient's room. This means that the chiropractor may need to work within the limitations of both the patient and the room and will definitely need to modify his or her treatment interventions.

Institutional Committees

Hospital and LTC institutions have various committees in which a chiropractic clinician can partake, i.e., medical advisory committees, professional advisory committees, accreditation committees, etc. As well, there are many interdisciplinary team committees in both hospitals and LTC facilities (e.g., pain and palliative care, skin and wound care) that may be of interest to the chiropractor. This is an effective way to forge relations with the other providers, gain insight into the institution, and be able to affect change from the inside.

Surgery

Learning the surgical procedures in an operating room (OR) can make one's observation much more meaningful and worthwhile. The surgical suite can be one of the most instructional experiences of a career.

It is absolutely necessary that sterile technique be used in the OR. Preparations for surgery involve the following:

- Don a pair of surgical scrubs after all clothing is removed (including T-shirts). Tuck the scrub top into the bottoms.
- Move from the locker room and obtain a mask, cap, and shoe covers. Men with beards should wear full caps. All hair must be covered.
- Before scrubbing, remove all jewelry and nail polish and put on the surgical mask when close to the scrub sinks. (A mask must be worn in all areas except the OR hallways, unless near the scrub sinks in the hallways.)
- If contamination occurs during scrubbing, begin the entire procedure over again. (The purpose of scrubbing is to remove bacteria from the skin of the hands and arms.) Check with the surgeon before deviating from standard scrubbing protocols.
- After completing the hand scrub, go back into the OR and dry hands. Always keep hands above elbows until fully gowned and gloved.
- After drying, hold arms out straight in front and allow a nurse to slip on the gown. Another nurse will tie the back string (remember, one's back is not sterile). The nurse will then hold out a surgical glove. Push hands through the gloves. Make sure the gloves are free of any holes. Double gloving may be necessary for patients with highly contagious diseases, such as AIDS and hepatitis. Finish this procedure by giving the front string of the gown to the nurse, turn in place, and then tie the strings together. The surgeon may now instruct that the powder be wiped off the gloves.
- After being fully scrubbed, gowned, and gloved, ascertain where one should be located and stand there with hands above waist in the praying position. Do not cross arms.
- If the surgeon makes a request, perform it precisely while remaining sterile. When moving around the OR, pass sterile areas with the front of the body and nonsterile areas with the back.

- If someone in the OR says you have been contaminated, accept that fact and do what is deemed necessary to ensure your sterility.
- When unscrubbed or nonsterile in the OR, remain at least one foot from any sterile areas and do not touch anything that is sterile.

Roles for the Chiropractor in the Institutional Setting

Chiropractors already have a significant role in the community, particularly as neuromusculoskeletal specialists. This role can be translated quite effectively into the mainstream institutional setting, with careful treading. Some options for the chiropractor include the creation of a primary care, Neuromusculoskeletal (NMS) Center or chiropractic clinic, as an ambulatory center within the hospital and/or integrating in various specialty departments including but not limited to:

- General or specialty pain clinics, chronic care and/or rehabilitation departments/programs

Table 5.1 Collaborative Roles for the Chiropractor

Medical Physician	Nursing Staff	Chiropractor	Physiotherapists/ Restorative Care Staff
PCP and general diagnosis Drug intervention: evaluate dosage, interactions, precautions, and adverse reactions Reassess dosages based on outcomes	Patient, family education Patient positioning, wound care, skin integrity, drug tx, relaxation Documentation of self-reported pain, identify pain behaviors and indicators, communication with family Pain outcome measures	PCP for NMS conditions (diagnosis and conservative care) Consultant to RNs, PTs (pt positioning, rehab) Spinal/extremity manipulation, acupuncture, taping/braces, neuro-rehab, nutraceuticals	Assessment of gait, stability, general functional status Exercise: cardiovascular, strength/resistance training, general mobility, gait endurance, ergonomics/occupational therapy, relaxation techniques Physical modalities: TENS, heat, cold, ultrasound therapy

- Urgent Care (non-critical care) or Emergency Care departments
- Spinal Health and Research Center

The objectives and goals for long-term care often center on supportive care; for example, supportive interventions for basic activities of daily living and general function and supportive pain measures. This is also true for chronic care hospital departments. A chiropractor's most effective role in this setting is involvement in an interdisciplinary pain and palliative care team. Potential collaborative roles in an interdisciplinary LTC pain management team are summarized in Table 5.1.

There is currently only a small percentage of chiropractors integrated in hospitals and LTC facilities in Canada and the United States. Chiropractors have certainly developed an important role in the community, serving approximately 15% of the population, but have had a tendency to shy away from mainstream institutions. Mainstream healthcare is where the largest percentage of patients are. Full functional integration of chiropractic services in mainstream healthcare could create a tremendous socioeconomic impact on the system, by having the means to effectively access patients and to identify and treat musculoskeletal pain conditions that are often detrimental to quality of life. Integration may also help to offset the financial burden to the healthcare system.

PART II

CLINICAL INVESTIGATIONS

There are in fact two things, science and opinion: the former begets knowledge, the latter ignorance.

Hippocrates

Chapter 6

History, Physical Examination, and Differential Diagnosis

Lawrence H. Wyatt, DC, DACBR, FICC

History

The history is the first step in the evaluation of any patient's chief complaint. It has been demonstrated that a good clinical history will lead the physician to the correct diagnosis the vast majority of the time. The art of history taking includes the ability to gather an appropriate description of the patient's complaints, to elicit information that has not been volunteered by the patient and to know that the patient does not have clinically essential matters that are left unstated.

The first step in taking a history is to be attentive. Too often the diagnosis is elusive because the physician fails to let the patient adequately explain the signs and symptoms he or she is experiencing. Another helpful hint is to ask the patient open-ended questions rather than questions that suggest a predictable response from the patient. Facilitating, while not leading the patient's responses, is critical. For example, it is better to ask, "Are you experiencing any pain anywhere else in your body?" than asking, "You aren't experiencing any pain in your legs, are you?" The latter suggests to the patient that a negative answer is expected. Questions should be phrased in terms that the patient fully understands; medical terminology should be avoided. Encouraging a patient to be an active participant in care begins with collaborating with him or her. For example, the question, "Are you experiencing any pain below your breastbone?" is better than, "Are you experiencing any substernal angina?"

Facilitation involves the use of both verbal and nonverbal cues, so the patient explains his or her problem in a narrative format rather than spending time answering your questions. Silence on the part of the physician while making eye contact with the patient allows the patient to narrate the problem. Paraphrasing what the patient said and repeating it can be very helpful in making the patient comfortable and will often elicit a more accurate and detailed response. It is also important to remember to record a negative response from a patient as "the patient denies leg pain" rather than "the patient has not had any leg pain." This distinction places the onus for accurate clinical reporting on the patient. Every attempt should be made to quantify historical findings (e.g., "four days" instead of "for a while").

Chief Complaint

The chief complaint is the reason for the patient's visit. Avoid interpreting the patient's response and, instead, record it *verbatim* when possible and enclose it in quotation marks. It may become apparent later during the examination that this complaint is not the patient's most serious problem, but it is the starting point of all good clinical workups.

A number of factors concerning the chief complaint must be obtained. These are included in the mnemonic OPPQRST and represent the events of the present illness.

- *Onset*—When did this complaint begin?
- *Provocative factors*—What worsens the complaint (e.g., movement, lying down)?
- *Palliative factors*—What relieves the complaint (e.g., aspirin, rest, lying on your side)?
- *Quality*—What type of pain is it (e.g., dull, achy, sharp, stabbing, gnawing, burning)?
- *Radiation*—Does the pain radiate to other areas of the body? How far and specifically to what region(s)?
- *Setting*—When does the complaint occur (e.g., when bending over, morning, night)?
- *Timing*—How long does the complaint last (e.g., 20 minutes, continuous, intermittent)?

As the patient answers these questions, it will become obvious that other follow-up questions are necessary to help the clinician collate all the information pertinent to the history of the present illness (HPI). Any dates and times included in the HPI should be accurate. Follow-up questions are helpful in confirming or denying what the patient has already said. After the follow-up questioning, the clinician may wish to repeat the HPI back to the patient for further confirmation.

During clinical history taking it is important to uncover clues that will guide you in formulating a working diagnosis and therapeutic regimen. Of critical importance in this search is to seek out clues in the history that the patient may be suffering from a serious illness. Table 6.1 lists items that should raise suspicion of a more serious condition.

General History

In taking the general history, the following components, represented by the mnemonic A.M.P.L.E., are reviewed. (Table 6.2)

Allergies

The presence of allergies to drugs, foods, and other substances should be noted. The exact reactions to allergens, including timing and eventual outcome, should be recorded.

Medications

Any medications the patient is currently taking, including analgesics and oral contraceptive agents, should be noted. The dosage, route of administration, and intended purpose of the drug(s) should also be charted. Any adverse reactions should be noted, with the type and severity of the reaction.

Past Medical History (PMH)

The mnemonic H.I.S.T.O.R.Y. is used in remembering the physical elements of the PMH.

- *Hospitalizations*—a chronological record of the patient's hospitalizations, with the reason for admission, treatment, and any complications. Obstetric history is also obtained here. The number of pregnancies (gravida), live births (para), and spontaneous or elective/therapeutic abortions (aborta) should be charted. A woman having had no children is nulliparous, having her first pregnancy is primiparous, and having had multiple children is multiparous. Any difficulties with pregnancies or labor and delivery should also be noted.
- *Injuries*—any trauma the patient has sustained, including date of trauma, treatment, and outcome for each event
- *Sugar Diabetes*—family or patient history of diabetes mellitus or any other diseases such as myocardial infarction, cerebrovascular accident, or liver, kidney, or lung disease, including dates, treatments, and any sequelae

Table 6.1 Historical Items Suggesting Serious Disease

General
Prior care without any relief (2)
Rapidly progressive symptoms
Cancer (2,3)
Insidious nontraumatic onset of pain
Night pain
History of previous cancer
Unexplained weight loss
Vertebrobasilar ischemia/aneurysm (4)
"Worst headache/neck pain I've ever had"
Vertigo
Blurred vision
Nausea and vomiting
Ataxia
Dysarthria
Infection
High grade fever
Substance abuse
Unstable neurologic lesion
Progressive neurologic findings
Loss of bowel and/or bladder control
Motor weakness
Bilateral anesthesia
Major trauma
Fall from >10 feet
Midline spine pain
Cardiovascular lesion
Substernal chest pain
Nondermatomal medial left arm pain
Shortness of breath
Loss of distal pulses
Cold extremities

Table 6.2 History Mnemonics

A-allergies
M-medications
P-past medical history
L-last meal, last menstrual period
E-events of the present illness
O-onset of problem
P-provocative factors
P-palliative factors
Q-quality of symptoms
R-radiation of symptoms
S-setting under which the symptoms occur
T-timing of symptoms
H-hospitalizations
I-injuries
S-sugar diabetes
T-tumors
O-operations
R-review of systems
Y-youth diseases

- *Tumors*—any history of cancer, including type of cancer, date of diagnosis, treatment, and outcome
- *Operations*—any surgical procedures, especially those related to the chief complaint, including date of and reason for surgery as well as clinical outcome and complications
- *Review of Systems (ROS)*—the review of each of the organ systems of the body (see Table 6.3)
- *Youth Diseases*—childhood diseases and immunizations are important, as they may offer the final clue to an elusive diagnosis

Table 6.3 Elements in the Review of Systems (ROS)

System	Symptom
General	Weight change, fatigue, anorexia, weakness, fever, chills, changes in activity
Skin	Rashes, eruptions, changes in warts or moles, pigmentation changes, bruising, itching, hair loss, nail changes
Head	Trauma, headaches, dizziness, lightheadedness
Eyes	Change in acuity of vision, use of corrective lenses, loss of vision, diplopia, photophobia, blurred vision, scotomata, pain, excessive lacrimation, redness, discharge
Ears	Changes in hearing, deafness, tinnitus, discharge, pain, vertigo, otitis
Nose	Rhinorrhea, epistaxis, allergies, airway obstruction
Mouth and throat	Ulcers, tooth pain/extractions, temporomandibular joint pain, gum bleeding, soreness, swelling, enlarged glands, sore throat, strep throat
Neck	Stiffness, lumps/swelling/masses, pain
Lungs	Cough (productive/nonproductive), hemoptysis, dyspnea, pain with respiration, wheezing, night sweats
Cardiac	Palpitations, chest pain, orthopnea, paroxysmal nocturnal dyspnea, ankle swelling, syncope
Vascular	Raynaud's phenomenon, intermittent claudication, hypertension, rheumatic fever
Breasts	Self-examination frequency/results, pain, nipple discharge, lumps/masses, skin dimpling
Gastrointestinal	Usual diet, dysphagia, regurgitation, dyspepsia, nausea, vomiting, belching, abdominal pain, cramps, hematemesis, stool color changes, diarrhea, constipation, change in bowel habits, jaundice, abdominal swelling
Genitourinary	Polyuria, nocturia, oliguria, dysuria, urgency, incontinence, urine color changes, hematuria, sexually transmitted diseases, dyspareunia, scotal mass (male), hernia
Endocrine	Polydypsia, polyphagia, temperature intolerance, tremors, goiter, alopecia, hirsutism, menstruation history, pregnancy history, dysmenorrhea, premenstrual syndrome, climacteric
Hematopoietic	Anemia, abnormal bleeding, lymph node enlargement/pain
Musculoskeletal	Bone/joint pain, swelling, joint deformity, trauma, restricted range of motion, weakness, atrophy
Neurological	Cranial nerve deficits, seizures, loss of consciousness, paralysis, tremors, ataxia, loss of balance, numbness, paresthesias
Psychological	Mood swings, depression, anxiety, phobias

Family History

A record of relatives' health, including disease history in living relatives and causes of death and ages at time of death of deceased family members (Figure 6–1), illustrates a typical family history tree.

Psychosocial History

Queries should be made regarding home and sex life as well as the patient's normal activities of daily living, especially with regard to how the present complaint may be interfering with any of those activities. Alcohol and drug use should also be documented. Cigarette smoking should be charted as the number of packs per day multiplied by the number of years smoking. The result will be a number of "pack years." This value better serves the clinician in that it better represents the amount the patient has smoked.

Last Menstrual Period/Last Meal

The day of onset of the last menstrual period is important for both the history and the assessment of the ability to X-ray the patient. This is explained in Chapter 10. In cases involving abdominal and thoracic complaints, the time and contents of the patient's last meal can be important.

Events of the Present Illness

The characteristics of the present illness are assessed by asking the patient a number of questions. These questions are outlined in the section in this chapter on chief complaint and are outlined by the mnemonic OPPQRST.

Figure 6–1 **Family History Tree**

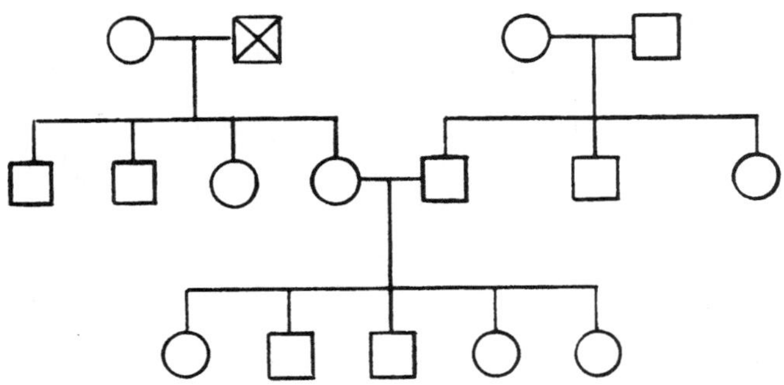

Note: □ = male; ○ = female; X = dead (cause of death and disease for each individual should be noted).

Physical Examination

The complement to the clinical history is the physical examination, an art that has been forsaken by many and replaced by advanced diagnostic testing. Most often the proper diagnosis can be ascertained from a good history and physical examination.

General Signs (Table 6.4)

The physical examination should begin as soon as the clinician sees the patient, with an overview of the body habitus and general health. Ideally, the patient should not have had alcohol, tobacco, caffeine, or performed vigorous exercise within 30 minutes of the exam. The examination room should be well-lit, quiet, and the patient should be appropriately gowned. The patient's height, weight, and body mass index (BMI) are recorded. (Table 6.5) BMI has been shown to be directly correlated with risk of death; as BMI increases, risk of death increases as well. (1) The amount of distress displayed by the patient, such as through facial

Table 6.4 General Physical Exam Signs

Body habitus	
Normal	Mesomorphic
Thin	Ectomorphic
Obese	Endomorphic
Height	
Weight	
Distress levels	
Normal	No apparent distress
Mild	Mild distress
Moderate	Moderate distress
Severe	Severe distress
Mental alertness	
Person	Who are you?
Place	Where are you?
Time	What time is it?
Situation	Why are you here?

Table 6.5 Optimum Body Mass Index (BMI)*†

Normal	18.5-24.9
Grade 1 obesity	25.0-29.9
Grade 2 obesity	30.0-30.9
Grade 3 obesity	>40.0

*weight (kg) divided by height (m) squared
†World Health Organization

grimacing, a limp, or protection of the affected part, should be noted. Also, whether a patient's stated age is in concert with his or her apparent age should be determined.

The patient's affect (e.g., overall emotional state) can be assessed by simply conversing with the patient and noting his or her alertness and orientation to time, place, identity, and the present situation (AOx4).

Vital Signs

Table 6.6 outlines normal and abnormal values of adult vital signs. Record data on the following vital bodily functions with the patient in a resting, nonagitated state, if possible.

- Temperature-oral, rectal, aural, or axillary
- Pulse rate and characteristics
- Respiratory rate and characteristics
- Blood pressure (BP)-supine, seated, and standing, if necessary

Clinical Pearls

- A patient who is febrile has an infection until proven otherwise.
- Supraventricular tachycardia can, at times, be controlled by having the patient perform a Valsalva maneuver until emergency assistance arrives.
- Any irregular pulse rate should be monitored for one full minute.
- Pulses can be regular (normal), regularly irregular (a regular pattern with periodic skipped beats), and irregularly irregular (chaotic with no distinguishable pattern). There are a number of abnormal pulse patterns which are outlined in Table 6.7.

Table 6.6 Adult Vital Signs and Sequelae

Temperature		
Oral	96.5 (35.9)-99.1 (37.3) degrees	
Axillary	95.5 (35.3)-98.1 (37.7) degrees	
Rectal/Aural	97.5 (36.4)-100.1 (37.8) degrees	
Pulse (resting)		
Regular rate, rhythm and amplitude		
Normal	60–100 beats per minute (bpm)	
Bradycardia	<60 bpm	
Tachycardia	>100 bpm	
Respirations (resting)		
Regular rate and rhythm, nonlabored		
Normal	12-20 per minute	
Bradypnea	<12 per minute	
Tachypnea	>20 per minute	
Blood Pressure (resting)*		
Finding	**Systolic**	**Diastolic**
Normal	<130	<80
Pre-hypertension	130-139	80-89
Systolic hypertension	>140	<90
Mild hypertension	140-159	90-99
Moderate hypertension	160-179	100-109
Severe hypertension	180-209	110-119
Hypertensive crisis	>210	>120

*Normal pulse pressure (systolic-diastolic) is ~30-40 mm Hg (see text for abnormalities)

- Respirations are counted after the pulse is noted but before the clinician's hand is removed from the patient's wrist to prevent the patient from voluntarily changing his or her respiratory rate.
- Abnormalities in respiration are outlined in Table 6.8.
- Incorrect BP cuff placement can result in inaccurate readings. The bottom of the cuff should be approximately one inch above the antecubital fossa with the bladder centered over the brachial artery.
- Incorrect BP cuff size can result in inaccurate readings. The cuff should be approximately 40% of the limb's circumference and 80% of the length of the brachium.

Table 6.7 Common Abnormal Pulses

Bradycardia (<60 bpm)
- Hypothyroidism
- Congestive heart failure (decompensated)
- Athletes
- Medications

Irregularly irregular pulse (chaotic with no distinguishable pattern)
- Premature ventricular contractions
- Atrial fibrillation

Pulsus alternans (alternation between small and large pulse amplitudes)
- Left-sided heart failure

Pulsus deferens (difference in pulse amplitude from right to left)
- Unilateral vascular obstruction

Pulsus paradoxus (inspiratory decrease in arterial pressure >10 mm Hg)
- Chronic obstructive pulmonary disease (emphysema, asthma)
- Right-sided heart failure
- Pericarditis/effusion
- Hypovolemia
- Pulmonary embolism
- Tricuspid stenosis

Regularly irregular pulse (associated with regularly spaced premature ventricular contractions)
- Bigeminal pulse-every other beat is of low amplitude
- Trigeminal pulse-every third beat is of low amplitude

Tachycardia (>100 bpm)
- Anemia
- Hyperthyroidism
- Hypovolemia
- Fever
- Exercise
- Congestive heart failure

Water-hammer pulse (bounding pulse with rapid ascent and descent)
- Aortic regurgitation
- Patent ductus arteriosus

Table 6.8 **Common Respiratory Abnormalities**

- Bradypnea (respiratory rate of <12/minute)
  - Athletes
  - Central nervous system disease
  - Electrolyte disturbances
  - Acid-base balance abnormalities
  - Pulmonary infection
  - Uremia
- Hyperpnea (deep, rapid, labored breathing)
  - Anxiety/hyperventilation
  - Exercise
  - Central nervous system disease
  - Metabolic acidosis (Kussmaul respiration)
- Hypopnea (shallow breathing)
  - Rib fracture
  - Pleurisy
- Orthopnea (dyspnea with recumbancy)
  - Congestive heart failure
  - Pulmonary edema
- Paroxysmal Noctural Dyspnea (sudden dyspnea during sleep)
  - Congestive heart failure
- Prolonged Exhalation
  - Chronic obstructive pulmonary disease
- Prolonged Inspiration
  - Chronic restrictive pulmonary disease
- Tachypnea
  - Exertion
  - Respiratory acidosis
  - Fever
  - Congestive heart failure
  - Pneumonia
  - Acute respiratory distress

- The diagnosis of hypertension (HTN) (>140/90) requires three separate measurements at least six hours apart.
- Most cases (90%) of HTN are considered essential HTN, with no identifiable cause. Causes such as renal disease or nervous system disease should be ruled out before making the diagnosis of essential HTN.
- Orthostatic hypotension is diagnosed by a fall of greater than 20 mm of Hg when the patient moves from a recumbent position to a standing position. (5) Common causes include central/peripheral nervous system lesions, venous pooling, heart failure, and side effects from medications.
- Pre-hypertension has been demonstrated to increase the risk of developing HTN two-fold. (6)
- Altered pulse pressure reading (< >30–40 mm Hg) is found with a number of pathologic conditions. (Table 6.9)
- Asymmetric BP readings can be a sign of unilateral vascular obstruction.

Table 6.9 **Common Pulse Pressure Abnormalities**

High (widened) pulse pressure (>40 mm Hg)
Isolated systolic HTN
Anemia
Stimulants (caffeine, medications)
Hyperthyroidism
Fever
Anxiety
Aortic regurgitation
Pregnancy
Low (narrowed) pulse pressure (<30 mm Hg)
Tachycardia
Congestive heart failure
Aortic stenosis
Pericarditis/pericardial effusion
Ascites

Skin

The temperature, color, and consistency of the skin along with the presence of any scars, tattoos, moles, unusual hair distribution, or rashes are noted. The presence of itching and tenderness are important signs for differential diagnosis.

Common skin lesions include macules (flat lesion, < 5 mm; freckle, rubella), papules (raised lesion, < 5 mm; measles), pustules (raised lesion, < 5 mm, filled with pus; furuncle), vesicles (raised lesion, < 5 mm, filled with serous fluid; herpes simplex), nodules (hard raised lesion, > 5 mm; granuloma), and bullae (raised lesion, > 5 mm, filled with serous fluid; blister).

Clinical Pearls

- Central cyanosis presents as blue discoloration of the skin of the lips, face and chest and is associated with cardiovascular diseases.
- Peripheral cyanosis presents as blue discoloration of the acral portions of the extremities and is most often associated with peripheral vascular disease.
- Jaundiced patients have a yellowing of the skin and sclera (icterus) and may also have itching.
- Generally speaking, benign skin lesions are tender, mobile, and do not bleed, while nontender, hard, immobile, bleeding lesions are malignant.
- Malignant skin lesions are typically painless (7). Any mole that changes in size, shape, or consistency is malignant until proven otherwise.

Head/Face

Examination of the head includes assessment of size and shape along with hair distribution and any visible skin lesions. Tender areas are also noted. The normal head is considered atraumatic normocephalic. Abnormal skull shapes include scaphocephaly (abnormally long skull; premature closure of sagittal suture), brachycephaly (abnormally wide forehead/skull; premature closure of coronal suture), plagiocephaly ("crooked skull"; deformed skull shape or premature closure of one side of the coronal suture), trigonocephaly (triangular-shaped forehead; premature closure of the metopic suture) and unexplained enlargement of the skull (Paget's disease).

The presence of any facial deformities suggestive of certain diseases is recorded. These include hypertelorism (eyes too far apart), hypotelorism (eyes too close together), micrognathia (abnormally small mandible), prognathism (abnormally large mandible), and cleft lip/palate (abnormal nonclosure of upper lip or portion/all of soft/hard palate). The anomalies in facial bone formation can occur singularly or as part of a congenital syndrome.

Clinical Pearls

- The bruits of intracranial tumors, aneurysms, and arteriovenous malformations can be auscultated with the bell of the stethoscope, oftentimes over the orbits. (8)
- Hypothyroid patients present with a "moon facies" and acromegalics have prognathism, a protruding mandible.

Eyes (Figure 6–2)

The eyes should be examined for any of the following:

- *Eyelids*—Inability to close the lids, edema, drooping (ptosis), and the presence of turned-in eyelid (entropion) or turned-out eyelid (extropion).
- *Lacrimal Apparatus*—Overflowing tears (epiphora) and blockage of the nasolacrimal duct, palpation of the lacrimal gland for size and tenderness.
- *Conjunctiva/Sclera*—Unusual scleral color and the presence of nodules. Is there any redness of the conjunctiva? The lower lid should be everted and the "redness" of the internal aspect of the lid estimated.

Figure 6–2 **Normal Retina of the Right Eye**

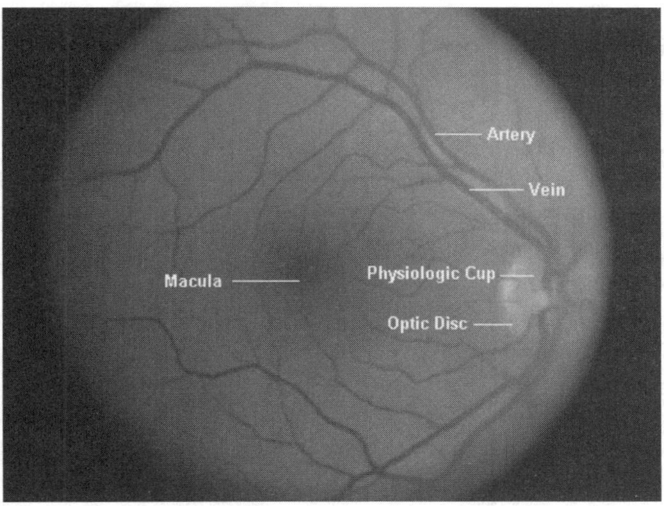

- *Pupil/Iris*—Unusual size or shape of the pupil and iris along with defects in the iris. Pupillary reflex is challenged for direct and consensual response. Any asymmetry in pupillary size is also noted. Pupillary abnormalities are identified in Table 6.10.
- *Extraocular Muscles*—The six cardinal positions of gaze (Figure 6–3); any nystagmus and its characteristics, any deviation of the eyes (strabismus). The motions of the eyes and their respective cranial nerve supply are represented by the formula *LR6 SO4 A03* (lateral rectus/CN VI, superior oblique/CN IV, all others/CN III).
- *Visual Acuity*—Acuity is checked with Snellen and Rosenbaum charts. Note if the vision was checked with or without corrective lenses.

Table 6.10 Pupillary Abnormalities

Pupillary Abnormalities
Anisocoria (pupillary inequality)
Physiologic, associated with aging
Migraine headache
Horner's syndrome
Cranial nerve III palsy
Eye trauma
Pontine hemorrhage
Mydriasis (pupillary dilation)
Stimulants (bilateral)
Antihistamines (bilateral)
Antidepressants (bilateral)
Increased intracranial pressure (bilateral)
Meiosis (pupillary constriction)
Parasympathomimetic drugs (bilateral)
Opiate overdose (bilateral)
White pupil reflex/leukocoria (white instead of red reflex when shining light into eye)
Retinoblastoma
Corneal opacity
Cataract
Retinal disease
Hyphema (blood in the anterior chamber)

Figure 6–3 **Cardinal Positions of Gaze and Ocular Muscle Movement**

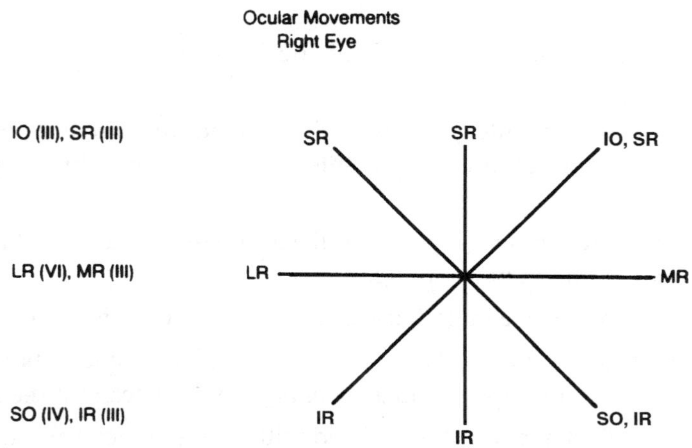

- *Visual Fields*—Fields are checked by the confrontation method. A general estimation of the size of each field is made and recorded.
- *Ocular Pressure*—A general estimation of pressure, made by palpating the globe. Any right-to-left asymmetry is noted. Elevated pressure is consistent with glaucoma.
- *Fundoscopic Examination*—Any defects in the red reflex (cataracts, etc.) and their position and shape. Are there any abnormalities of the anterior or posterior chambers, retina, optic disc, macula, or microvasculature?

Clinical Pearls

- Yellow sclera is consistent with icterus (jaundice); blue sclera with osteogenesis imperfecta.
- Eyelid abnormalities include xanthelasma (yellowish, flat, lid deposits; hyperlipidemia), ptosis (lid drooping; cranial nerve III (true ptosis)), cranial nerve VII (pseudoptosis), entropion (lower lid turned inward (may irritate conjunctiva/cornea)), extropion (lower lid turned outward (excessive tearing)), hordeolum (sty; infection of an eyelash follicle) and chalazion (meibomian gland infection).
- Abnormalities of the globe (eyeball) include pterygium (abnormal overgrowth of conjunctiva which covers a portion of the iris), conjunctivitis

("pink eye"; contagious viral/bacterial infection of the conjunctiva), subconjunctival hemorrhage (traumatic well-outlined area of blood under the conjuctiva), exophthalmos (protrusion of the globes; hyperthyroidism, retro-globar tumor, normal variant in blacks and Mediterraneans).

- Pallor of the internal aspects of the lower eyelids is consistent with anemia.
- Arcus senilis (white/gray deposits around the circumference of the cornea) is normal in older patients but may indicate hyperlipidemia in younger patients.
- An Argyll Robertson pupil (syphilis) is one that is small and responds to accommodation but not to light.
- Unequal pupil size in geriatric patients (anisocoria) is not uncommon.
- Emmetropia is normal far and near vision; hyperopia is farsightedness (cannot see close up); myopia is nearsightedness (cannot see far away).
- Presbyopia is hyperopia associated with aging; typically seen in patients over 40.
- Paralysis or palsy of an extraocular muscle should lead to a search for intracranial pathology as the primary concern. (9)
- A patient with mydriasis and/or visual field loss (nasal?, peripheral?, total?) who sees halos around lights should be evaluated for glaucoma. (10)
- A swollen optic disc (papilledema) suggests an increase in intracranial pressure and pseudotumor cerebri. (11)
- Black spots on the retina are suspicious for retinitis pigmentosa.
- Arterioles are smaller than venules; arterioles reflect light better than venules.
- Diabetic retinopathy causes microaneurysms (red spots on retina; earliest sign of retinopathy), retinal hemorrhages (red dots similar to microaneurysms), cotton-wool spots (poorly defined yellowish retinal lesions), nerve fiber retinal layer infarcts, venous beading (retinal ischemia), and macular edema.
- Hypertensive retinopathy causes arteriovenous nicking (compression of the venule beneath a thickened arteriole), increased arteriolar light reflex, decreased size of arterioles, cotton-wool spots (poorly defined yellowish retinal lesions; retinal infarcts), shiny retina and papilledema.
- Optic neuritis is often an early sign of multiple sclerosis.

- Loss of temporal vision bilaterally (bitemporal hemianopsia) is consistent with a parasellar lesion compressing the optic chiasm.
- A simple test for myopia is for the patient to look at the vision charts through a pinhole. If vision improves, the patient is myopic.

Ears

External Examination

Examination of the ears begins with inspection of the pinna, tragus, and antitragus for any visible lesions (gouty tofus). A slight tug should be placed on the outer ear and any pain (otitis externa) and its location noted. The presence and type of discharge (cerumen, pus) from the external auditory canal is also important.

Otoscopic Examination

The largest speculum that will fit comfortably into the external auditory canal should be used. The external auditory canal is examined for any wax buildup (cerumen), foreign bodies, or lesions (otitis externa (swimmer's ear)). The tympanic membrane is checked for normal light reflex (five o'clock in the right ear and seven o'clock in the left ear), any defects (perforated membrane), scars, fluid behind the membrane (otitis media), and infection of the membrane itself (tympanitis). The normal tympanic membrane is a pinkish gray color. A sharp tap on the mastoid process is a quick check for mastoiditis.

Auditory Examination

Weber's test, the Rinne's test, watch ticking, and finger rubbing are ways to evaluate hearing. If impairment is found, audiometry is indicated to define the loss as sensorineural or conductive in nature.

Clinical Pearls

- Pull the pinna up and back to straighten the external auditory canal for insertion of a speculum.
- Presbycusis is hearing loss associated with aging.
- Chalky white deposits in the pinna are classically associated with gout.
- Cauliflower ear (external ear appears unusually shaped) is often the result of repeated trauma (e.g., wrestlers).
- A blue-black discoloration of the external ear is found in alkaptonuria (ochronosis (deposition of homogentisic acid into connective tissues)).
- Pain with movement of the pinna is consistent with otitis externa (swimmer's ear).

- The external auditory canal is a relatively common location for psoriasis.
- The most common cause of hearing loss is cerumen (wax) buildup in the external canal. Other common causes include prolonged exposure to loud noises, Meniere's disease (deafness, tinnitus, vertigo, nausea, and vomiting), acoustic neuroma, ototoxic antibiotics (erythromycin, kanamycin, neomycin), and recurrent otitis media.
- Pure conductive hearing loss is demonstrated by lateralization of sound to the affected ear on Weber's test, with bone conduction > air conduction on Rinne's test.
- Pure sensorineural hearing loss is evidenced by lateralization of sound to the unaffected ear on Weber's test and air conduction > bone conduction on Rinne's test.
- Otitis media is evidenced by retro-membranous effusion or air-fluid levels with an intact tympanic membrane; effusion may be serous or purulent.

Nose

The normal midline position of the septum is checked, as is the presence of any nasal discharge (acute coryza, allergic rhinitis, purulent discharge of bacterial infection). Speculum examination includes evaluation for obstruction (polyp), deformity (deviated nasal septum), lesions (ulcers, cancer), mucosal color (normally pink), and tenderness. Finally, sinusitis may be suggested by tapping on the skin over each of the frontal and maxillary sinuses. The sinuses may then be transilluminated for detection of fluid/air-fluid levels.

Clinical Pearls

- A pale, bluish discoloration of the nasal mucosa is indicative of hay fever (allergic rhinitis).
- Nasal polyps are seen with asthma, aspirin sensitivity, and cystic fibrosis (12).
- The most common cause of nosebleeds (epistaxis) is nose picking, although allergic rhinitis, HTN, infection and bleeding disorders should also be considered. (13)

Throat

The teeth, lips, and gums are assessed for lesions that can signal systemic illness. The oropharynx is inspected for redness (streptococcal pharyngitis (e.g., strep throat)), lesions (oropharyngeal cancer), and tonsillar swelling (tonsillitis). The gag reflex (cranial nerves IX, X) is also tested with a tongue depressor. Ask the patient to stick out his or her tongue to test the integrity of cranial nerve XII. A search for cervical lymphadenopathy should also be made. Benign lymph nodes are tender, mobile, and generally soft to firm. Malignant lymph nodes are generally nontender, immobile, and hard.

Clinical Pearls

- If you wish to suppress the gag reflex to examine the oropharynx and palate, have the patient inhale slowly while you insert a tongue depressor.
- Oral candidiasis is classically associated with diabetes mellitus and acquired immune deficiency syndrome (AIDS). (14)
- Oral candidiasis lesions are painful and bleed when scraped away.
- Leukoplakia is painless, does not bleed when scraped away, and is considered a precancerous lesion and should therefore be biopsied.
- The uvula deviates to the unaffected side with cranial nerve X lesions.
- The tongue deviates to the affected side with cranial nerve XII lesions.

Thorax/Lungs

Inspection

Asymmetry and abnormal shapes (Table 6.11) of the thorax are noted as well as unilateral inspiratory insufficiency. The respiratory rate is noted (normal=12–20/minute). Any alteration in the breathing pattern is also recorded. Skin lesions (vesicles (herpes zoster)) and café au lait spots (neurofibromatosis) are also noted. Inspection for blue discoloration of the extremities (peripheral cyanosis) or lips, face, and chest (central cyanosis) should also be performed.

Palpation

Chest expansion (normal=2.5–5.0 cm) and any paradoxical motion suggestive of a flail chest (multiple concurrent rib fractures) should be charted. Also noted should be any palpable tenderness (rib fracture, intercostal neuralgia) crepitus (rib fracture, subcutaneous emphysema) or deformity (rib fracture, pectus excavatum, pectus carinatum). Tactile fremitus is also performed.

Percussion

Check for normal diaphragmatic excursion (2–5 cm). Percussion in each of intercostal spaces is also conducted and the type of percussion note charted. The percussive note in chronic obstructive pulmonary disease (COPD) and pneumothorax is hyperresonant, and flat to dull in pneumonia and atelectasis.

Table 6.11 Abnormalities in the Shape of the Thorax

- Barrel chest
  - Increased anterior to posterior diameter of thorax (>1/2 width of thorax)
  - Associated with chronic obstructive pulmonary disease
- Gibbus deformity
  - Sharp angular kyphosis in thoracic spine
  - Associated with trauma and tuberculous spondylitis
- Pectus carinatum
  - Pigeon-chest
  - Sternum bows outward
  - Developmental anomaly
  - Occasionally seen with Marfan's syndrome and rickets
  - Normally of no clinical significance
- Pectus excavatum
  - Funnel-chest
  - Valley in the chest at the region of the sternum
  - Developmental anomaly
  - Of no particular clinical significance, unless cardiac compression is a concern

Auscultation

Begin with the posterior chest and listen in a systematic manner comparing right to left for asymmetry. Note any adventitious sounds such as crackles (rales), rhonchi, wheezes, or pleural friction rub. (Table 6.12) Also listen for an increase in the exhalation phase of respiration suggestive of COPD or during the inhalation phase, suggestive of chronic restrictive pulmonary disease. If indicated, perform egophony (a spoken "eeee" is heard as "aaaa" through the stethoscope), whispered pectoriloquy (a patient's whisper can be heard through the stethoscope), and bronchophony (louder and clearer spoken sounds heard through the stethoscope) tests that, when positive, are suggestive of pulmonary fluid.

Clinical Pearls

- Use the bell of the stethoscope to auscultate to lung apices and the diaphragm for the remainder of the examination.
- Emphysema patients are acyanotic and tachypneic (pink puffers) and have a barrel-shaped chest.

Table 6.12 Adventitious Lung Sounds

Crackles (Rales)
Crackling, high-pitched late inhalation sounds
Do not clear with coughing
Associated with pulmonary edema, bronchiectasis, and late pneumonia
Pleural friction rub
A dry, scratchy, grating, high-pitched inhalation sound
Associated with pleurisy
Rhonchi
Crackling, rumbling low-pitched inhalation/exhalation sounds
Clear with coughing
Associated with mucous plugs in bronchi with asthma and chronic bronchitis
Wheezes
Whistling, squeaking, high-pitched exhalation sound
Associated with bronchiolar narrowing
Can be associated with asthma or emphysema

- Chronic bronchitis patients are cyanotic and overweight (blue bloaters).
- Congestive heart failure patients may demonstrate Cheyne-Stokes respiration (Figure 6–4).
- Clubbing of the digits can be seen with chronic lung diseases. (15)

Heart and Great Vessels

Peripheral Examination

Inspection

The cardiovascular examination begins with a check for cyanosis and clubbing (16) of the digits. The precordium is inspected for any abnormal bulges or pulsations and also for the position of the apical impulse. If indicated, the jugular venous pulse is examined in the patient's neck by noting the height of the pulse above the level of the sternal notch.

Palpation

The radial and carotid pulses are then palpated for rate, rhythm, and character, and the BP is checked. The remainder of the peripheral pulses are then checked. Palpation is then used to confirm inspection findings, find any thrills

Figure 6–4 Cheyne-Stokes Respiration

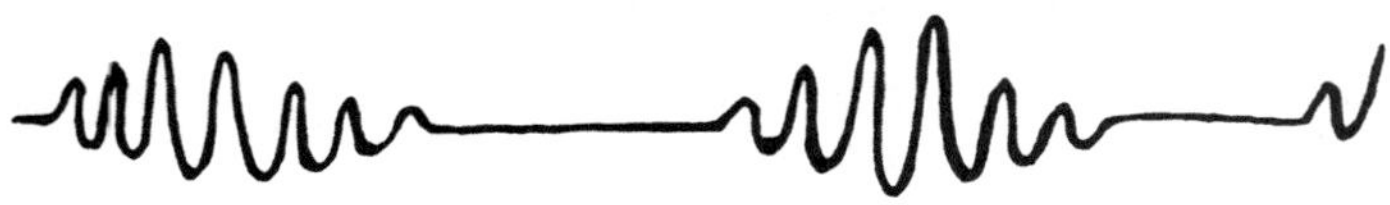

("palpable" murmurs), and locate the point of maximum intensity of the apical impulse, which is normally in the left 5th intercostal space at the midclavicular line.

Percussion
Percussion of the heart is usually deferred but it can be used to outline its borders. Cardiac size is better estimated with a chest X-ray or echocardiography. (17)

Auscultation
Each of the five auscultatory areas (Figure 6–5) are examined. The heart sounds (S1, S2), systole, diastole, and any adventitious sounds, such as pericardial friction rubs, are identified. (Table 6.13) Murmurs should be classified as to coarse and fine, timing, quality, intensity, and area of maximum intensity and radiation. Special maneuvers may also be used to accentuate murmurs. Figure 6–6 outlines the more common cardiac murmurs and Table 6.14 describes the grading system for murmurs.

Clinical Pearls

- Listen to the heart with both diaphragm and bell, as low pitch sounds are best heard with the bell and high pitch sounds with the diaphragm.
- A split of the S2 heart sound, particularly on inspiration, is usually of no clinical concern.
- A third heart sound (S3) may be normal, but a fourth sound (S4) is considered pathologic, usually indicating congestive heart failure. S3 is heard in early diastole while S4 is heard in late diastole.
- Systolic murmurs are often physiologic in young, thin patients.
- A diastolic murmur should never be considered normal.
- The normal jugular venous pulse is <5 cm above the sternal notch. An elevated pressure is consistent with right heart failure.
- Left heart failure causes pulmonary signs and right heart failure causes peripheral signs.

Figure 6–5 **Areas for Cardiac Auscultation**

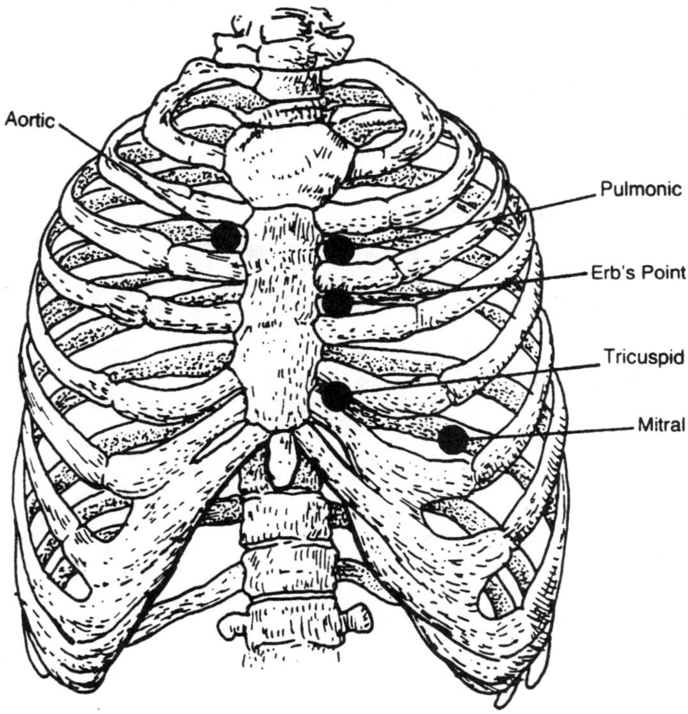

- Pressure on the liver while the patient lies supine can produce an increase in the visible jugular pulse (hepatojugular reflux).

Abdomen

Examination of the abdomen is performed in a different order than other physical examination procedures; inspection, auscultation, percussion, palpation. This prevents the bowel sounds from being disturbed by palpation being performed too early in the examination.

Inspection

The shape (scaphoid) and size (distension) of the abdomen and umbilicus (umbilical hernia), and the presence of any dilated veins (caput medusa), skin lesions, scars (laparoscopy, laparotomy), and striae (stretch marks, adrenal

Table 6.13 Adventitious Cardiac Sounds

Ejection click
- Clicking noise heard during early systole
- Aortic and pulmonic valve stenosis
- Mitral prolapse (non-ejection click)

Opening snap
- Snapping noise heard during early diastole
- Not affected by respiration
- Mitral valve stenosis
- Can be confused with S2

Pericardial friction rub
- Scratching noise heard during systole/diastole
- Pericarditis

S3
- Heard in early diastole, low-pitched
- Patient in left lateral decubitus position
- May be normal or congestive heart failure

S4
- Heard in late diastole, low-pitched
- Congestive heart failure

disease) are noted. A check should also be made for any visible peristalsis (early bowel obstruction) or abnormal pulsations (aneurysm).

Auscultation

All four quadrants of the abdomen are auscultated for bowel sound quantity (normal=3–30/minute) and quality. The regions of abdominal vasculature (abdominal aorta, renal arteries, splenic artery) should be checked for the presence of bruits, which are consistent with abnormal flow from atherosclerosis or aneurysm and venous hums (venous obstruction, hepatic hemangioma). Figure 6–7 graphically displays the normal position of abdominal vessels.

Percussion

The percussion notes (Table 6.15) in each quadrant and over abdominal viscera are noted. The presence of shifting dullness with patient movement from right to left lateral decubitus positions is associated with ascites.

Figure 6–6 Common Cardiac Murmurs

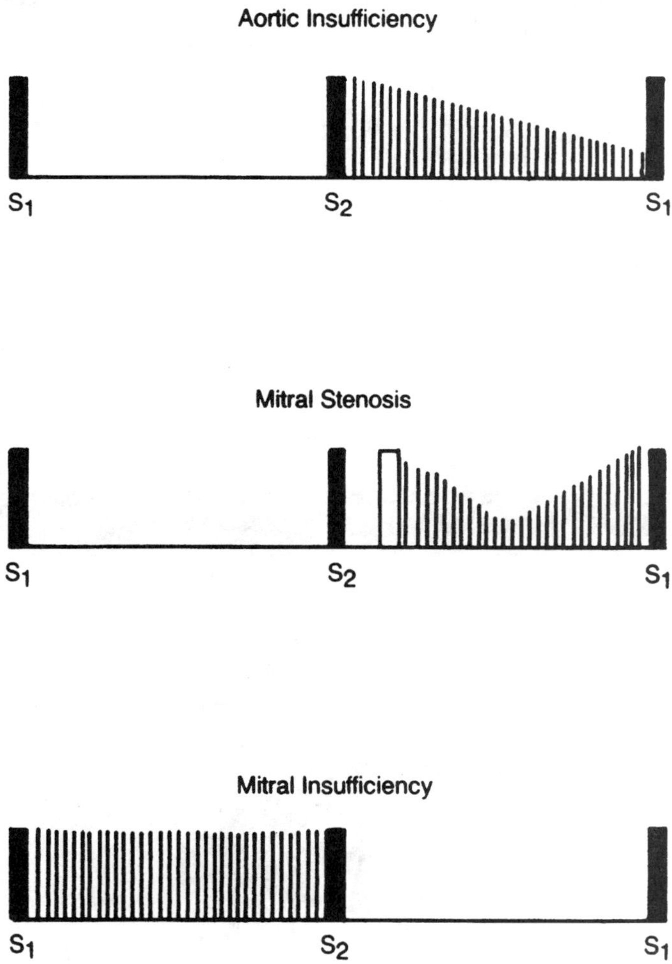

Palpation

The abdomen is palpated, tender quadrant last, for guarding, rigidity, organomegaly, tenderness, and the presence of a mass. Masses are characterized as to position, size, shape, consistency, and location. A fluid wave across the abdomen is consistent with ascites. Palpation for the abdominal aorta is a

Table 6.14 Murmur Grading System

Grade	Explanation
1	Barely audible
2	Soft but distinctly audible
3	Loud but no thrill
4	Loud with thrill
5	Loud with palpable thrill
6	Heard with stethoscope off chest

Figure 6–7 Normal Abdominal Vasculature

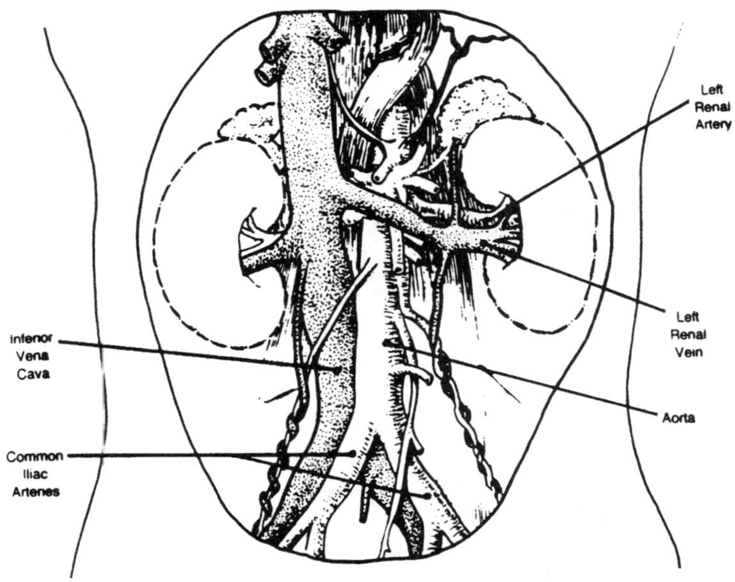

Table 6.15 Abdominal Percussion Notes

Dull
Liver
Spleen
Full bladder
Abdominal mass
Resonant
Normal bowel
Hyperresonant/tympanitic
Bowel obstruction
Adynamic ileus

mandatory portion of this examination. Examination for hernia may also be performed at this juncture.

Clinical Pearls

- Appropriate draping of the patient is important for patient modesty. The gown should cover those areas not being currently examined.
- A ticklish patient may be palpated with the patient's hand below the examiner's hand.
- Flexing the hips and knees while supine is the best position for examining the abdomen.
- Abdominal guarding is voluntary; **rigidity is involuntary and suggests peritonitis.**
- Lateral displacement of the fingers when palpating the abdominal aorta is consistent with aneurysm.
- The presence of a hard, **nontender, immovable, left supraclavicular lymph node** (Virchow's node) is often seen with **metastatic gastrointestinal malignancy and lymphomas.**
- Iliac artery aneurysms often accompany abdominal aortic aneurysms (AAA). (18)
- Approximately 10% of patients over 65 have an AAA. (18)

- Palpation of the popliteal fossa is mandatory in a patient suspected of having an abdominal aortic aneurysm, as many of these patients also have popliteal artery dilatation. (19)

Extremities

Inspection
A check is made for any visible ulcers (diabetes mellitus), varicosities, edema (peripheral vascular disease, cardiovascular disease, renal disease), atrophy (nerve compression), or deformity (fracture, dislocation). Comparing right to left for symmetry is the best way to examine the extremities.

Palpation
Palpation of the joints for swelling (trauma, arthritis), lumps and bumps (degenerative joint disease, gouty arthritis), tenderness, and redness (infection, inflammatory arthritis) is performed. Any muscular tenderness (strain) or tenderness to palpation of tendons (tendinitis, tear) or ligaments (sprain, tear) is noted. The presence of any lymphadenopathy should also be noted. Generally speaking, malignant lymph nodes are hard, nontender, and immobile while benign lymph nodes are tender, mobile, and soft to firm in texture.

Percussion
This study is usually deferred.

Auscultation
Auscultation is reserved for any areas suspicious for vascular disease, tumor, or fracture.

Special Tests/Signs in Physical Examination

The following list of tests and signs is commonly used in physical examination to help with differential diagnosis of some of the more common patient complaints. They are listed in alphabetical order.

- *Battle's Sign*—Demonstrates retroauricular ecchymosis associated with basilar skull fracture. (20)
- *Chvostek's Sign*—Tapping over the region of the facial nerve causes spasm of the facial muscles. This reaction is seen with hypocalcemic tetany. (21)
- *Clubbing (digital)*—Bulbous enlargement of the tips of the fingers seen most often with lung cancer, although it may be seen with many chronic diseases. (22)

- *Cullen's Sign*—Periumbilical ecchymosis consistent with intraperitoneal bleeding, most often from pancreatitis. (23)
- *Homans' Sign*—Calf pain while squeezing the calf and forcibly dorsiflexing the foot. This sign is, at times, consistent with thrombophlebitis and/or deep vein thrombosis. (24)
- *Koplik's Spots*—Small punctuate lesions on the buccal mucosa consistent with early measles.
- *Levine's Sign*—When a patient having a myocardial infarction or angina pectoris clenches the fist and holds it at the sternal region while complaining of pain in that region. (25)
- *McBurney's Sign*—Tenderness at the site one-third the distance from the anterior superior iliac spine to the umbilicus, suggestive of appendicitis. (26)
- *Murphy's Punch Test*—A sharp punch at the costovertebral angles that elicits pain in a patient with renal disease.
- *Murphy's Sign*—Sharp pain on deep inspiration and palpation of the inferior edge of the liver. Consistent with cholecystitis. (27)
- *Myxedema*—Diffuse non-pitting edema with skin thickening seen classically in the pre-tibial region, but also seen in the face, neck, ears, and upper trunk. Often associated with thyroid disorders, but also seen in stasis dermatitis.
- *Nail Pitting*—Small pits in fingernails, often associated with psoriasis.
- *Obturator Sign*—When flexion and external rotation of the right hip causes pain in the right lower quadrant, suggestive of appendicitis. (28)
- *Psoas Sign*—When extending and elevating the right leg with the patient prone produces pain in the right lower quadrant; found in patients with appendicitis. (28)
- *Raccoon Eyes*—Periorbital ecchymosis in a patient with a possible skull fracture. (29)
- *Raynaud's Phenomenon*—Skin in the fingertips, toes, nose, and ears turns from white to blue to red in cold conditions. It is a sign of vascular disease.
- *Rust's Sign*—When patient supports head with both hands, as in cases of cervical spine trauma. This sign is consistent with a spinal fracture.
- *Splinter Hemorrhages*—Longitudinal hemorrhages in the nail beds consistent with subacute bacterial endocarditis.

- *Strawberry Tongue*—Raised lingual papillae through a white base on the tongue giving the appearance of the skin of a strawberry. Associated with scarlet fever.

Differential Diagnosis of Common Signs and Symptoms

Abdominal Pain

Right Upper Quadrant: gallbladder disease (cholecystitis, cholelithiasis (stones)), cholangitis, hepatic disease (hepatitis, cirrhosis), peptic ulcer disease, pancreatitis, thoracic aortic aneurysm, pulmonary disease (pleurisy, embolism, pneumonia), cardiac disease (angina, myocardial infarction, cardiomyopathy), appendicitis (retroperitoneal appendix location), pyelonephritis

Left Upper Quadrant: thoracic aortic aneurysm, esophagitis, gastritis, gastroesophageal reflux disease (GERD), peptic ulcer disease, pancreatitis, pulmonary disease (pleurisy, embolism, pneumonia), cardiac disease (angina, myocardial infarction, cardiomyopathy), pyelonephritis

Right Lower Quadrant: appendicitis, irritable bowel syndrome, abdominal aortic aneurysm, cholecystitis (especially with perforation), Crohn's disease, perforated peptic ulcer, urinary tract infection, cecal volvulus, pelvic inflammatory disease, ovarian disease (cyst), ectopic pregnancy

Left Lower Quadrant: abdominal aortic aneurysm, diverticulitis, ulcerative colitis, Crohn's disease, irritable bowel syndrome, urinary tract infection, sigmoid volvulus, pelvic inflammatory disease, ovarian disease (cyst), ectopic pregnancy

Diffuse: early appendicitis, mesenteric thrombosis, gastroenteritis, irritable bowel syndrome, pancreatitis, renal colic, peritonitis

Ascites

Portal hypertension (secondary to alcoholic cirrhosis most commonly), congestive heart failure, peritonitis, pancreatitis, tumors (e.g., metastatic seeding), hypoproteinemia (e.g., terminal cancer patients)

Chest Pain

Poorly localized, dull, deep pain: angina pectoris, myocardial infarction, aortic aneurysm, pulmonary embolism, pulmonary hypertension
Substernal, pressure/pain/discomfort: angina pectoris, myocardial infarction, GERD, esophagitis

Specific, sharp pain: pleurisy, pulmonary embolism, pneumothorax, pericarditis, rib fracture, costochondritis (Tietze's syndrome), cholecystitis, pancreatitis

Constipation

Dehydration, lack of exercise, low fiber diet, irritable bowel syndrome, colon cancer (pencil-thin stools), medications (narcotic analgesics), laxative abuse, hemorrhoids, anal fissure, inflammatory bowel disease, poor bowel hygiene, fecal impaction, neurologic disorders, hypothyroidism, depression

Cough

Acute: upper respiratory infection, pneumonia, allergies, pharyngitis, asthma, GERD
Chronic: chronic bronchitis, emphysema, bronchiectasis, smoking, bronchogenic carcinoma, pharyngeal/laryngeal carcinoma, tuberculosis

Diarrhea

Acute: infectious gastroenteritis (viral, fungal protozoal), food poisoning, antibiotics, medications (parasympathomimetics), ulcerative colitis, Crohn's disease, irritable bowel syndrome, food intolerance, appendicitis, diverticulitis
Chronic: Crohn's disease, ulcerative colitis, irritable bowel syndrome, diverticulitis, carcinoma (alternating diarrhea and constipation), malabsorption syndromes, lactose intolerance, hyperthyroidism, Addison's disease, AIDS

Dysphagia

Achalasia, esophageal motor dysfunction, progressive systemic sclerosis (scleroderma), esophageal cancer, esophageal webs, esophageal stricture, globus hystericus, diabetic neuropathy, dermatomyositis, brain stem infarction

Dyspnea

Upper respiratory infection, tracheal tumors, chronic obstructive pulmonary disease, allergies, asthma, pulmonary edema, pneumothorax, angina pectoris, myocardial infarction, congestive heart failure, atelectasis, pulmonary embolism, pulmonary infarction, anxiety, rib fracture, pleurisy, chronic restrictive lung diseases

Dysuria

Lower urinary tract infection, urinary tract stones, benign prostatic hypertrophy, cystitis, pyelonephritis, prostate carcinoma, bladder cancer, dehydration

Edema, Peripheral

Congestive heart failure, renal failure, hypothyroidism, hepatic cirrhosis, malnutrition, thrombophlebitis, lymphatic obstruction (cancer)

Fever of Unknown Origin

Urinary tract infection, tuberculosis, fungal infections, endocarditis, abscess, malignancy (e.g., lymphoma, leukemia), connective tissue diseases, medications, temporal arteritis

Heartburn (Pyrosis)

GERD, reflux esophagitis, gastritis, hiatus hernia, peptic ulcer disease, cholecystitis, progressive systemic sclerosis (scleroderma) affecting the esophagus, overeating, food intolerance

Hematemesis

Swallowed blood (e.g., mouth lesion, hemoptysis), esophageal varices, esophageal cancer, gastric cancer, peptic ulcer disease, Mallory-Weiss syndrome

Hematuria

Genitourinary tumors (benign and malignant), trauma (including intercourse, masturbation), urinary tract infection, false positives (hemoglobinuria, myoglobinuria), nephrolithiasis, menstruation, vigorous exercise ("runner's hematuria")

Hemoptysis

Pulmonary infections, pulmonary embolism/infarct, bronchogenic carcinoma, pneumonia, pulmonary edema, chronic obstructive pulmonary disease (e.g., chronic bronchitis, bronchiectasis), chest trauma, inhaled foreign body

Hepatomegaly/Splenomegaly

Cirrhosis, alcoholic hepatitis, infectious hepatitis, congestive heart failure, chronic granulomatous diseases (amyloidosis, sarcoidosis), anemias, infectious mononucleosis, hemachromatosis, hepatocellular carcinoma

Jaundice

Hepatitis, cirrhosis, cholecystitis/cholelithiasis, drug-induced hyperbilirubinemia, hepatocellular carcinoma, hemolysis, pregnancy, neonatal jaundice

Lymphadenopathy

Infection (bacterial, fungal, viral), malignancy (metastasis, lymphoma), sarcoidosis, AIDS, drug-induced (Dilantin), connective tissue diseases

Melena

Swallowed blood (e.g., mouth lesion, hemoptysis), esophageal varices, esophageal cancer, gastric cancer, peptic ulcer disease, Mallory-Weiss syndrome

Oliguria/Anuria

[oliguria= < 500 cc urine/day, anuria= < 100 cc urine/day]

Congestive heart failure, shock, volume depletion (e.g., hemorrhage), renal artery stenosis, glomerulonephritis, acute tubular necrosis, renal failure, medications (e.g., amphotericin B), ureteral obstruction (bilateral), benign prostatic hypertrophy, prostatic carcinoma, bladder cancer, neurogenic bladder (e.g., cauda equina syndrome)

Weight Loss, Unexplained

[> 10% body weight in 6 months]

Anorexia, malignancy, hyperthyroidism, anxiety, medications (e.g., amphetamines), parasites, malabsorption syndromes, depression, severe cardiac disease, severe liver disease, terminal illness, AIDS

Wheezing

Asthma, emphysema, chronic bronchitis, foreign body, tracheal stenosis, upper respiratory infection, congestive heart failure, pulmonary embolism, atelectasis, anaphylaxis, myocardial infarction

References

1. Calle, E.E., Thun, M.J., Petrelli, J.M., Rodriguez, C., & Heath, C.W., Jr. Body-mass index and mortality in a prospective cohort of US adults. *The New England Journal of Medicine.* 1999;341:1097–1105.
2. Slipman, C.W., Patel, R.K., Botwin, K., Huston, C., Zhang, L., Lenrow, D., & Garvan, C. Epidemiology of spine tumors presenting to musculoskeletal physiatrists. *Arch Phys Med Rehabil.* 2003;Apr;84(4):492–495.
3. Deyo, R.A., & Diehl, A.K. Cancer as a cause of back pain: frequency, clinical presentation, and diagnostic strategies. *J Gen Intern Med.* 1988;3:230–238.

4. Bassi, P., Lattuada, P., & Gomitoni, A. Cervical cerebral artery dissection: a multicenter prospective study (preliminary report). *Neurol Sci.* 2003;May;24 Suppl 1:S4–7.
5. Mathias, C.J. Orthostatic hypotension: causes, mechanisms, and influencing factors. *Neurology.* 1995;45(4 Suppl 5):S6–11.
6. Vasan, R.S., Larson, M.G., Leip, E.P., et al. Assessment of frequency of progression to hypertension in nonhypertensive participants in the Framingham Heart Study: A cohort study. *Lancet.* 2001;358:1682–1686.
7. Negin, B.P., Riedel, E., Oliveria, S.A., Berwick, M., Coit, D.G., & Brady, M.S. Symptoms and signs of primary melanoma: important indicators of Breslow depth. *Cancer.* 2003;Jul 15;98(2):344–348.
8. Shaaf, M., Cagle, S.K., & Farris, B.K. "Mickey Mouse" aneurysm presenting with cranial bruit: case report. *Neurosurgery.* 1994;Sep;35(3):509–12; discussion 512. Eskridge, J.B. Extraocular motor dysfunction associated with tumors. *Optom Clin.* 1993;3(3): 135–160.
9. Goldberg, I. Relationship between intraocular pressure and preservation of visual field in glaucoma. *Surv Ophthalmol.* 2003;Apr;48 Suppl 1:S3–7.
10. Kosmorsky, G. Pseudotumor cerebri. *Neurosurg Clin N Am.* 2001;Oct;12(4):775–797, ix.
11. Bateman, N.D., Fahy, C., & Woolford, T.J. Nasal polyps: still more questions than answers. *J Laryngol Otol.* 2003;Jan;117(1):1–9.
12. Jackson, K.R., & Jackson, R.T. Factors associated with active, refractory epistaxis. *Arch Otolaryngol Head Neck Surg.* 1988;Aug;114(8):862–865. Dreizen, S. Oral candidiasis. *Am J Med.* 1984;Oct 30;77(4D):28–33.
13. Dickinson, C.J. Lung diseases associated with digital clubbing. *Clin Exp Rheumatol.* 1992;May–Jun;10 Suppl 7:23–25.
14. McDonnell, J.K. Cardiac disease and the skin. *Dermatol Clin.* 2002;Jul;20(3):503–511, vii.
15. Righetti, A., Crawford, M.H., O'Rourke, R.A., Daily, P.O., & Ross, J., Jr. Echocardiographic and roentgenographic determination of left ventricular size after coronary arterial bypass graft surgery. *Chest.* 1977 Oct;72(4):455–458.
16. Steckmeier, B. Epidemiology of aortic disease: aneurysm, dissection, occlusion. *Radiologe.* 2001;Aug;41(8):624–632. Review. German.
17. Diwan, A., Sarkar, R., Stanley, J.C., Zelenock, G.B., & Wakefield, T.W. Incidence of femoral and popliteal artery aneurysms in patients with abdominal aortic aneurysms. *J Vasc Surg.* 2000;May;31(5):863–869.
18. Alvi, A. Battle's sign in temporal bone trauma. *Otolaryngol Head Neck Surg.* 1998; Jun;118(6):908.
19. Krogh, L., Wynne, J.M., & Cywes, S. The value of Chvostek's sign in tetany. *S Afr Med J.* 1968;Aug 17;42(32):846–847.
20. Clarke, S., Barnsley, L., Peters, M., Morgan, L., & Van der Wall, H. Hypertrophic pulmonary osteoarthropathy without clubbing of the digits. *Skeletal Radiol.* 2001;Nov; 30(11):652–655. Epub 2001 Sep 22.

21. Chung, M.A., Oung, C., & Szilagyi, A. Cullen's sign: it doesn't always mean hemorrhagic pancreatitis. *Am J Gastroenterol.* 1992;Aug;87(8):1026–1028.
22. Kennedy, D., Setnik, G., & Li, J. Physical examination findings in deep venous thrombosis. *Emerg Med Clin North Am.* 2001;Nov;19(4):869–876.
23. Marik, P.E., & Shem, M. The "clenched fist" sign of myocardial ischemia. *S Afr Med J.* 1989;May 6;75(9):451–452.
24. McBurney, Charles (1845–1913). Point, sign, and incision. *JAMA.* 1966;Sep 26; 197(13):1098–1099.
25. Singer, A.J., McCracken, G., Henry, M.C., Thode, H.C. Jr., & Cabahug, C.J. Correlation among clinical, laboratory, and hepatobiliary scanning findings in patients with suspected acute cholecystitis. *Ann Emerg Med.* 1996;Sep;28(3):267–272.
26. Wagner, J.M., McKinney, W.P., & Carpenter, J.L. Does this patient have appendicitis? *JAMA.* 1996;Nov 20;276(19):1589–1594.
27. Kral, T., Zentner, J., Vieweg, U., Solymosi, L., & Schramm, J. Diagnosis and treatment of frontobasal skull fractures. *Neurosurg Rev.* 1997;20(1):19–23.

Chapter 7

Orthopedics

Lawrence H. Wyatt, DC, DACBR, FICC

Introduction

Orthopedics is the study of the skeletal system and related structures and the diseases that affect that system. Orthopedic evaluation is an integral part of the examination of every chiropractic patient. Although many of the tests used are nonspecific, in many cases a combination of positive findings can lead the physician to a diagnosis. Studies have concluded that orthopedic tests for low back pain have limited value once root tension signs have been excluded. (1)

It should be remembered that the best clinical yield from an orthopedic test occurs when the test or maneuver reproduces or aggravates the patient's chief complaint. It is critical to understand the proper application of interpretation of these tests. (2) If performing the test causes pain different from the chief complaint, then the pain and its characteristics should be noted, but the test, in most cases, should not be considered positive.

Another important aspect of orthopedic evaluation is the absence of an important finding, the so-called "pertinent negative." The absence of positive findings with certain tests suggests that certain disease processes do not exist. For this reason, if a test is found to be negative, it should be noted as such.

Useful Orthopedic Tests/Signs

This section of tests and signs is by no means exhaustive but is instead a compilation of those most germane to chiropractic practice. They are organized by body region.

General Spine Tests

Dejerine's Triad

The production of spine pain with or without radiation into an extremity while coughing, sneezing, or having a bowel movement is suggestive of a intra-canalicular space occupying lesion compressing the cord or nerve roots.

Figure 7–1 Libman's Test

- Examiner applies pressure with the thumbs to the mastoid process
- Gauges the patient's pain response

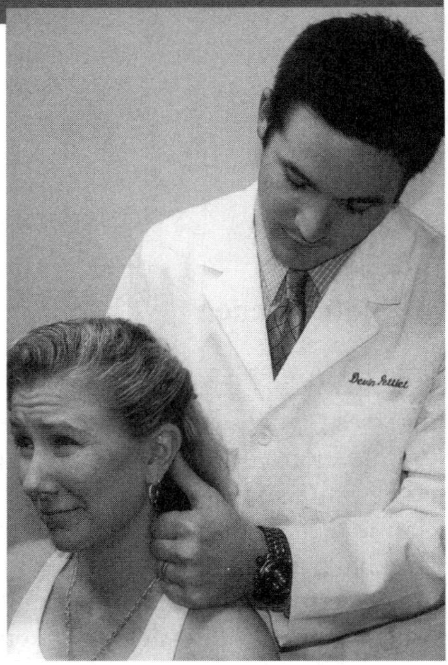

Figure 7–2 Spinous Percussion

- Examiner taps spinous processes with reflex hammer

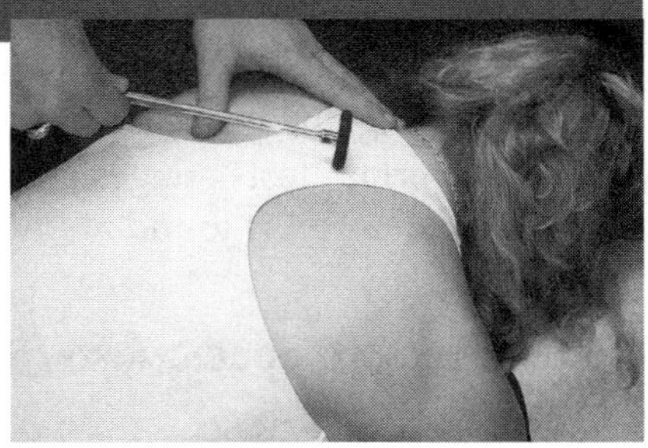

Malingering Tests

Figure 7–3 **Burn's Bench Test**

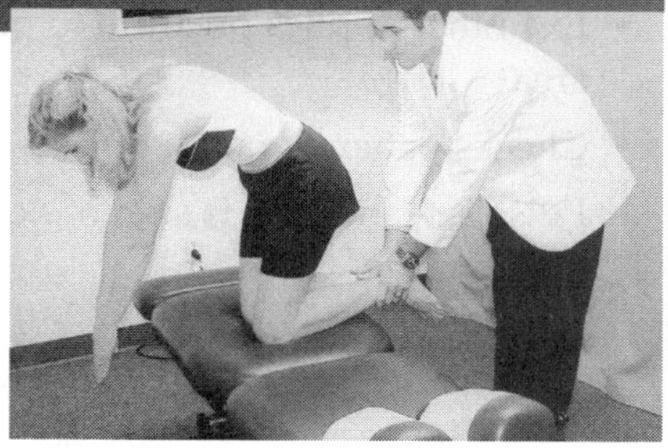

- Patient kneels on table, leans forward
- Examiner supports heels
- Positive indicates low back pain

Figure 7–4 **Hoover's Sign**

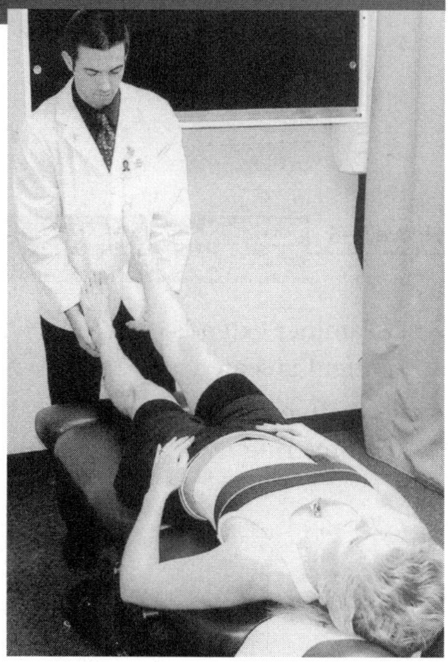

- Patient raises affected limb
- Negative response to feeling pressure under the nonaffected heel suggests malingering

Figure 7–5 **Mankopf's Test**

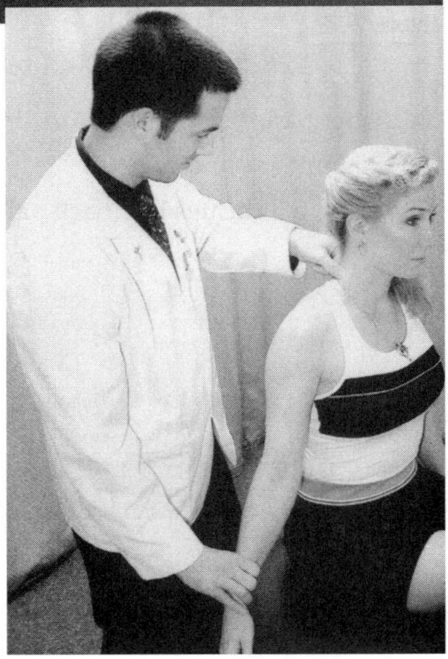

- Examiner applies pressure to painful area
- Checks patient's radial pulse
- Pulse rate increase is sign of non-malingering

Figure 7–6 **Seated Straight Leg Raise Test**

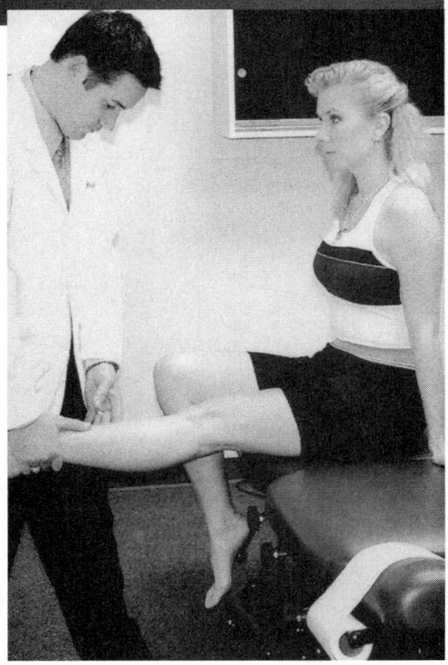

- Examiner extends each knee while patient is seated
- Negative reaction is sign of malingering

Cervical Spine Tests

Figure 7–7 **Bakody's Sign**

- Patient holds hand of painful arm on top of head
- This is a sign of cervical radiculopathy

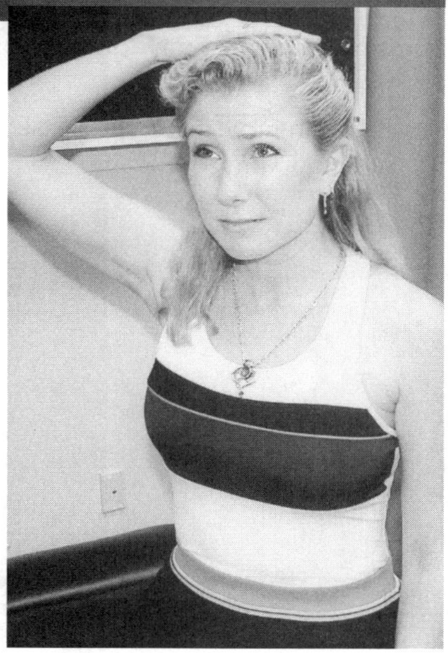

Figure 7–8 **Brudzinski's Sign**

- Patient's head is forcibly flexed while in a supine posture
- Positive findings are consistent with meningeal irritation

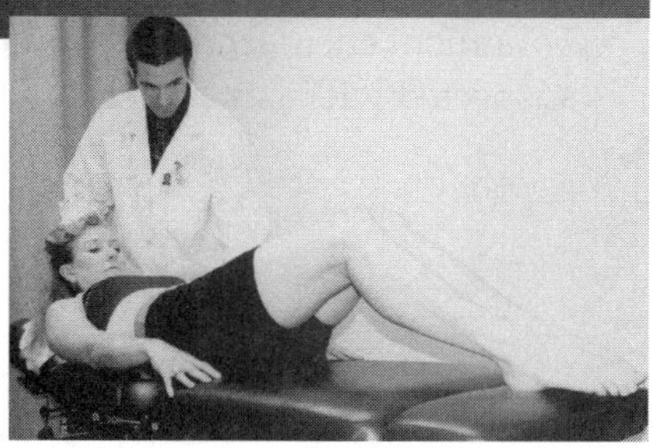

Figure 7–9 Cervical Compression Test

- Direct axial compression is accomplished by pushing down on top of patient's head
- Pain can indicate facet disease, radiculopathy, or sprain

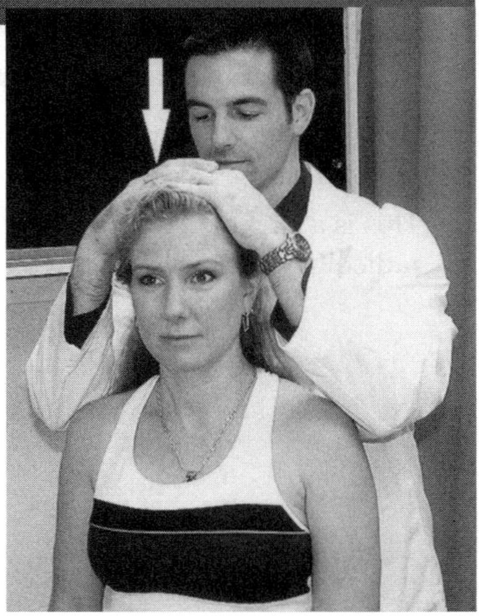

Figure 7–10 Cervical Distraction Test

- Axial distraction of the head away from the shoulders is performed
- Pain indicates myofascial disorders
- Foraminal encroachment should be suspected with pain relief

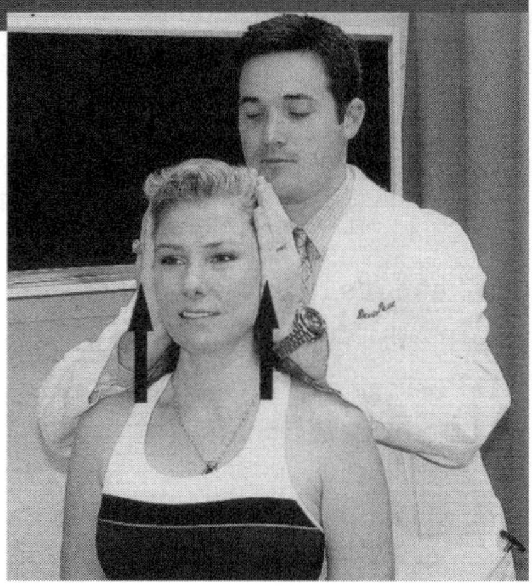

Figure 7–11 **Lhermitte's Sign**

- Forward neck flexion causes pain down the spine
- This sign can be found with multiple sclerosis, meningitis, and spinal cord compression

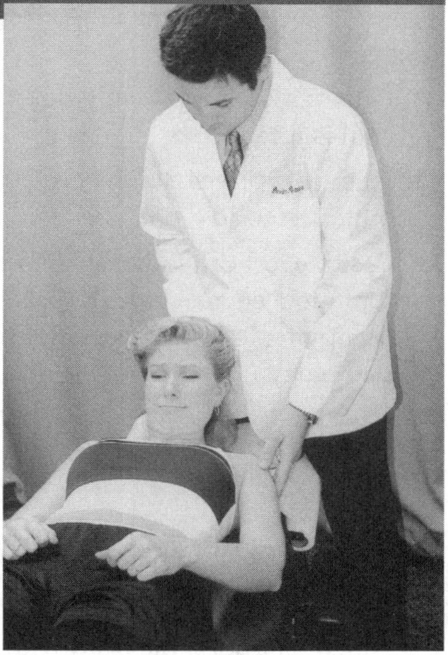

Figure 7–12 **Linder's Sign**

- While patient is supine, examiner forces head, neck, and trunk into flexion
- This sign is consistent with nerve root tension or meningeal irritation

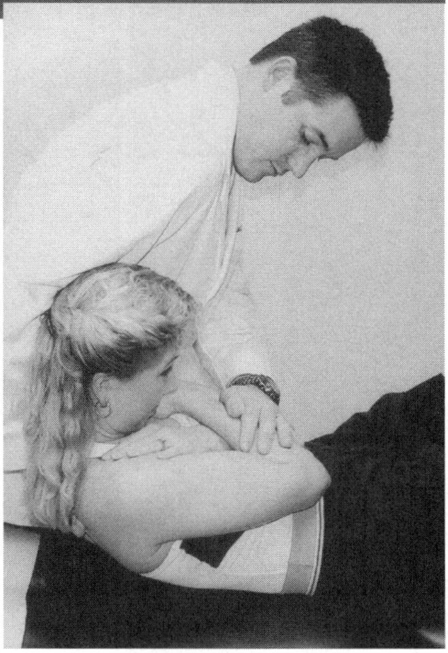

Figure 7–13 **Maximum Cervical Compression Test**

- Patient's neck is laterally flexed and chin is rotated
- Examiner places downward pressure on top of head
- Positive test can indicate neural foraminal encroachment, space-occupying lesion, or posterior joint pathology

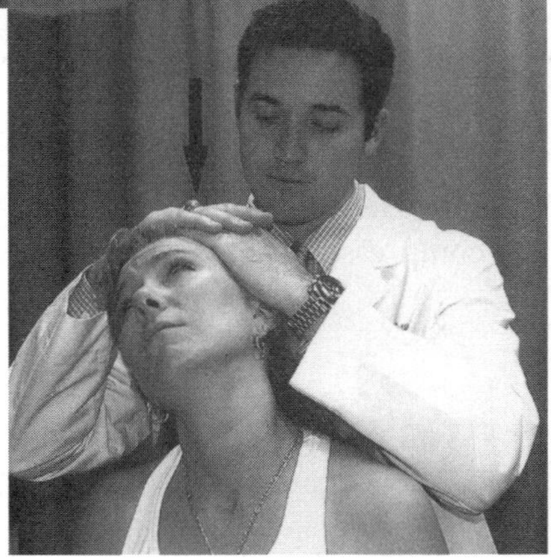

Figure 7–14 **Rust's Sign**

- Patient supports the head with both hands
- Indicates cervical spine fractures

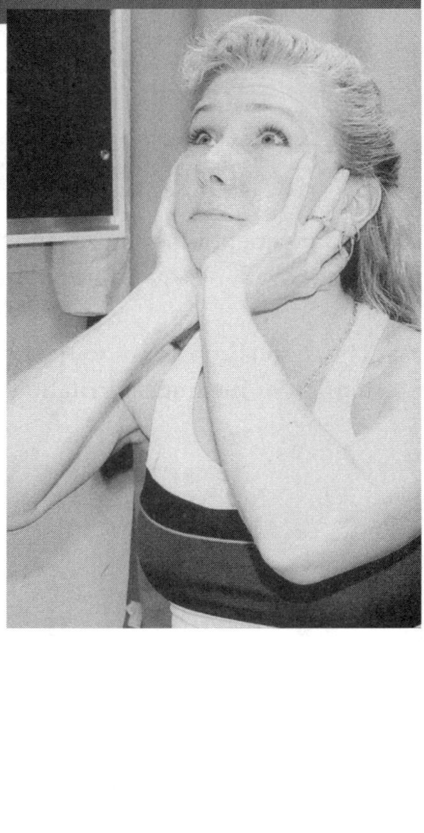

Figure 7–15 Shoulder Depression Test

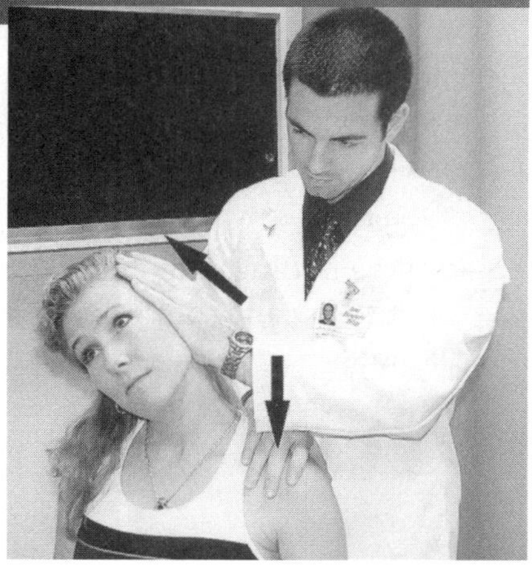

- While the patient is seated, the head is laterally flexed and the shoulder is depressed
- Test may produce pain with number of lesions including brachial neuropathy or cervical radiculopathy

Figure 7–16 Soto-Hall Test

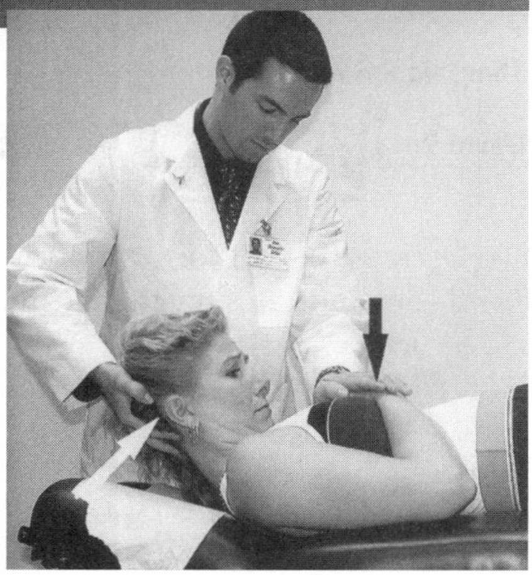

- While the patient is in supine position, patient's neck is flexed by examiner
- Examiner prevents flexion of rest of the spine
- Positive findings have been associated with compression fractures

Figure 7–17 **Spurling's Maneuver**

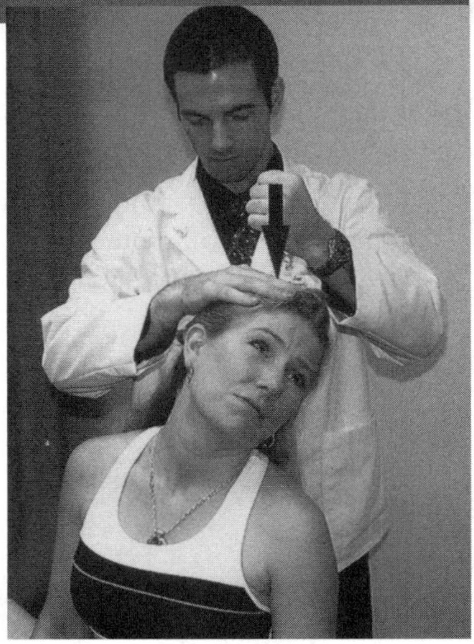

- Patient's head is maximally rotated and extended
- Downward pressure is placed on top of the head
- Positive findings can indicate nerve root tension and/or posterior joint disease

Thoracic Spine Tests

Figure 7–18 **Adam's Position**

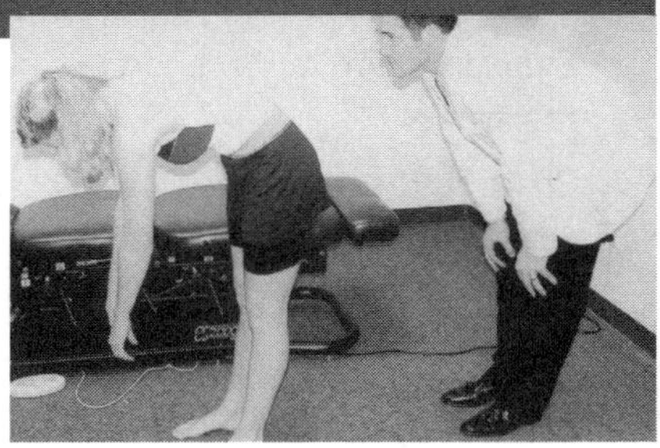

- Decrease of scoliosis with forward flexion indicates functional and not structural cause

Lumbar Spine Tests

Figure 7–19 **Apparent Leg Length**

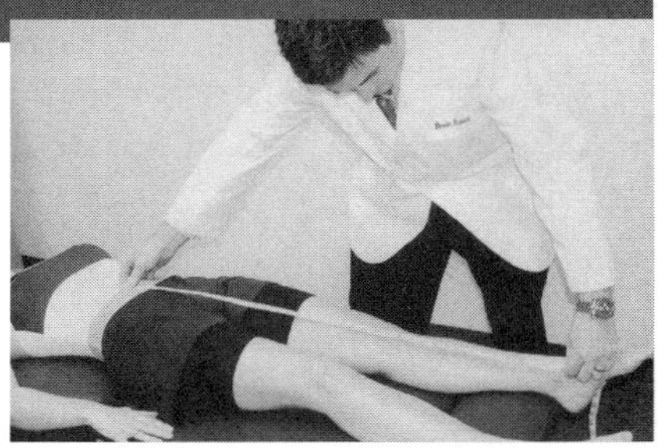

- Measurement from umbilicus to medial malleolus should be equal bilaterally
- Test is nonspecific for functional leg length inequality

Figure 7–20 **Bechterew's Test**

- Straight leg maneuver is performed with patient seated
- The test is positive when pain radiates down the leg and suggests nerve root tension

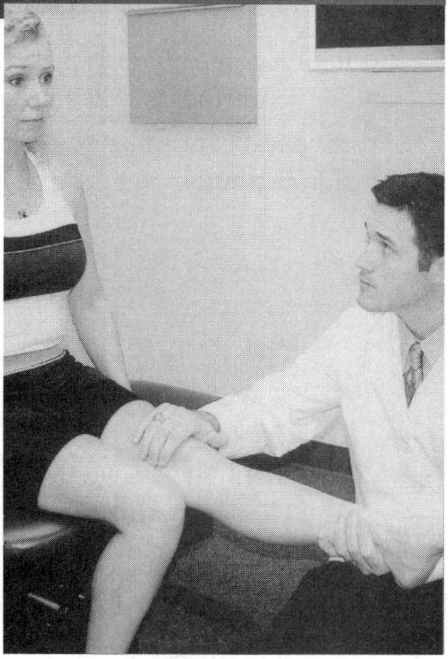

Figure 7–21 **Bowstring Sign**

- Patient's leg is taken to the point of pain with a straight leg maneuver
- Knee is then slighted flexed and foot allowed to rest on examiner's shoulder
- Pressure is placed in popliteal fossa
- Suggests radiculopathy

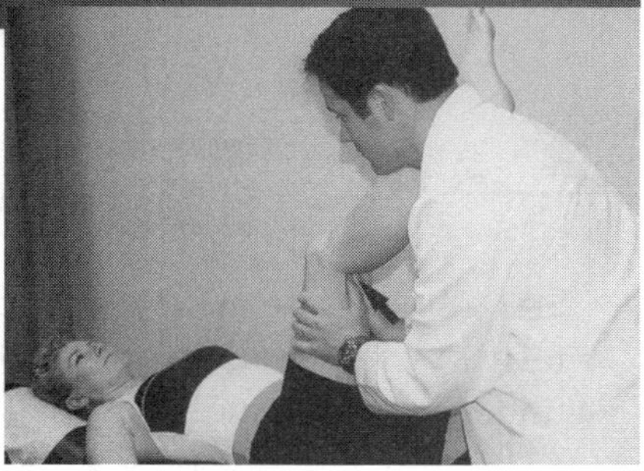

Figure 7–22 Bragard's Test

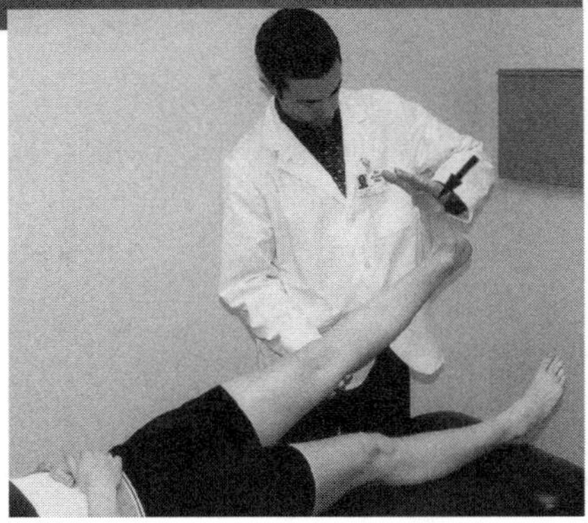

- Straight leg maneuver is performed and patient's foot is dorsiflexed
- Positive test confirms nerve root tension/irritation

Figure 7–23 Ely's (Heel-to-Buttock) Test

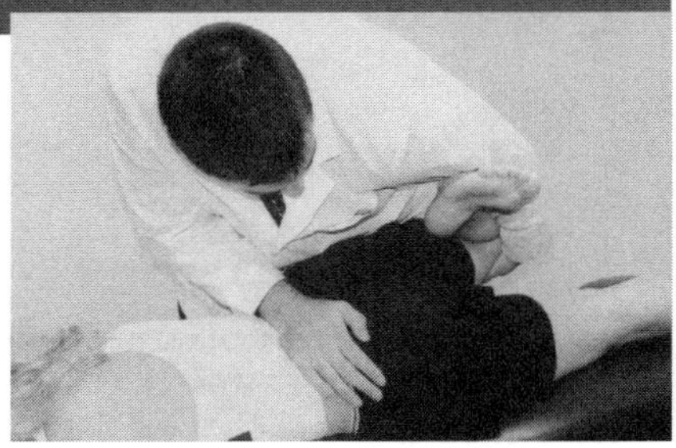

- With patient in prone position, knee is flexed and thigh is hyperextended
- Lesions and muscle irritation will cause positive findings

Figure 7–24 Goldthwait's Test

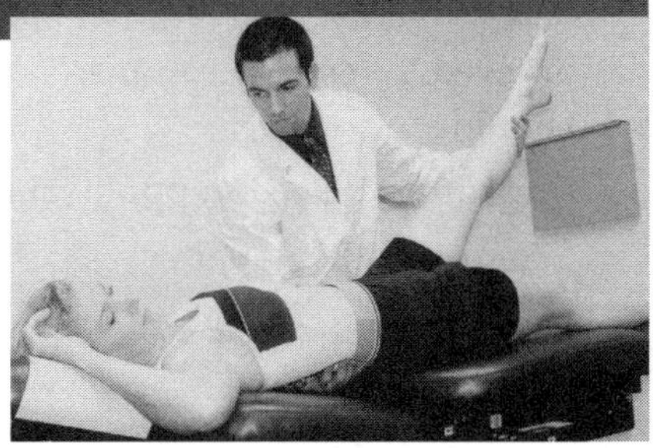

- Straight leg raise maneuver is performed while examiner places hand under lumbar spine
- If pain is felt before lumbar spine moves, sacroiliac lesion is suspected
- If pain occurs after lumbar spine moves, lumbar spine lesion is suspected

Figure 7–25 Kemp's Test

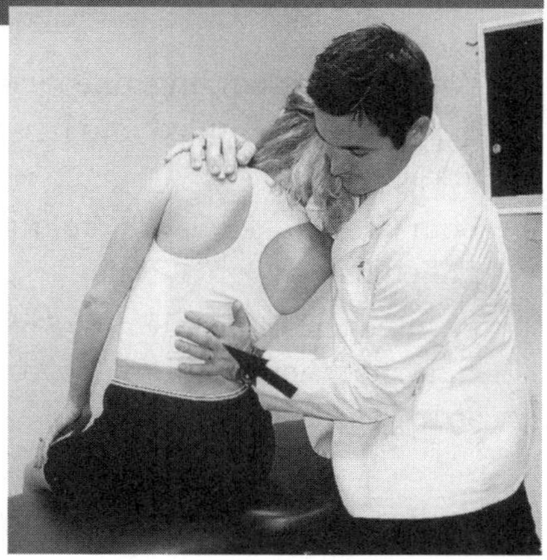

- Lumbar spine is laterally flexed, rotated, and extended while patient is seated
- Examiner attempts to exaggerate this posture
- Painful with facet disease, disc lesions

Figure 7–26 Kernig's Sign

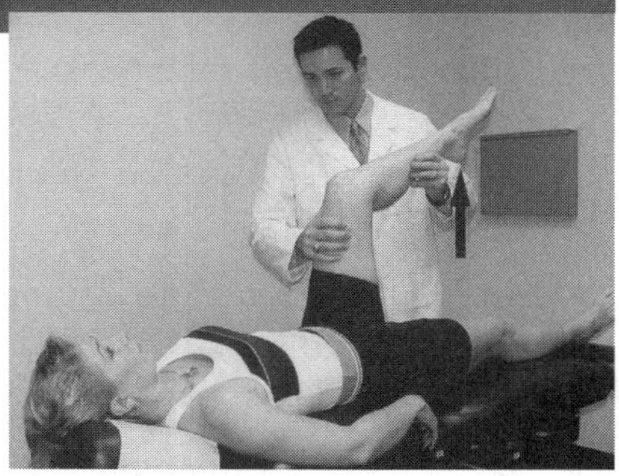

- While the patient is supine, patient's knee and hip on one side are flexed to 90 degrees
- Knee is fully extended
- Positive test indicates either meningitis or a radiculoneuropathy

Figure 7–27 Lewin's Test

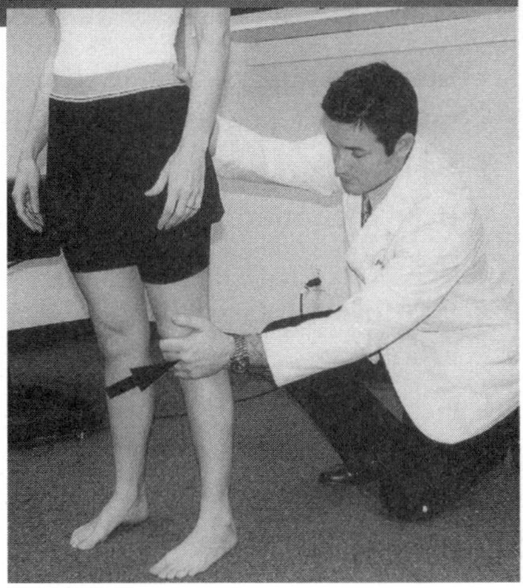

- With patient standing, one knee at a time is rapidly pulled into hyperextension
- Both knees together are rapidly pulled into hyperextension
- Positive test can show nerve root tension, peripheral neuropathy, or hamstring spasm

Figure 7–28 Lumbar Shear Stability

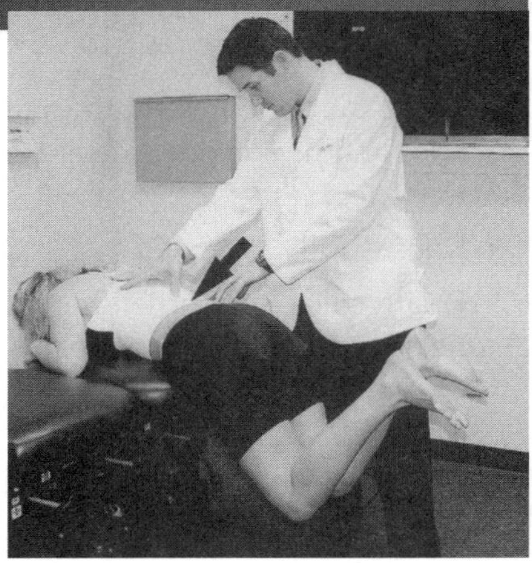

- Patient lies prone with relaxed torso on table
- Feet touch floor and hips and knees are bent
- Direct anterior pressure is applied to spinous processes
- Patient raises feet off floor
- Decrease in pain suggests erector spinae muscles are stabilizing the painful segments

Figure 7–29 Milgram's Test

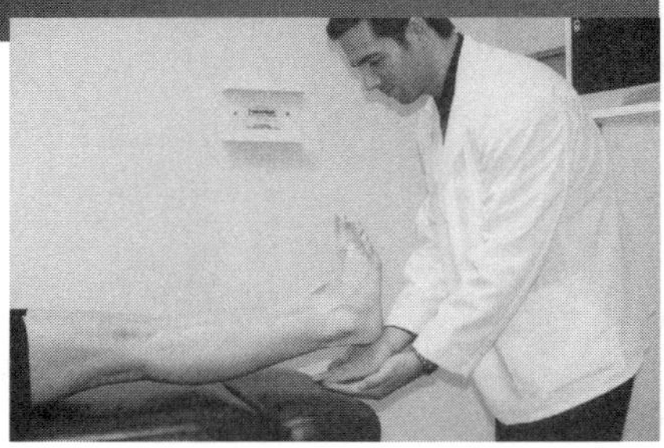

- While patient is supine, both feet are lifted off the table
- Attempt is made to hold the feet approximately six inches off the table
- Non-specific test for low back pathology

Figure 7–30 Minor's Sign

- Patient uses arms to rise from a seated position
- Flexes hips to protect lower back
- Motion found in patients with nerve root tension

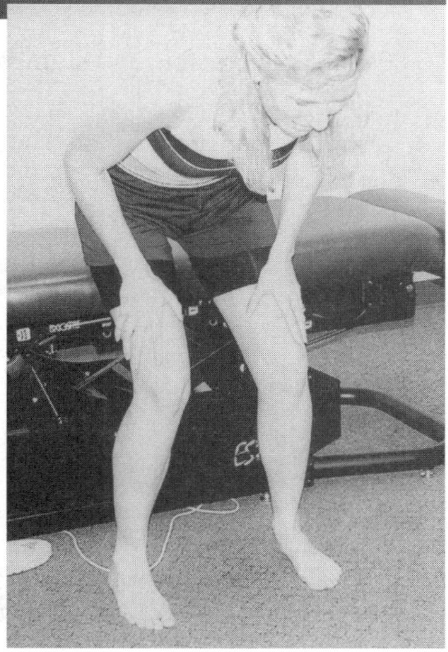

Figure 7–31 Neri's Bowing Test

- Patient attempts to flex forward from standing position without bending knees
- Bent knees are sign of nerve root tension, peripheral neuropathy, or hamstring spasm

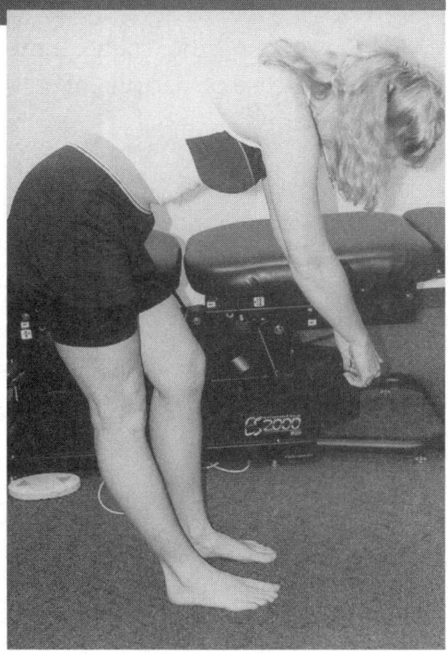

Figure 7–32 Sitting Slump Test

- Patient sits on table and slumps forward
- Examiner performs a seated straight leg raise test
- Radiating leg pain may indicate nerve root compression or adhesions

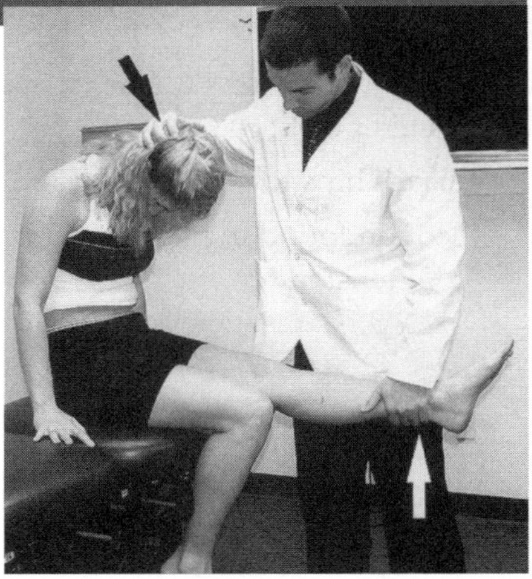

Figure 7–33 Straight Leg Raise

- With patient supine, leg on affected side is raised with knee fully extended
- This is nonspecific test for lumbar spine disease or peripheral neuropathy

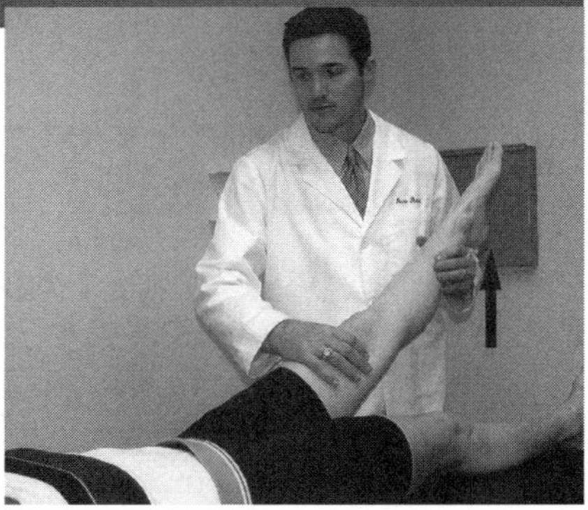

Figure 7–34 Tripod Sign

- Seated patient leans back
- Supports upper body with arms while legs are being extended
- Posture is considered positive for low back pain

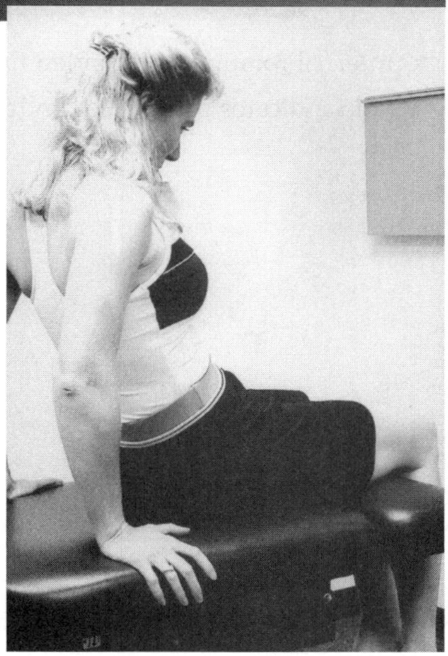

Pelvic Tests

Figure 7–35 Beatty's Maneuver

- Patient lies on uninvolved side
- Abducts involved thigh upward while hip is flexed
- Test is suggestive of piriformis syndrome

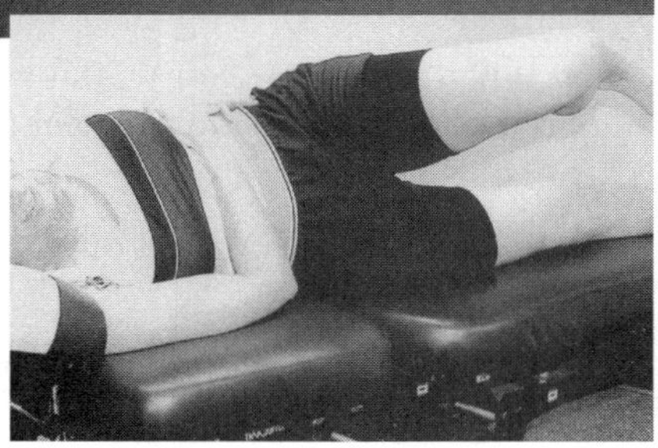

Figure 7–36 Freiberg Test

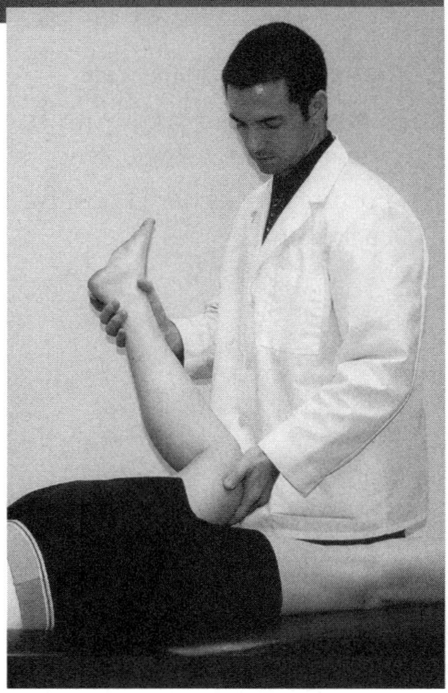

- Internal rotation of extended thigh
- Pain indicates piriformis syndrome

Figure 7–37 Gaenslen's Test

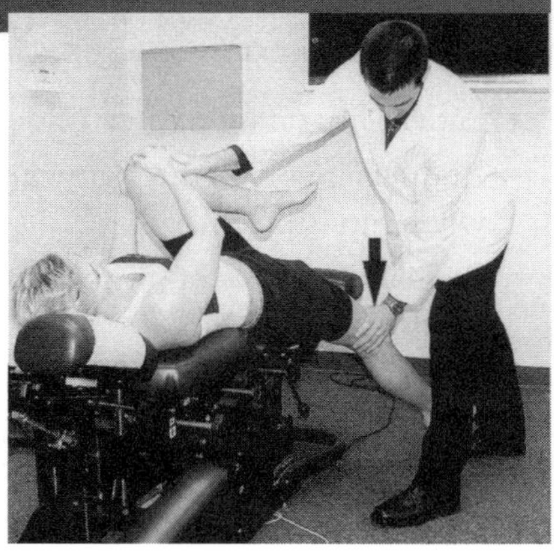

- While in supine position, patient holds unaffected side in knee- and hip-flexed position
- Affected side is lowered off side of table
- Pressure is placed on knee of extended leg
- Positive findings are consistent with sacroiliac lesion

Figure 7–38 Iliac Compression

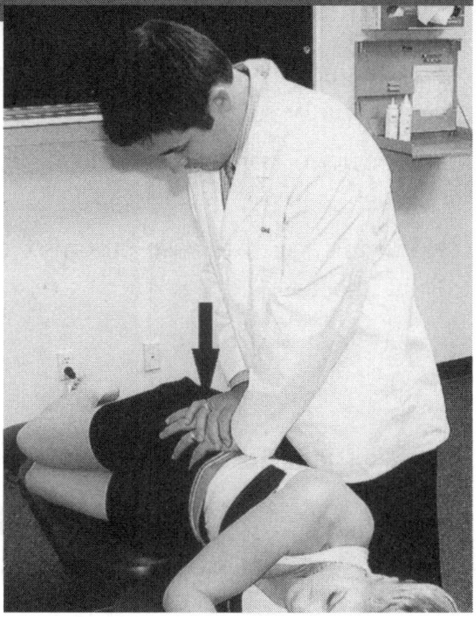

- With patient in side posture, downward pressure is placed on pelvis
- Positive findings indicate either pelvic or sacroiliac disease

Figure 7–39 Pace Test

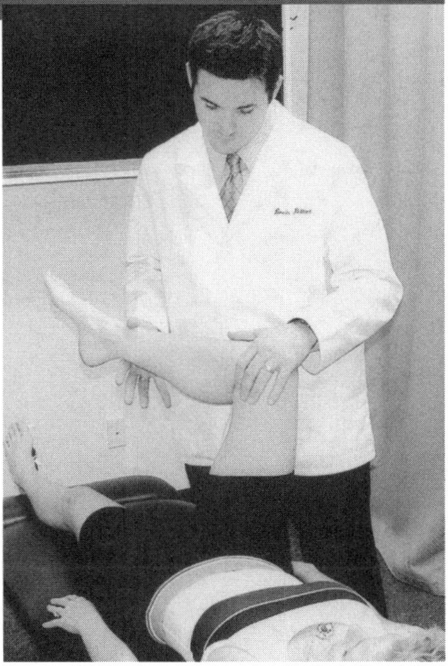

- Resisted abduction/external rotation of hip is made
- Pain with weakness is suggestive of piriformis syndrome

Figure 7–40 Patrick-FABER Test

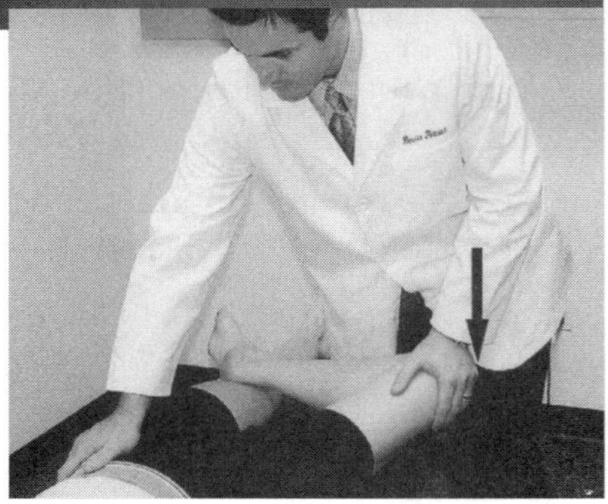

- Affected hip is flexed, abducted, and externally rotated
- Abduction pressure is placed at the knee
- Pain is accurate assessment of sacroiliac disease

Thoracic Outlet Tests

Figure 7–41 Adson's Test

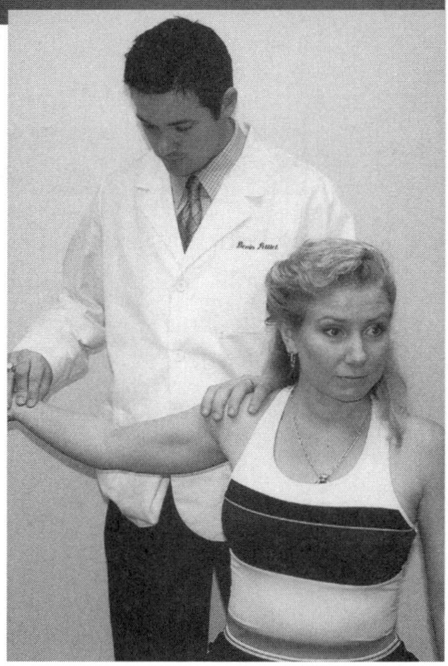

- Arm at the shoulder is elevated
- Lost radial pulse indicates thoracic outlet neurovascular compression syndome

Figure 7–42 **Allen's Test**

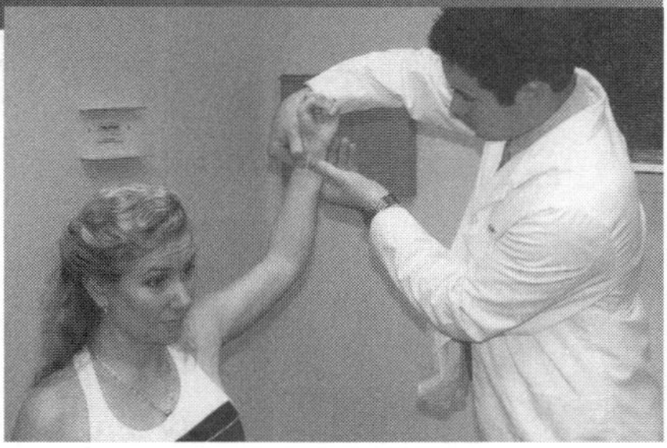

- Arm, with a clenched fist, is elevated
- Radial and/or ulnar artery insufficiency suggests a positive test

Figure 7–43 **Costoclavicular Tests**

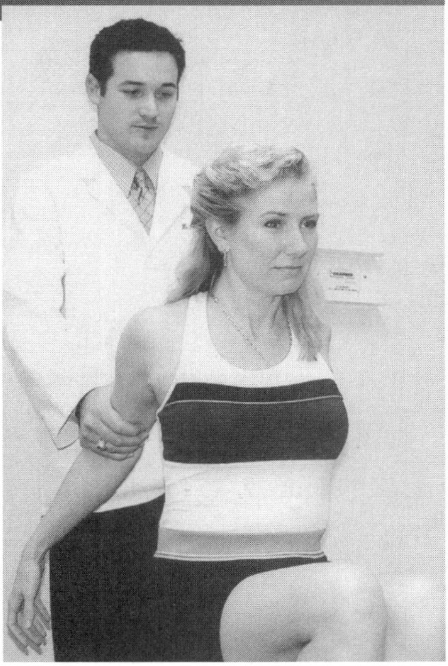

- Procedure pulls shoulders downward and backward
- Produces signs and symptoms of thoracic outlet syndrome

Figure 7–44 **Wright's Hyperabduction Test**

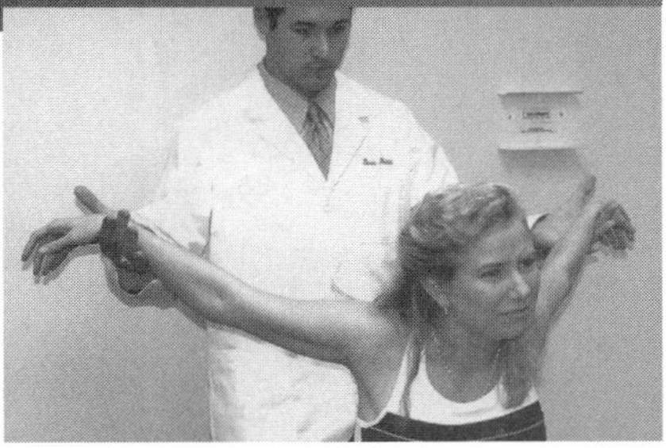

- Extended arm is hyperabducted
- Radial pulse should remain intact at same degree bilaterally
- Loss of pulse consistent with thoracic outlet neurovascular compression syndromes

Shoulder Tests

Figure 7–45 Apley's Scratch Test A

- Patient places tips of fingers of non-painful arm behind back
- Attempts to touch inferior and superior angles of opposite scapula
- Pain suggests shoulder pathology

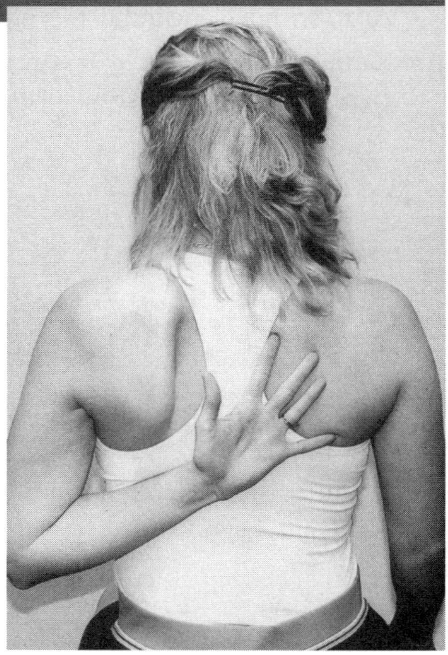

Figure 7–46 Apley's Scratch Test B

- See Figure 7–45 for description

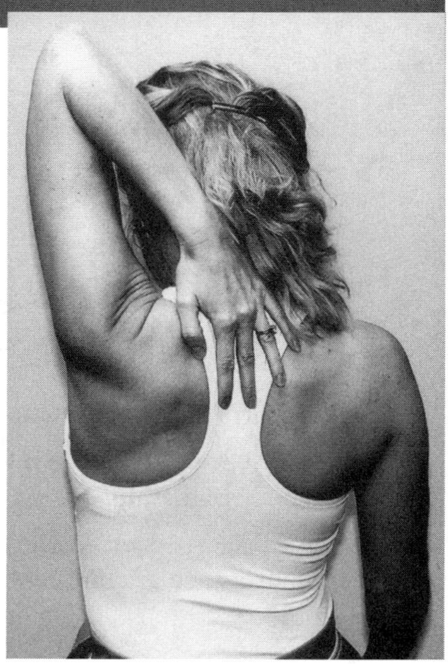

Figure 7–47 Apprehension Test

- Examiner places patient's shoulder in 90° of abduction
- Applies anterior pressure at posterior aspect of shoulder joint
- Patient's apprehension suggests shoulder pathology

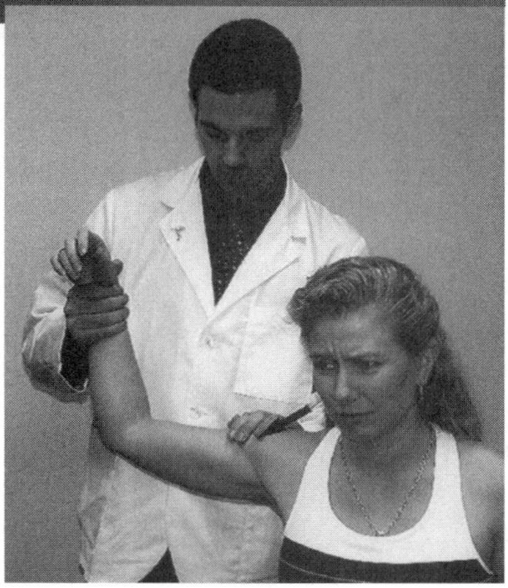

Figure 7–48 Beer Can Test

- Patient's arm is abducted to 90° at his side
- Pronates wrist as if emptying can of beer
- Pain/weakness sign of supraspinatus musculotendinous disease

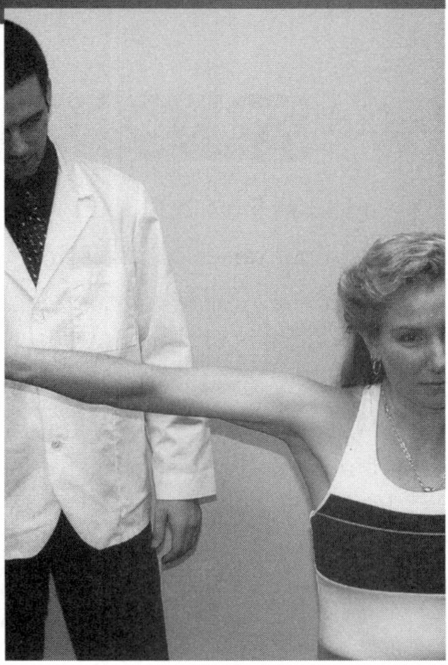

Figure 7–49 Codman's Sign

- Patient's arm is passively abducted above horizontal and relased
- Pain indicates rotator cuff tear/rupture

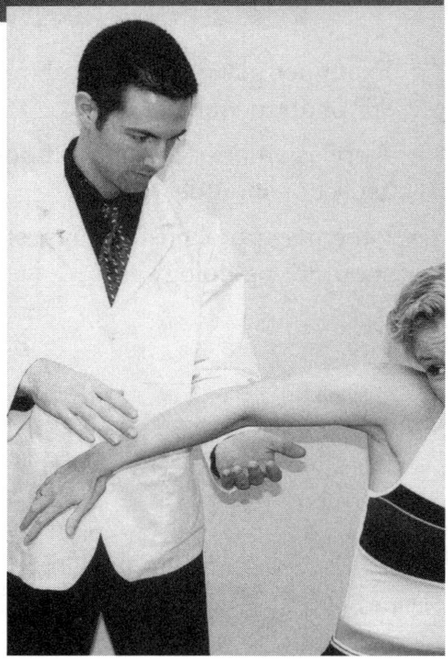

Figure 7–50 Crank Test

- Patient's elbow is flexed to 90°
- Examiner raises patient's arm to 180°
- Examiner applies compression along the long axis of the humerus
- Internally and externally rotates humerus
- Pain is relatively specific for labral lesions

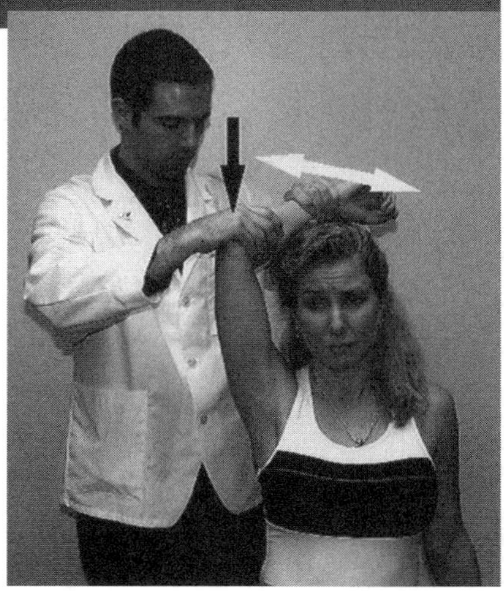

Figure 7–51 **Dugas' Test**

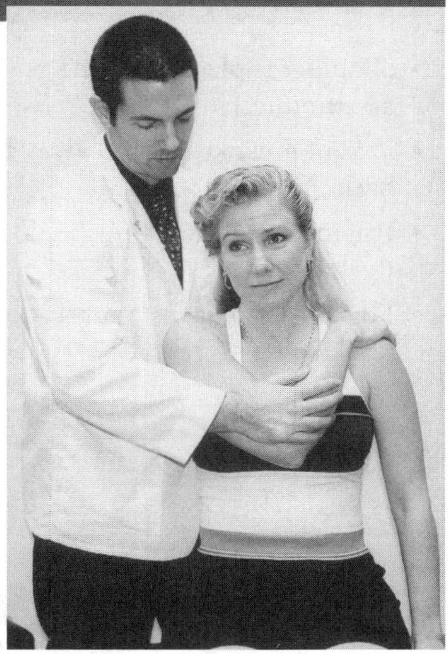

- Patient places hand of affected side on opposite shoulder
- Inability to maintain this posture is significant for shoulder dislocation

Figure 7–52 **Gerber Lift-off Test**

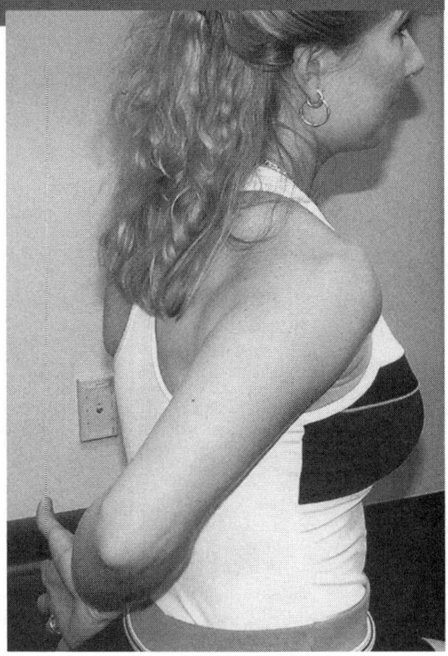

- Hand is placed 5–10 cm from back
- Palm is facing outward and elbow flexed at 90°
- Shoulder is placed passively in internal rotation and slight extension
- Test is positive when patient cannot hold this position and suggests subscapularis dysfunction

Figure 7–53 **Gerber Push-with-Force Test**

- Shoulder is placed in same position as lift-off test
- Patient must keep hand away from back
- Patient should resist push in palm of the hand
- Positive test suggests subscapularis tendinitis

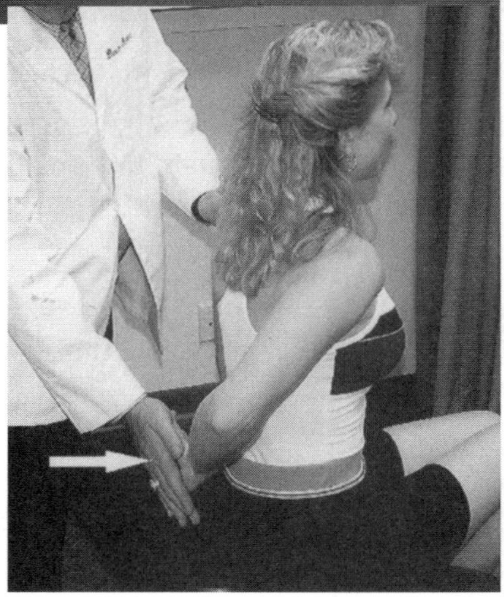

Figure 7–54 **Infraspinatus Isolation Test**

- Shoulder is positioned at 0° of elevation and 45° of internal rotation
- Shoulder external rotation is resisted
- Test is positive if it produces pain and suggests infraspinatus dysfunction

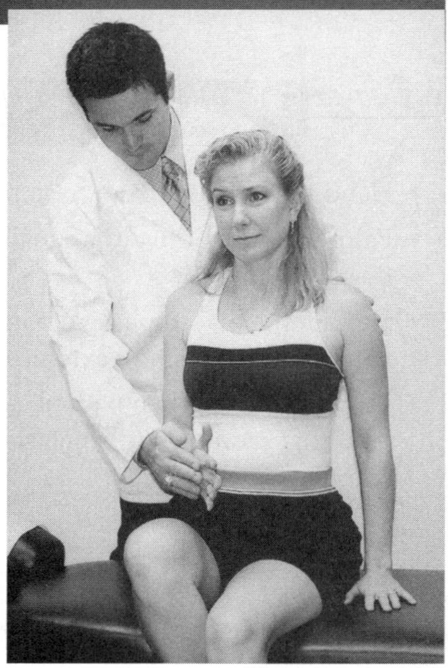

Figure 7–55 Jobe Test

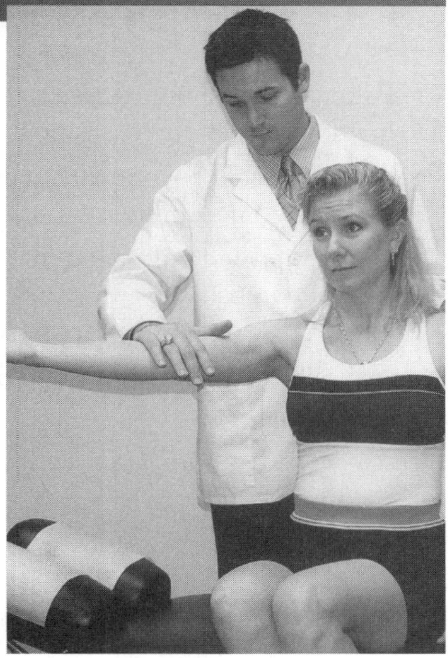

- Shoulder is held in 30° of flexion and abducted to 90°
- Humerus is parallel with scapula
- Abduction is resisted
- Pain suggests supraspinatus tendinitis

Figure 7–56 Neer Impingement Test

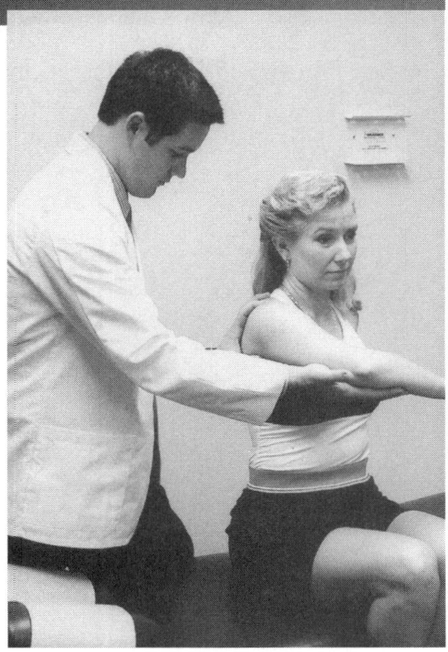

- With examiner standing behind patient, shoulder is flexed passively
- Shoulder may also be positioned in internal rotation
- Pain is suggestive of supraspinatus impingement

Figure 7–57 **O'Brien's Test—Thumbs Down Position**

- Patient flexes shoulder to 90° with hand in thumb down position
- Tries to raise it beyond 90° against resistance from examiner
- Test is repeated with hand in supinated position
- Pain in hand in thumbs down position relatively specific for anterior labral disease

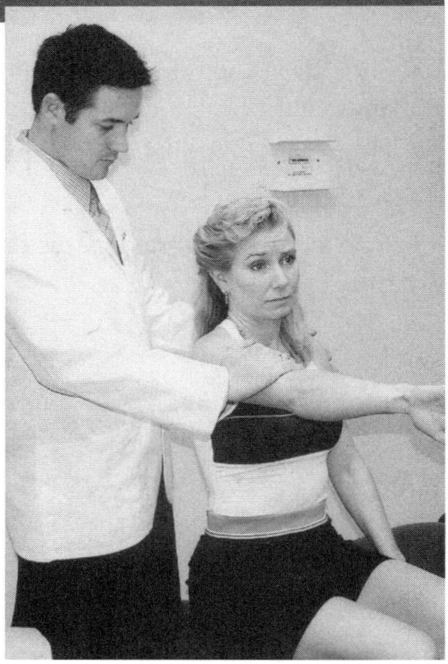

Figure 7–58 **O'Brien's Test—Supinated Position**

- See Figure 7–57 for description

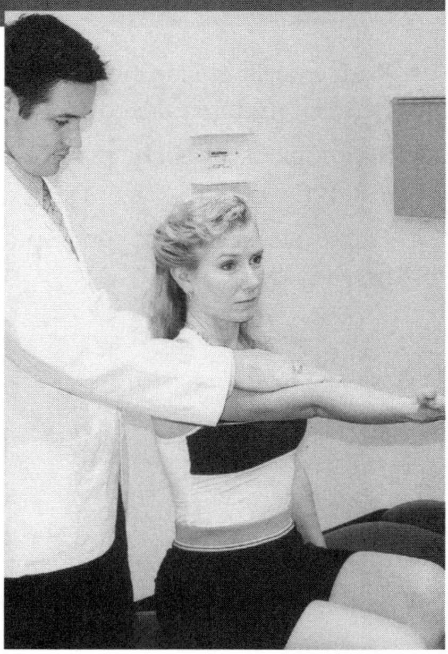

Figure 7–59 Patte Test

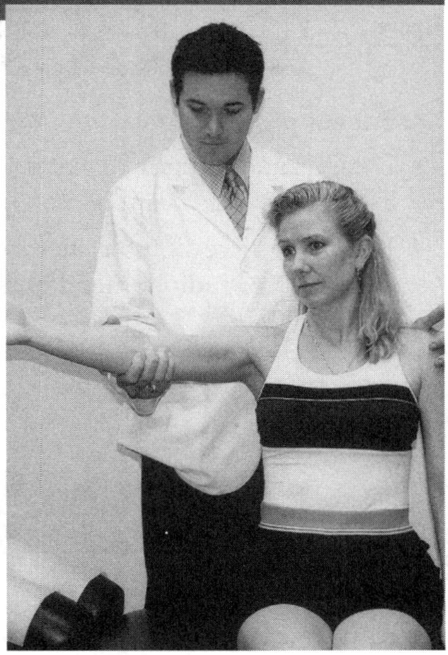

- Shoulder is placed at 90° abduction, neutral rotation and in plane of scapula
- Examiner holds elbow of patient and external rotation is resisted
- Positive test produces pain and suggests infraspinatus and teres minor/posterior rotator cuff disease

Figure 7–60 Yergason's Test

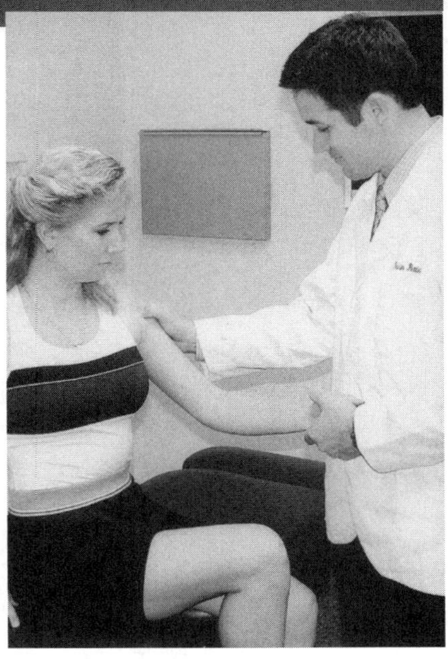

- Patient is seated with elbow at 90° flexion
- Resisted pronation and supination of wrist are performed
- Pain in bicipital groove is positive test and suggests biceps tendinitis/subluxation

Elbow Tests

Figure 7–61 Cozen's Test

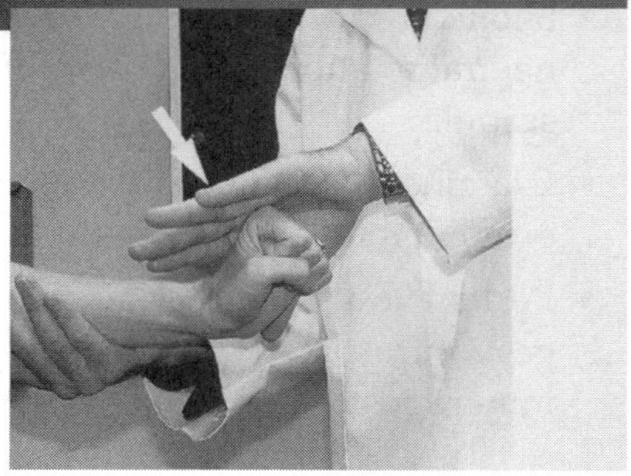

- Patient pronates forearm
- Extends and radially deviates wrist while resistance is applied
- Pain is positive sign for lateral epicondylitis or radiohumeral bursitis

Figure 7–62 Mill's Test

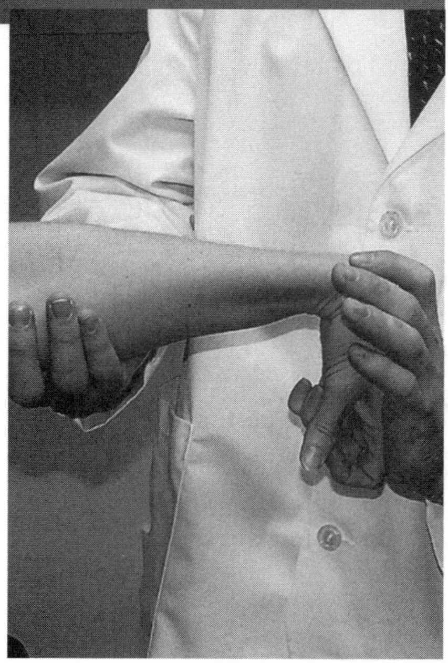

- Arm is pronated with fully extended elbow, flexed wrist, and fingers
- Pain indicates lateral epicondylitis

Figure 7–63 **Tinel's Sign at the Elbow**

- Tapping ulnar nerve in cubital tunnel
- Pain suggests cubital tunnel syndrome

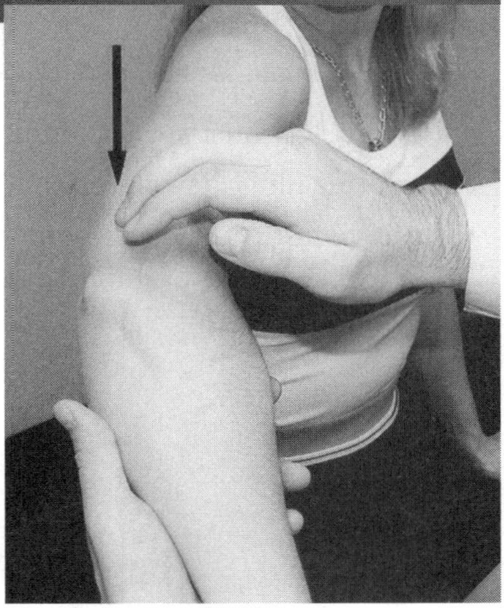

Figure 7–64 **Valgus Stress of the Ulnar (Medial) Collateral Ligament**

- Elbow is slightly flexed
- Determines ligamentous stability of ulnar and radial ligaments

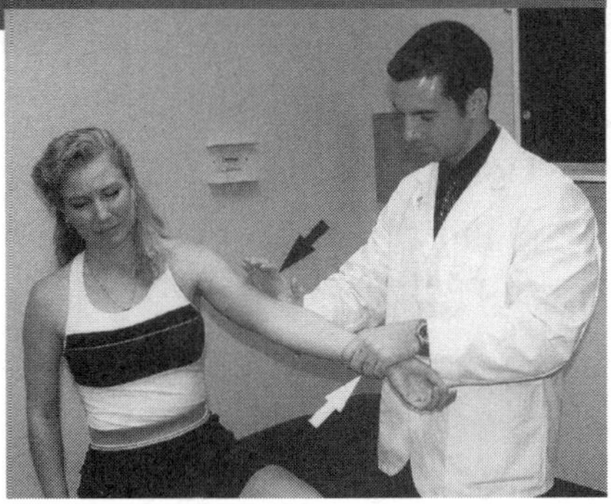

Figure 7–65 **Varus Stress of the Radial (Lateral) Collateral Ligament**

- See Figure 7–64 for description

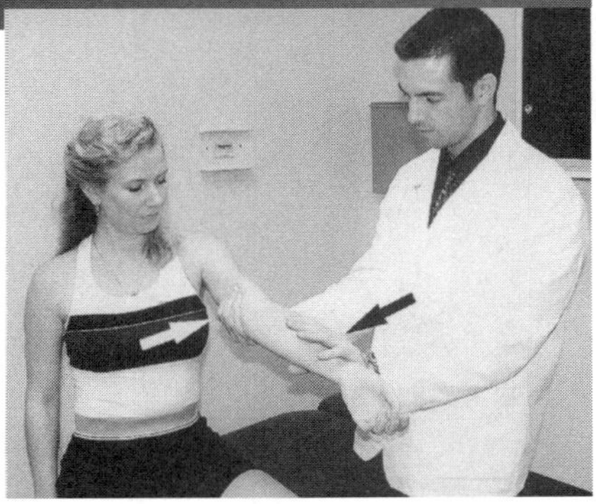

Wrist/Hand Tests

Figure 7–66 Finkelstein's Test

- Patient closes fist around thumb
- Performs ulnar deviation at wrist
- Positive test is consistent with stenosing tenosynovitis of thumb extensor/abductor tendons

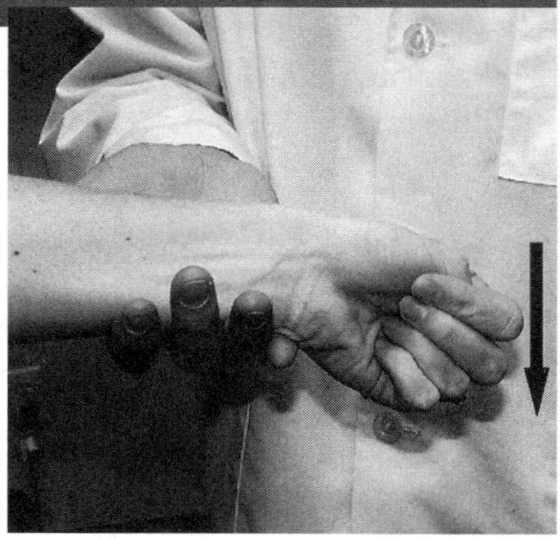

Figure 7–67 Phalen's Test

- Patient places dorsum of both hands together until wrists are fully flexed
- Holds this position for 30–60 seconds
- Numbness and/or pain suggests carpal tunnel syndrome

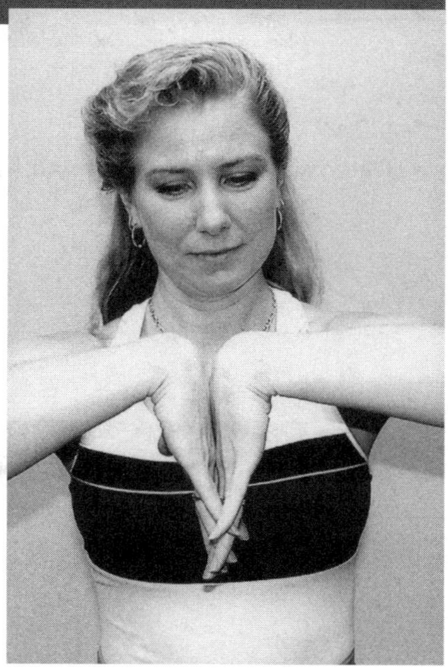

Figure 7–68 **Prayer Sign (Reverse Phalen's Test)**

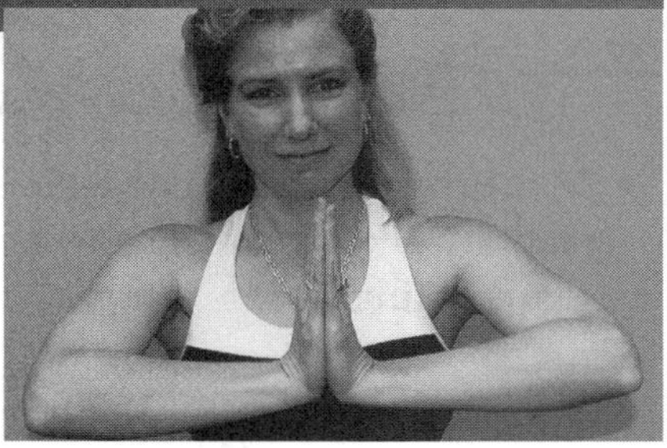

- Patient places palmar surfaces of both hands together until wrists are fully extended
- Holds this position for 30–60 seconds
- Numbness and/or pain suggests carpal tunnel syndrome

Figure 7–69 **Snuff Box Palpation**

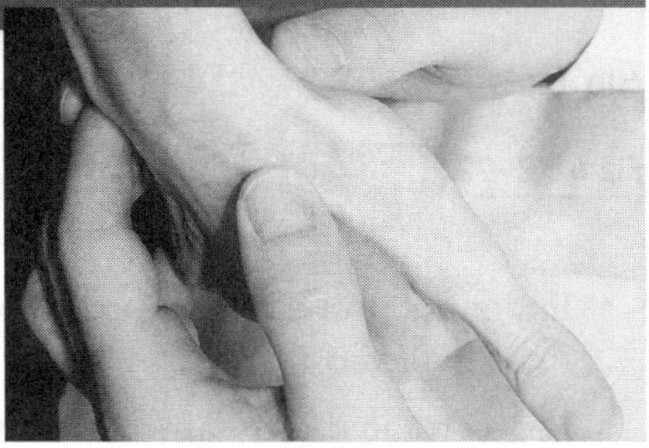

- Scaphoid fracture may be result of tenderness with palpation of anatomical snuff box

Figure 7–70 **Tinel's Sign at the Wrist**

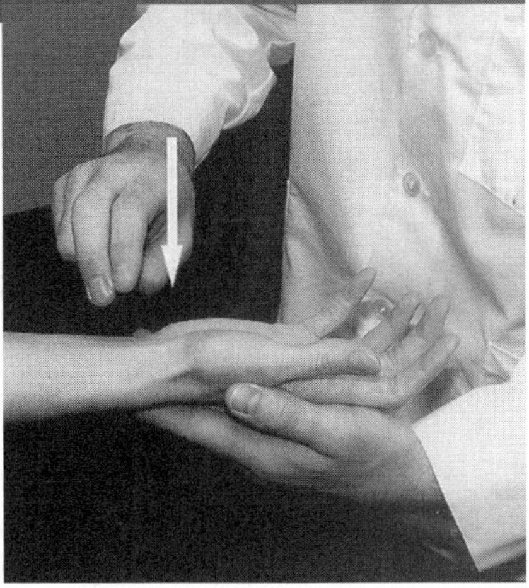

- Tapping ventral surface of wrist
- Pain or numbness suggests carpal tunnel syndrome

Hand Tests

Figure 7–71 Valgus and Varus Stress

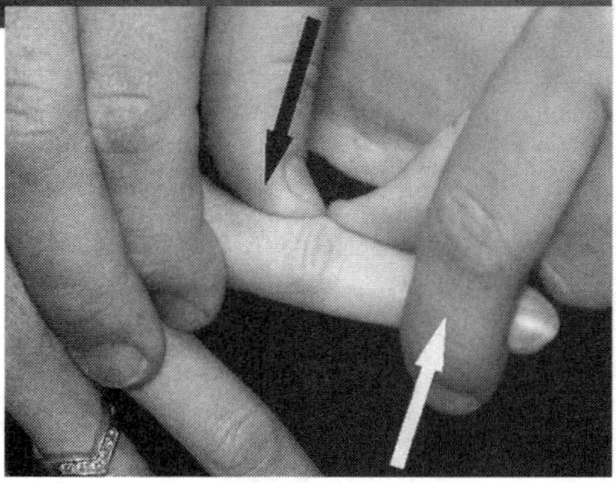

- Maneuvers to determine ligamentous stability of collateral ligaments of joints of fingers

Hip Tests

Figure 7–72 Hibbs' Test

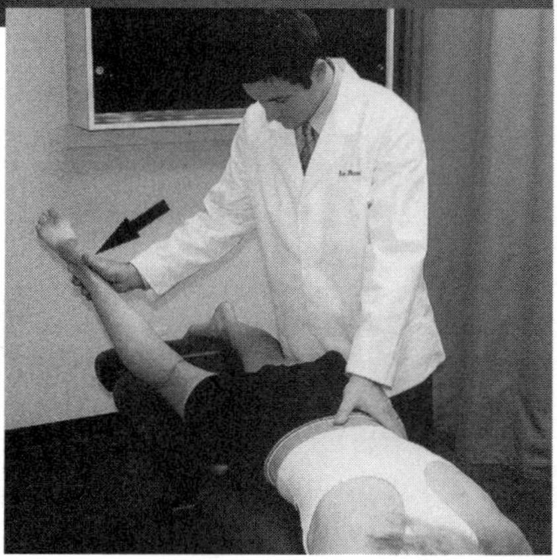

- Patient is prone and opposite side knee is flexed to 90°
- Leg is rotated outward while opposite side of pelvis is stabilized
- Test may be positive for sacroiliac and hip disease

Figure 7–73 **Ober's Test**

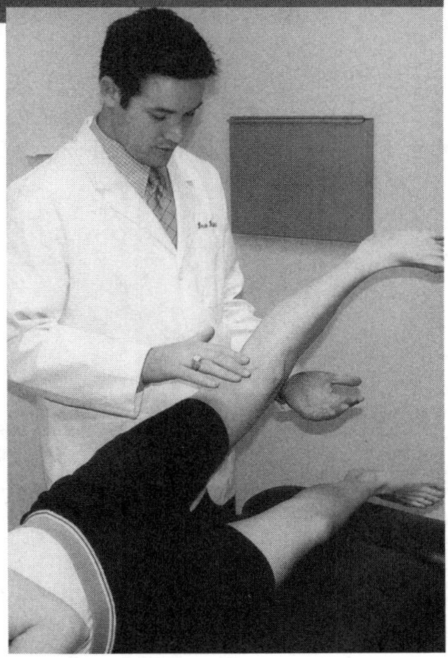

- Patient lies in side posture
- Leg is abducted at hip
- Leg should fall back to neutral position after examiner releases grasp on leg
- Test is considered positive if leg remains passively abducted and suggests contraction of the tensor fascia lata

Figure 7–74 **Patrick-FABER Test (Figure Four Test)**

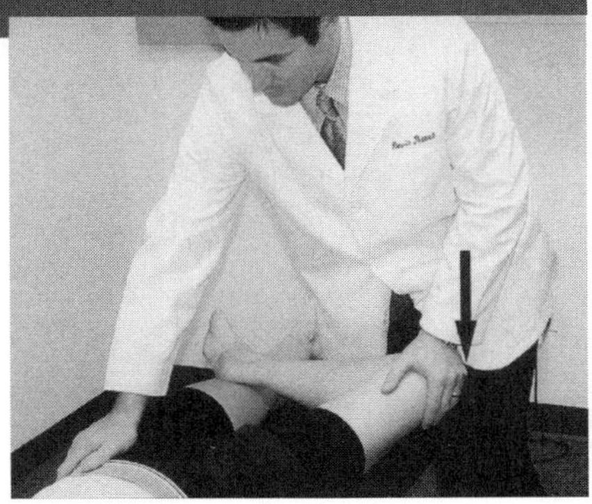

- Affected hip is flexed, abducted, and externally rotated
- Further abduction pressure is placed at knee
- Pain in sacroiliac joint/accurate assessment of sacroiliac disease

Figure 7–75 Thomas Test

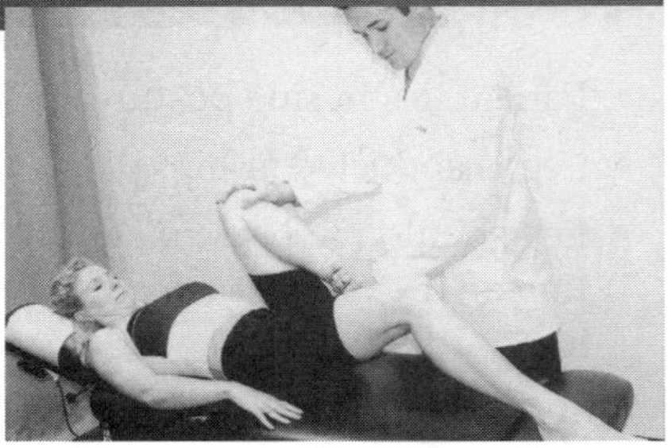

- Examiner fully flexes knee and hip on unaffected side
- Knee of affected leg will passively flex
- Positive findings indicate hip flexion contracture

Figure 7–76 Trendelenburg's Test

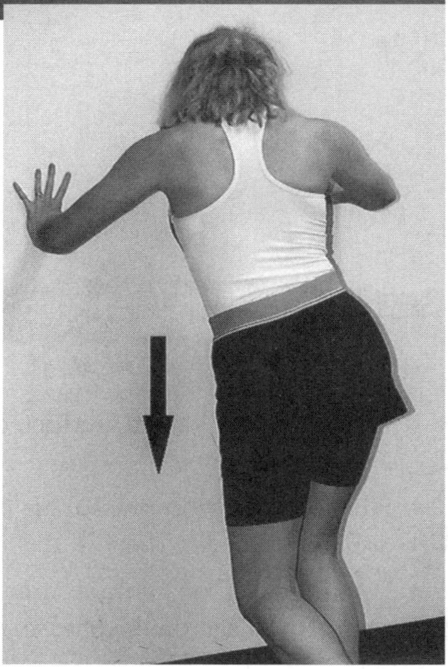

- Patient stands and lifts one foot off floor
- Pelvis on same side will elevate as well
- Test is considered positive if pelvis fails to elevate

Figure 7–77 **Yeoman's Test**

- With patient in prone position, examiner fully flexes knee to buttock
- Hyperextends hip while placing pressure on sacroiliac joint
- Pain is consistent with sacroiliac joint disease

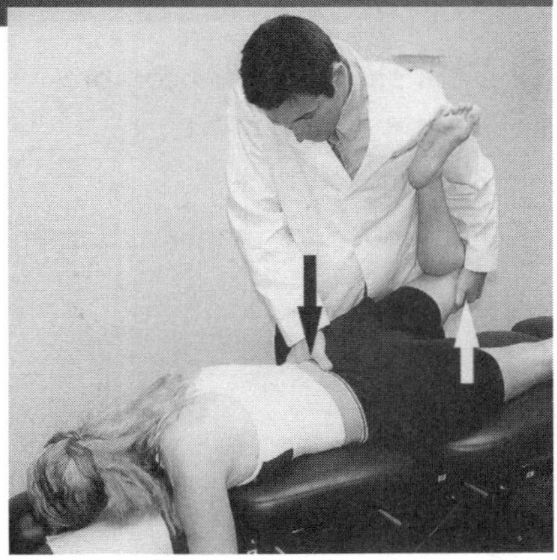

Knee Tests

Figure 7–78 **Anterior Drawer Sign of the Knee**

- Tibia is distracted anteriorly
- Estimation of stability compared to other side
- Excessive motion indicates tear of anterior cruciate ligament with instability

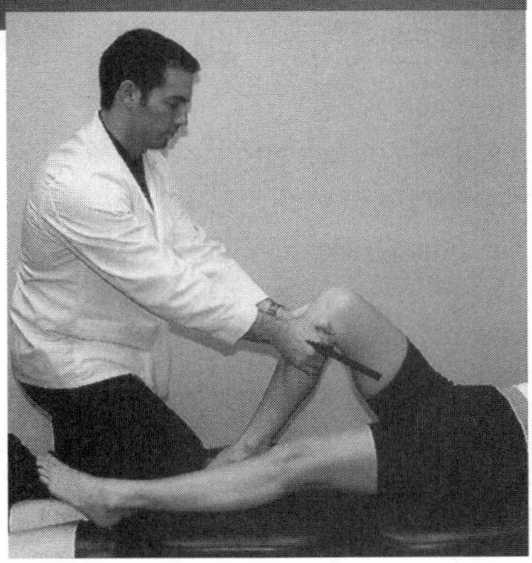

Figure 7–79 Apley's Compression Test

- With patient prone, compress lower leg into knee joint
- Knee flexed to 90°
- Pain indicates meniscal damage

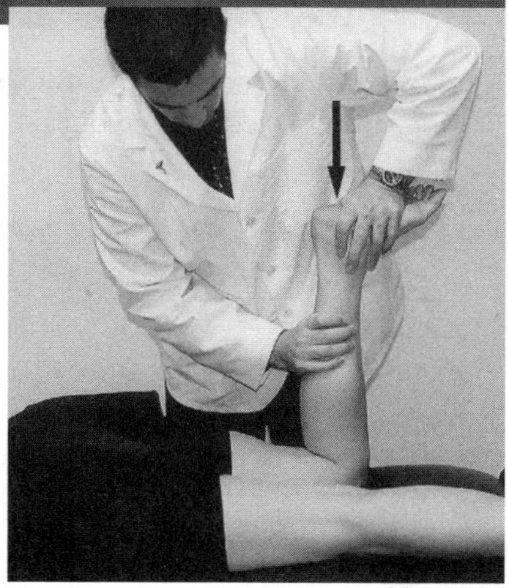

Figure 7–80 Apley's Distraction Test

- With patient prone, distract lower leg from knee
- Pain indicates ligamentous damage

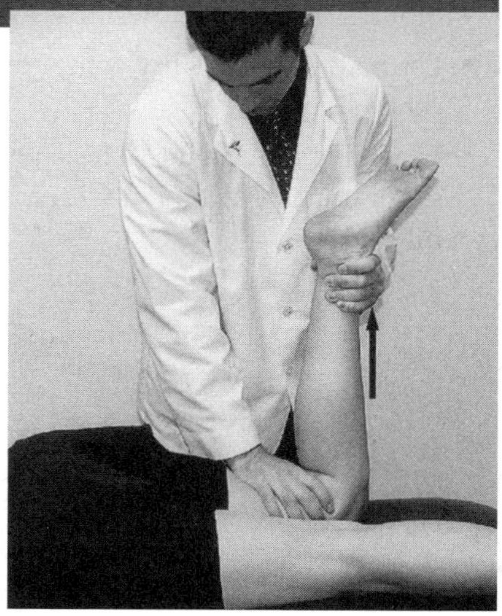

Figure 7-81 Lachman's Test

- One hand places anterior distraction on upper tibia
- Other hand places posterior distraction of distal femur
- Used to diagnose anterior cruciate ligament tear

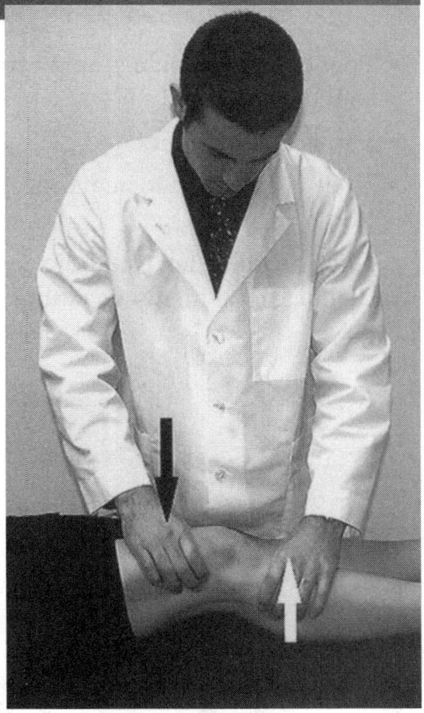

Figure 7-82 Medial-lateral Grind Test

- Leg is subjected to varus and valgus stress in both flexion and extension
- Grinding sensation felt by examiner suggests meniscus tear

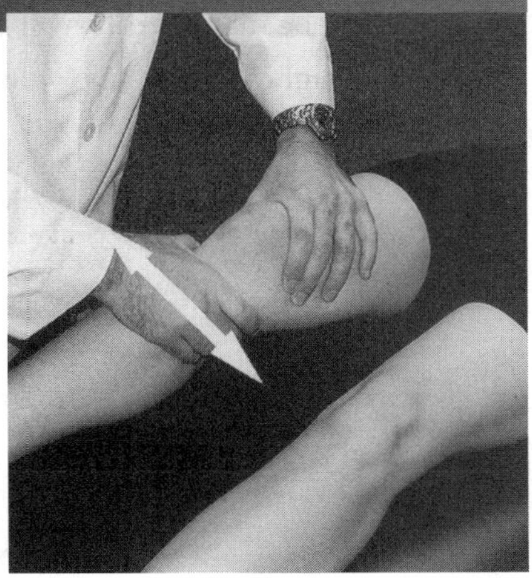

Figure 7–83 McMurray's Test

- Foot of affected side is approximated to buttock
- Hip is externally rotated
- Knee is extended to anatomical position
- Click heard or felt can indicate medial or lateral meniscus pathology

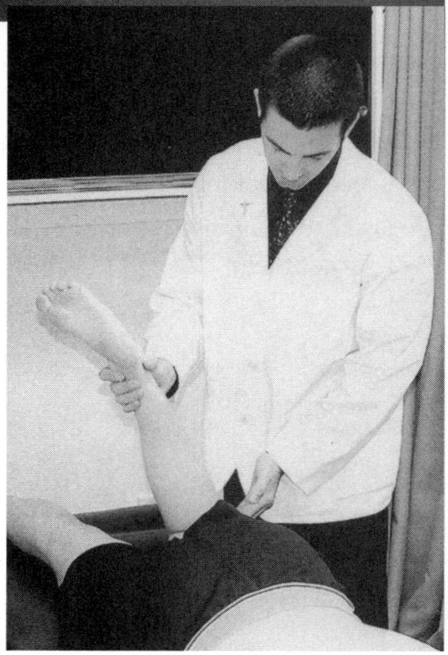

Figure 7–84 Pivot Shift Test

- Knee is medially rotated
- Tibia may be displaced forward
- Test has highest predictive value for anterior cruciate ligament tear

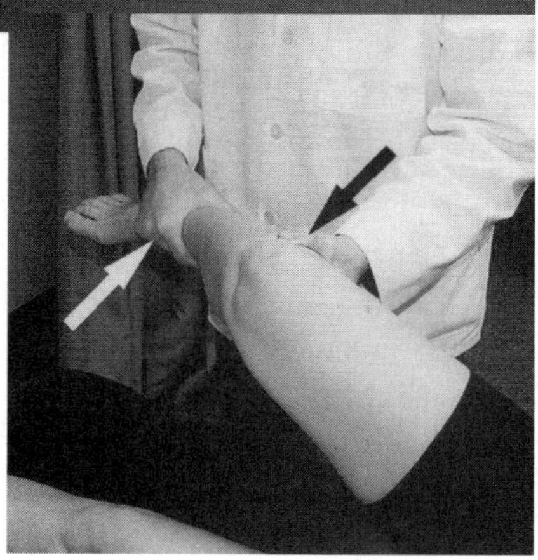

Ankle/Foot Tests

Figure 7–85 Anterior Drawer Sign of the Ankle

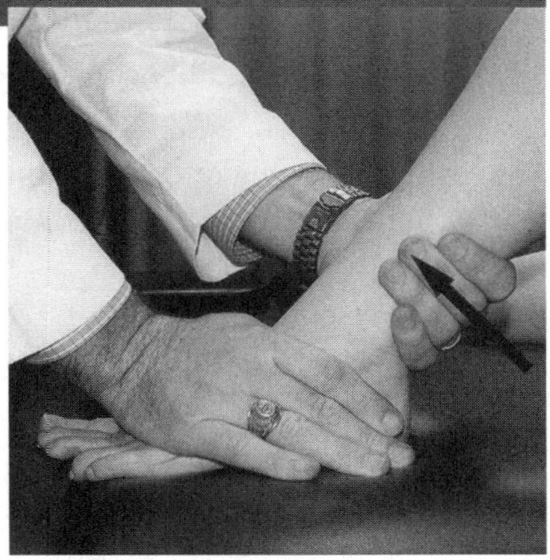

- Heel is distracted anteriorly
- Estimation of stability compared to other side
- Excessive motion indicates ligamentous rupture with instability

Figure 7–86 Morton's Test

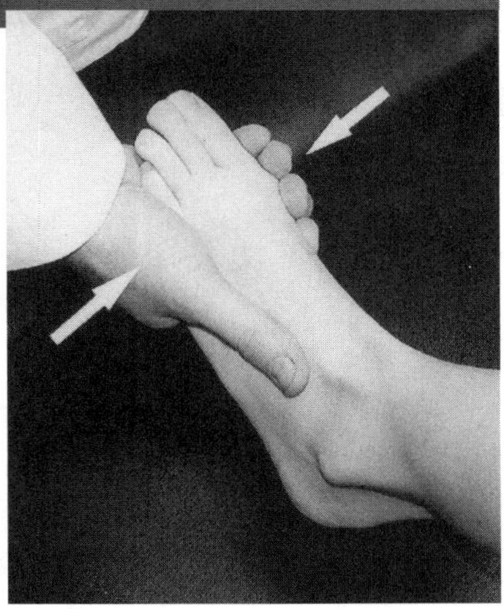

- Doctor squeezes metatarsal heads together
- Pain suggests neuroma or fracture

Figure 7–87 Posterior Drawer Sign of the Ankle

- Heel is distracted posteriorly
- Estimation of stability compared to other side
- Test indicates ligamentous rupture with instability

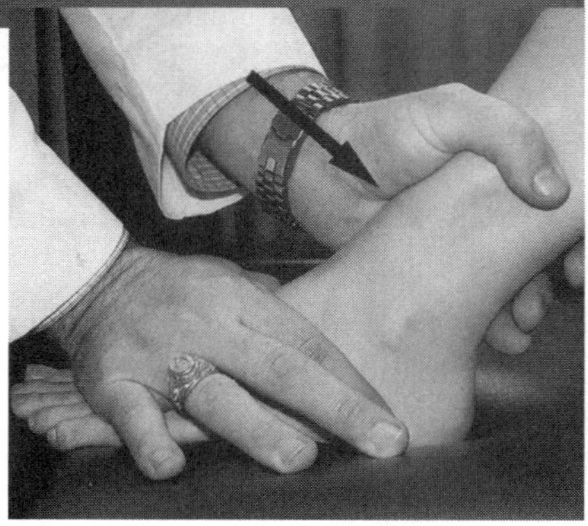

Figure 7–88 Thompson's Test

- With patient prone, examiner squeezes calf muscles
- No plantarflexion of the foot indicates Achilles's tendon rupture

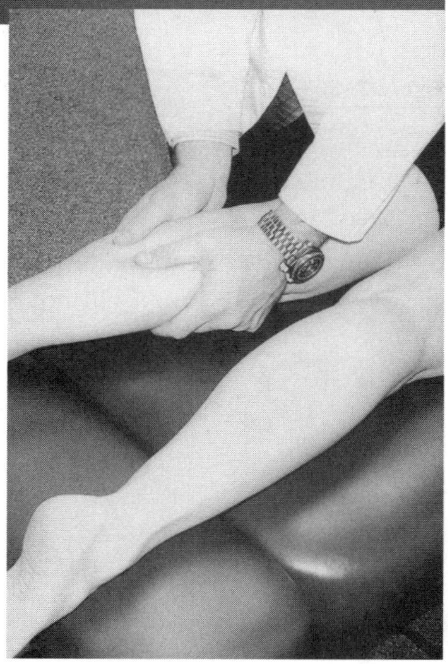

Figure 7–89 Valgus and Varus Stress

- Used to determine ligamentous stability of medial and lateral ligaments of the ankle

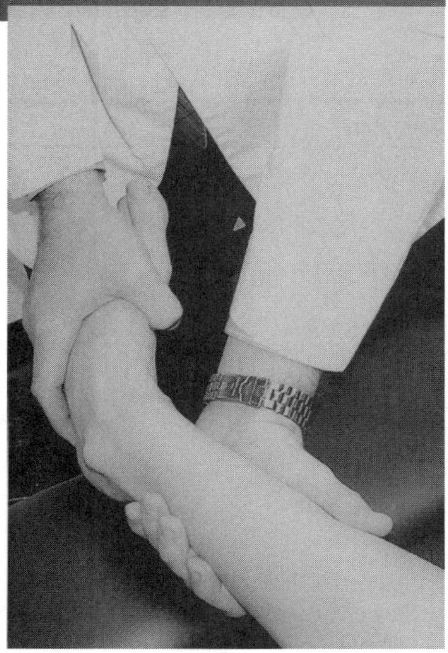

Range of Motion

The assessment of joint range of motion is an especially important portion of the orthopedic examination for chiropractic clinicians. Restoration of joint range of motion is a major goal of therapy in most cases. Table 7.1 contains a list of the ranges of motion for the various joints of the body. Range of motion is most accurately measured with a goniometer.

Spinal intersegmental range of motion is addressed in the chapter on manipulation.

Scoliosis Evaluation

In recent studies, it has been demonstrated that scoliosis has a major impact on the general lifestyle of patients afflicted with this condition. (3) These changes include poorer general health, decrease in vitality, and difficulty in social functioning along with the presence of co-morbid conditions such as low back pain and hypertension. Accurate evaluation of these patients is, therefore, critical.

Table 7.1 Normal Ranges of Motion (in degrees)

Body Part	Motion	Range of Motion
Ankle	Dorsiflexion	15–20
	Plantarflexion	40–50
	Inversion	05
	Eversion	05
Cervical Spine	Extension	40–50
	Flexion	40–50
	Lateral bending	40–50
	Rotation	40–60
Elbow	Flexion	140–150
	Extension	00
Fingers	Flexion	
Distal interphalangeal joint		70–90
Proximal interphalangeal joint		90–100
Metacarpophalangeal joint		85–95
	Extension	00–05
Forearm	Pronation	60–80
	Supination	80–90
Forefoot	Eversion	15–20
	Inversion	30–35
Hip	Abduction	45–50
	Adduction	20–30
	Extension	25–35
	Flexion	110–120
	Rotation (external)	40–50
	Rotation (internal)	30–40
Knee	Extension	00–10
	Flexion	85–95
	Lateral bending	15–25
	Rotation	25–35

Table 7.1 Normal Ranges of Motion (in degrees) *(continued)*

Body Part	Motion	Range of Motion
Shoulder	Abduction	170–180
	Adduction	40–50
	Extension	40–50
	Flexion	170–180
	Rotation (external)	80–90
	Rotation (internal)	70–90
Toes (First metatarsophalangeal joint)		
	Extension	70–90
	Flexion	40–45
Wrist	Extension	60–70
	Flexion	70–80
	Radial deviation	15–20
	Ulnar deviation	25–30

The Scoliosis Research Society defines scoliosis as "lateral deviation of the normal vertical line of the spine which, when measured by X-ray, is greater than ten degrees. Scoliosis consists of a lateral curvature of the spine with rotation of the vertebrae within the curve." (4) Any curvature below 10° should not be termed a scoliosis, as this term engenders horrific images in the minds of children and adults alike. Accurate representation of the size, magnitude, sequelae, available treatments, and prognosis for lateral spinal curvatures is essential.

Only a thorough evaluation of patients with scoliosis can accurately assess which of the many types of available therapy will best fit the needs of the patient. Proper evaluation includes an appropriate history, physical examination, and radiography of the spine.

Etiology

The etiology of scoliosis is just as important as the degree of deformity in determining appropriate treatment and prognosis. The myriad types of scoliosis are outlined in Table 7.2. By far, the most common form of scoliosis is idiopathic, representing approximately 80% of cases.

Table 7.2 Epidemiology of Scoliosis

Type	Epidemiology
Congenital	Failure of spinal segmentation/formation at birth
Hysterical	Associated with psychological disorder
Idiopathic	No cause determined
Neuromuscular	Secondary to neurologic or muscular disorder
Pathologic	Spinal tumors
Infantile	Develops before age 3
Juvenile	Develops between ages 3–10
Adolescent	Develops between puberty and skeletal maturity
Adult	Develops after skeletal maturity

History

Family history should be assessed for a history of scoliosis. The cause of the scoliosis should be sought, especially if it is a dysplastic cause, such as neurofibromatosis or Marfan's syndrome. The patient should then be examined for any findings of these syndromes.

Physical Examination

The evaluating physician should measure the lateral and posterior curvatures of the spine, as well as the rib hump, shoulder, and pelvic heights. These measurements will serve as reference points for future examinations and for charting the progression or regression of the curvatures.

Examination of the thorax is of paramount importance in scoliosis patients. Some patients with severe curvatures (>75°) suffer from cardiovascular and pulmonary disease secondary to reduced thoracic cage volume. Cardiac and lung auscultation, along with chest expansion measurements, should be performed and routinely monitored on all scoliosis patients.

An entire head-to-toe physical examination, including a neurologic assessment, should also be completed, with special emphasis on the rate of growth, if the patient is not a skeletally mature adult. In addition, inspection of the skin for café au lait spots, fibromas, skin dimples, herald patches of hair, and any cutaneous sinuses or fistulae should be performed.

The Adam's test should be performed to ascertain the nature and extent of trunk asymmetry. This test is performed by assessing for postural asymmetry in both the standing and forward-flexed positions. The knees should be extended and the arms outstretched during this maneuver. Changes in the characteristics of thorax symmetry in these two positions are then charted. It is worth mentioning that erector spinae muscle asymmetry may mimic the findings of a lateral spinal curvature with the Adam's test. Diagnostic imaging helps in this assessment. In addition, a number of nonradiographic tools are available for the evaluation of scoliosis, including plumb line analysis and a scoliometer to measure rib hump size.

Follow-up examinations are imperative in charting the patient's progress, especially with thoracic adolescent idiopathic scoliosis, which is the most often progressive form. These assessments may be performed as often as is necessary if, in the clinical judgment of the physician, it will be of benefit to the patient, but they are typically spaced at 4–6 month intervals.

Radiographic Examination

Full spine anteroposterior and sometimes lateral radiographic examination of the spine is essential in any patient suspected of having scoliosis. The lateral and anteroposterior curvatures of the spine are measured and recorded for future reference. (Figures 7–90 and 7–91) An estimation of the patient's skeletal age is also made. (Figure 7–92) This measurement will assist in the prediction of any future progression of the curvature(s).

Treatment

The treatment of scoliosis varies from simple exercises to surgical intervention. The aches and pains associated with most small curvatures seen in chiropractic general practice can be managed with manipulation, mobilization, exercise, stretching, and muscle stimulation. None of these modalities has been consistently scientifically validated as to curve regression or cessation of curve progression. Careful observation, bracing, and surgery are the most effective options for progressive curvature management and are dependent upon the patient's skeletal maturity, whether the adolescent growth spurt has occurred yet and size and location of the curvature. Proper brace requisition and fitting are best accomplished by referral to an orthotist with instructions from the treating physician. Referral to an orthopedic surgeon with a spine and/or scoliosis specialty can be utilized in those patients who have a high risk of progression or those who may suffer visceral organ compromise from the curvature and attendant postural abnormalities. Surgical instrumentation has been demonstrated to be effective when patients are properly selected. Specific treatment options are outlined in Table 7.3.

Figure 7–90 **Cobb Method of Scoliosis Measurement**

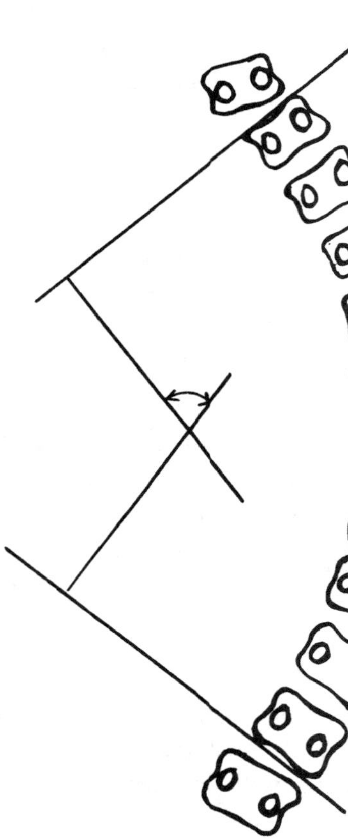

Effectiveness of the various treatments for scoliosis varies. Manipulation (5) and electrical stimulation (6) have not been consistently shown to be beneficial. The results claimed by those who utilize these techniques have been primarily anecdotal. (7) The results for therapeutic exercise have been equivocal (8, 9) with some studies demonstrating effectiveness and others failure. Manipulation has been shown to have a beneficial effect on back pain associated with scoliosis, however. (10)

Thoracic and lumbar orthoses have demonstrated good success in some studies. Van Rhijn et al. (11) showed a 70% success rate, where success was defined as less than six degrees of progression during the study period. Some cur-

Figure 7–91 Risser-Ferguson Method of Scoliosis Measurement

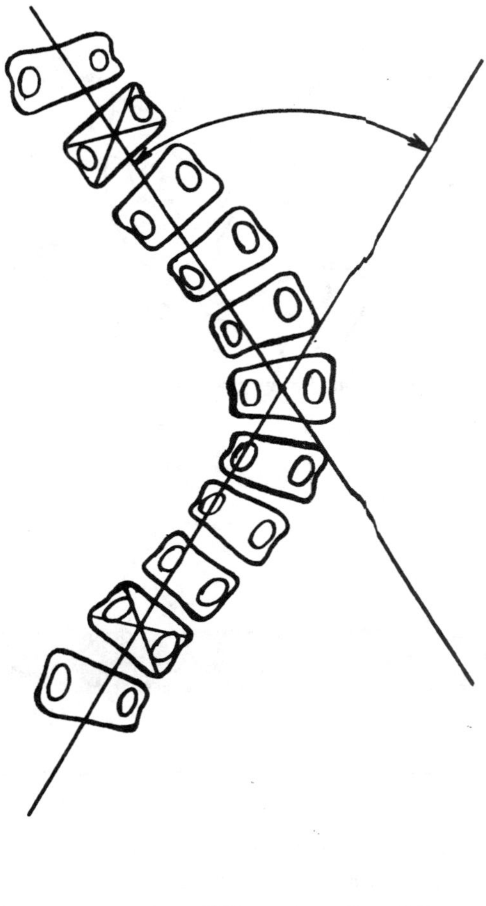

vatures in this study even regressed. Some studies (12) suggest that there is no difference in the natural history of adolescent idiopathic scoliosis and those who are treated with underarm orthoses. Others recommend bracing for only 16 hours per day. (13) Brace compliance is often poor, only 38% in one study. (14) Indicators of a good clinical outcome from bracing are demonstrated by assessing for a reduction in the Cobb angle and vertebral rotation after the brace is fitted. Patients who do not have these reductions typically have brace failure and many require surgery. (15)

Both anterior and posterior approaches to surgical instrumentation are available, and the results are similar in both instances. (16) Surgery for scoliosis is not

Figure 7–92 **Risser's Sign of Skeletal Maturation**

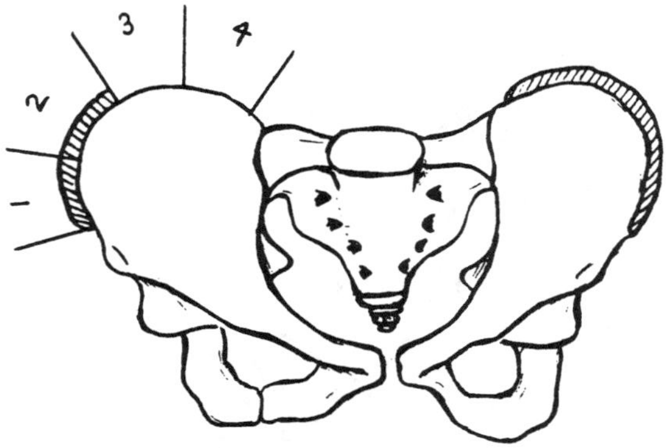

Note: After grade 4 and the apophysis fuses, skeletal growth has ceased.

Table 7.3 **Scoliosis Treatment Options**

Observation
- Curvatures <25° in patients who are almost skeletally mature
- Curvatures <45° in patients who are skeletally mature
- Reevaluate every 4–6 months including radiography

Spinal Orthosis
- Curvatures 25–40° in patients with skeletal growth remaining
- Attempt to stop curve progression; regression is unlikely
- Type of brace and time-in-brace are variable according to protocols

Surgical Instrumentation
- Curvatures >50° in previously untreated patients
- Curvatures >50° in patients with poor orthosis results
- Patients with visceral complaints related to the scoliosis
- Instrumentation is often accompanied by arthrodesis

without negative sequelae, however. In one series, approximately 20% of patients required re-operation to remove the appliances after an initial primary instrumentation was intolerable secondary to late operative site pain. (17) The literature also demonstrates a decrease in the incidence in back pain in patients who have a surgical arthrodesis for scoliosis over those who do not have an arthrodesis, but the incidence of back pain was higher in both scoliosis groups than in a control group. (18)

Danielsson et al. compared bracing to surgery and found that patients who had surgical instrumentation lost a mean of 3.5° of correction, and those patients who were braced progressed a mean of 7.9°. (19)

Curvature Progression

Peterson and Nachemson determined a number of factors that accurately predict the progression of a scoliosis. The findings that suggested that curvature progression would occur were a Risser sign of zero or one, a curvature apex above T12, and an imbalance of ten millimeters or less. (20)

Spondylolisthesis

Spondylolisthesis (SL) is the abnormal anterior translation of a vertebral body associated with lesions or deformity of the posterior arch of the involved vertebra. It has a prevalence of approximately 5% of the general population.

It has been somewhat of an enigma for all the health care disciplines for many years. Treatment regimens vary from rest to forms of radical surgery. As yet, no one has arrived at any definitive conclusions as to the etiology, let alone, treatment of SL.

This section will discuss theories regarding pathogenesis, proper diagnosis, and chiropractic treatment as well as surgical management of SL.

Clinical Findings

Most patients with this condition are asymptomatic and are unaware of its existence. Symptoms are most common in young people, while symptoms in adults from SL are unusual unless there is a history of previous back pain. Patients most often complain of achy low back pain that is exacerbated by motion, particularly extension and rotation. Occasionally, a patient with SL will complain of radiculopathy-type symptoms. In these cases, a search for nerve root compression in the neural foramen should be undertaken.

Physical examination findings include a possible "step-defect" at the level *above* the SL from the anterior translation associated with this lesion that brings the cephalad vertebra forward. Most patients will also have hamstring "tightness" on palpation. Pain with palpation of the lower lumbar spine can also be found.

Pathogenesis

There are five basic etiologies for SL (21).

Spondylolytic SL is the most common form. There is a reported incidence of slightly over 5% by age 18. In this form, there is a stress fracture at the pars interarticularis of the vertebral arch, which results in anterolisthesis of the involved vertebra. This type of SL occurs most commonly at L5 but may also be seen anywhere throughout the spine. Grade I slippage is the most common, representing approximately three-fourths of cases. It is interesting to note that although pars defects are half as common in girls as in boys, high-grade slippage is four times more common in girls. Pain, when present, is usually located in the caudal portion of the lumbar region. There may or may not be radiation into the buttock(s) and leg(s). Radiographic features that tend to correlate with low back symptoms include anterolisthesis of greater than 25%, spondylolysis or spondylolisthesis at L4, and/or early disc degeneration at the lumbosacral level. It is generally agreed that in most cases, over 90% of the slippage has already occurred at the time of initial examination. Further slippage is exceedingly unusual after skeletal maturation.

Degenerative SL, on the other hand, does not involve fracture of any portion of the vertebral body. Its presentation is that of an anterolisthesis of a vertebral body at the level of a degenerated disc and many times unusual facet joint morphology and facet arthrosis. There is a conspicuous absence of pars defects with this form of SL.

Traumatic SL is usually reserved for fractured pedicles at C2 from severe hyperextension injuries of the neck. This form of SL may present to the chiropractic office. Care should be taken to rule out its presence in a trauma patient before any manipulation is performed, lest neurologic sequelae possibly result.

Pathologic SL occurs when there is some pathologic condition of the posterior spinal elements that results in a SL. This type of spondylolisthesis must be investigated aggressively to ascertain the nature and extent of the disease causing the SL.

Congenital/dysplastic SL is uncommon. In this type of SL, the facets do not prevent any anterolisthesis of the L5 vertebra. This type comprises approximately 15–20% of treated cases with a 2:1 female-to-male ratio.

Diagnosis

The diagnosis of SL is usually straightforward when radiography is employed; the main question is the etiology of the SL. The presence or absence of pars defects characterizes spondylolytic and degenerative types, respectively. Oblique radiographic views confirm this distinction. Traumatic SL occurs most commonly in the cervical spine and is associated with severe hyperextension injuries.

Grading of SL is outlined in Table 7.4.

If there is a possibility of instability, then flexion and extension radiographic views and hanging or compression radiography may be helpful. Additional anterolisthesis during these special maneuvers may be suggestive of instability and may require referral if the patient is significantly affected or incapacitated by the pain or has neurologic defects.

Treatment

Lumbar stabilization is the goal of therapy in patients with SL.

Therapeutic exercise has been evaluated by a number of studies. Although the only two that were included in a recent systematic review suggested benefits from exercise, the exercise regimens differed. The authors conclude that more research into exercise as a therapy is needed. (22) Similar findings have been seen with other physical medicine modalities such as orthoses (anti-lordotic posture) and stretching.

Surgery, including decompression and/or fusion, is also performed, many times without success (23) although an endoscopic approach to foraminal decompression is showing some promise. (24) Surgery should be reserved for patients who fail to respond to conservative care and are enduring long-standing uncontrolled pain and/or radiculopathy or myelopathy, particularly children who have not yet reached skeletal maturity and have more of a propensity for further slippage and neural compromise.

It may be necessary to limit participation in contact sports or those sports, such as gymnastics, that require a great deal of lumbar hyperextension, for those children at higher risk of slippage and neurologic sequelae.

Table 7.4 Spondylolisthesis Grades

Grade	Slippage
I	1–25% slippage
II	26–50% slippage
III	51–75% slippage
IV	76–100% slippage
V*	>100% slippage

*Also known as spondyloptosis

Manipulation appears to be as effective in patients with SL as those without this condition (25) and is therefore a viable conservative approach to care.

Screening Orthopedic Examinations

After the patient's chief complaint is recorded and established as either an orthopedic or a neurologic problem, a screening examination may be performed to help the clinician isolate the area of the problem so that a more detailed examination of that area may be performed. It should be remembered that these screening examinations in no way specifically isolate the diagnosis. It should also be remembered that visceral pathology can refer pain to any area of the musculoskeletal system. There are two screening exams: the upper body and lower body screening examinations.

Upper Body Screening Examination (with patient sitting)

- Inspection
  —Head and neck
  —Shoulders
  —Elbows
  —Wrists
  —Hands
- Shoulder range of motion
  —Active abduction with end of range pressure (EORP)
  —Active extension with adduction with EORP
- Cervical spine
  —Active ranges of motion
  —Passive motion with EORP
  —Resisted range of motion (Table 7.5)
  —Vertebrobasilar artery patency tests
- Dermatomes/sensory
  —Pinwheel examination (with two instruments)
  —Sensation of pins/needles/numbness/tingling

Table 7.5 Upper Body Muscle Testing
Cervical flexion/extension
Elbow flexion
Shoulder rotation/abduction
Wrist flexion/extension
Finger squeeze

- Reflexes
  - —Biceps brachialis (C5)
  - —Brachioradialis (C6)
  - —Triceps (C7)
- Detailed evaluation of area of involvement suggested by the screening examination

Lower Body Screening Examination

- Patient standing
  - —Posture
  - —Deep knee bend (tests all joints of lower extremity)
  - —Tandem gait (away from examiner) (ataxia?)
  - —Heel walk (toward examiner) (L4/5)
  - —Toe walk (away from examiner) (L5/S1)
- Patient sitting
  - —Thoracolumbar spine
    - Inspection
    - Active range of motion with EORP
    - Passive range of motion with EORP
  - —Orthopedic tests
    - Valsalva Maneuver
    - Internal rotation of the hip

—Neurologic tests

Dermatomes (bilateral with pinwheels)

Reflexes

—Knee jerk (L3/4)

Ankle jerk (S1)

- Patient supine

—Orthopedic tests

Sciatic nerve stretch tests

Patrick FABER test

—Hip evaluation

Active range of motion with EORP

Passive range of motion with EORP

—Knee evaluation

Active range of motion with EORP

Passive range of motion with EORP

Valgus/varus stress

—Ankle evaluation

Active range of motion with EORP

Passive range of motion with EORP

Anterior/posterior drawer sign

—Reflexes

Knee jerk, ankle jerk

Babinski response (upper motor neuron lesion)

Shin tracing with heel (cerebellar integrity)

- Patient prone

—Gluteal mass inspection

—Orthopedic tests

Femoral nerve stretch tests

Internal/external hip rotation

Spring test (S1 joint)

—Resisted muscle testing (Table 7.6)

- Detailed evaluation of the area of involvement suggested by the screening examination

Table 7.6 **Lower Body Muscle Testing**

Lumbar flexion/extension
Hip flexion/extension
Knee flexion/extension
Ankle dorsiflexion/plantar flexion
Great toe extension

Table 7.7 **Angular Deformities of the Skeleton**

Spine
- Hyperlordosis–abnormal accentuation of an anterior sagittal spinal curve
- Hypolordosis–abnormal flattening of an anterior sagittal spinal curve
- Hyperkyphosis–abnormal accentuation of a posterior sagittal spinal curve
- Hypokyphosis–abnormal flattening of a posterior sagittal spinal curve

Hips
- Coxa Valga–increased angle of femoral inclination; may be traumatic, congenital, bone-softening diseases
- Coxa Varum–decreased angle of femoral inclination; may be traumatic, congenital, bone-softening diseases

Knees
- Genu Valgum–lateral angulation of the tibia at the knee resulting in "knock-knees"
- Genu Varum–medial angulation of the tibia at the knee resulting in "bowed legs"

Feet
- Pes Planus–loss of the longitudinal arch of the foot; "flat foot"; often biomechanical in etiology
- Pes Cavus–accentuation of the longitudinal arch of the foot; "cave foot"; often associated with neurologic disorders

Elbow
- Cubitus Valgum–increased elbow carrying angle
- Cubitus Varum–decreased elbow carrying angle

Deformities of the Skeleton

Table 7.7 outlines some of the more common deformities of bones and joints in the axial and appendicular skeleton.

References

1. Walsh, M.J. Evaluation of orthopedic testing of the low back for nonspecific lower back pain. *J Manipulative Physiol Ther.* 1998 May;21(4):232–236.
2. Malanga, G.A., Andrus, S., Nadler, S.F., & McLean, J. Physical examination of the knee: a review of the original test description and scientific validity of common orthopedic tests. *Arch Phys Med Rehabil.* 2003 Apr;84(4):592–603.
3. Schwab, F., Dubey, A., Pagala, M., Gamez, L., & Farcy, J.P. Adult scoliosis: a health assessment analysis by SF-36. *Spine.* 2003 Mar 15;28(6):602–606.
4. Scoliosis Research Society. http://www.srs.org/homepage.htm.
5. Lantz, C.A., & Chen, J. Effects of chiropractic intervention on small scoliotic curves in younger subjects: a time-series cohort design. *J Manipulative Physiol Ther.* 2001. 24:385–393.
6. Durham, J.W., Moskowitz, A., & Whitney, J. Surface electrode stimulation versus brace in treatment of idiopathic scoliosis. *Spine.* 1990. 15(9):888–892.
7. Tarola, G.A. Manipulation for the control of back pain and curve progression in patients with skeletally mature idiopathic scoliosis: two cases. *J Manipulative Physiol Ther.* 1994 May;17(4):253–257.
8. Carman, D., Roach, J.W., Speck, G., Wenger, D.R., & Herring, J.A. Role of exercises in the Milwaukee brace treatment of scoliosis. *J Pediatr Orthop.* 1985 Jan–Feb;5(1):65–68.
9. Weiss, H.R., Weiss, G., & Petermann, F. Incidence of curvature progression in idiopathic scoliosis patients treated with scoliosis in-patient rehabilitation (SIR): an age- and sex-matched controlled study. *Pediatr Rehabil.* 2003 Jan–Mar;6(1):23–30.
10. Nykoliation, J.W., Cassidy, J.D., Arthur, B.E., & Wedge, J.H. An algorithm for the management of scoliosis. *J Manipulative Physiol Ther.* 1986 Mar;9(1):1–14.
11. Van Rhijn, L.W., Veraart, B.E., & Plasmans, C.M. Application of a lumbar brace for thoracic and double thoracic lumbar scoliosis: a comparative study. *J Pediatr Orthop B.* 2003 May;12(3):178–182.
12. Goldberg, C.J., Dowling, F.E., Hall, J.E., & Emans, J.B. A statistical comparison between natural history of AIS and brace treatment in skeletally immature adolescent girls. *Spine.* 1993. 18(7):902–908.
13. Green, N.E. Part-time bracing of adolescent idiopathic scoliosis. *JBJS.* 1986. 68-A:738–742.
14. Karol, L.A. Effectiveness of bracing in male patients with idiopathic scoliosis. *Spine.* 2001. 26:2001–2005.

15. Upadhyay, S.S., Nelson, I.W., Ho, E.K., Hsu, L.C., & Leong, J.C. New prognostic factors to predict the final outcome of brace treatment in adolescent idiopathic scoliosis. *Spine.* 1995 Mar 1;20(5):537–545.
16. Rhee, J.M., Bridwell, K.H., Won, D.S., Lenke, L.G., Chotigavanichaya, C., & Hanson, D.S. Sagittal plane analysis of adolescent idiopathic scoliosis: the effect of anterior versus posterior instrumentation. *Spine.* 2002 Nov 1;27(21):2350–2356.
17. Cook, S., Asher, M., Lai, S.M., & Shobe, J. Reoperation after primary posterior instrumentation and fusion for idiopathic scoliosis. Toward defining late operative site pain of unknown cause. *Spine.* 2000 Feb 15;25(4):463–468.
18. Parsch, D., Gaertner, V., Brocai, D.R., & Carstens, C. The effect of spinal fusion on the long-term outcome of idiopathic scoliosis. A case-control study. *J Bone Joint Surg Br.* 2001 Nov;83(8):1133–1136.
19. Danielsson, A.J., & Nachemson, A.L. Radiologic findings and curve progression 22 years after treatment for adolescent idiopathic scoliosis: comparison of brace and surgical treatment with matching control group of straight individuals. *Spine.* 2001. 26:516–525.
20. Peterson, L.E., & Nachemson, A.L. Prediction of progression of the curve in girls who have adolescent idiopathic scoliosis of moderate severity. Logistic regression analysis based on data from The Brace Study of the Scoliosis Research Society. *J Bone Joint Surg Am.* 1995 Jun;77(6):823–827.
21. Wiltse, L.L., Newman, P.H., & Macnab, I. Classification of spondylolysis and spondylolisthesis. *Clin Orthop.* 1976;117:23–29.
22. McNeely, M.L., Torrance, G., & Magee, D.J. A systematic review of physiotherapy for spondylolysis and spondylolisthesis. *Man Ther.* 2003 May;8(2):80–91.
23. Adam, F.F. Surgical management of isthmic spondylolisthesis with radicular pain. I*nt Orthop.* 2003 Jul 3.
24. Knight, M., & Goswami, A. Management of isthmic spondylolisthesis with posterolateral endoscopic foraminal decompression. *Spine.* 2003 Mar 15;28(6):573–581.
25. Mierau, D., Cassidy, J.D., McGregor, M., & Kirkaldy-Willis, W.H. A comparison of the effectiveness of spinal manipulative therapy for low back pain patients with and without spondylolisthesis. *J Manipulative Physiol Ther.* 1987 Apr;10(2):49–55.

Chapter 8

NEUROLOGY

Lawrence H. Wyatt, DC, DACBR, FICC

Introduction

Neurology is the study of diseases that affect the nervous system. For many years, the beneficial and detrimental effects of manipulation on the human nervous system have been investigated by researchers.

It is known that complications, particularly involving post-manipulative inflammation, vascular damage, hemorrhage, and ischemic neurological sequelae may occur with chiropractic manipulation in extremely rare instances. (1) These sequelae range from continued pain to quadriplegia and, in some extremely rare cases, death.

This chapter outlines the neurologic evaluation of patients presenting to the chiropractic physician. Emphasis is placed on diagnostics and the evaluation of the patient for neurologic contraindications to manipulation.

The neurologic evaluation of a patient is divided into four separate parts: location of the lesion, etiology of the lesion, treatment of the lesion, and contraindications to manipulation because of the lesion.

Location of the Lesion

An important aspect of neurologic diagnosis is locating the lesion. In most instances, the location of the lesion defines treatment and helps define any contraindications to manipulation.

The cerebral cortex is responsible for several activities. Among the most important are consciousness, speech, and motor and sensory functions. Alterations in these functions should suggest a cortical lesion.

The subcortical region contains the internal capsule, basal ganglia, and the thalamus. This region can be considered a relay station for the higher command functions performed by the cerebral cortex and the lower distribution pathway of the spinal cord. The internal capsule directly relays motor and sensory function, the basal ganglia is responsible for the fine adjustment of movements, and the thalamus is the sensory relay point. Signs and symptoms related to the above noted functions should suggest a subcortical lesion.

The cerebellum, in conjunction with the basal ganglia, helps to refine motor activity. Abnormalities in motor coordination suggest a lesion in these regions.

The brainstem contains the origin of the cranial nerves and contains the primitive functions of living—the breathing center and vasomotor center—and modulates the interaction between the cerebellum and the rest of the central nervous system (CNS). Patients presenting with cranial nerve lesions therefore often have intracranial lesions, although peripheral neuropathy of the cranial nerves also occurs.

The first step in locating the lesion is to decide whether it involves the CNS or peripheral nervous system. Is the lesion an upper motor neuron lesion (UMNL) or lower motor neuron lesion (LMNL)? (Table 8.1).

Deep Tendon Reflexes

Hyperreflexia, secondary to loss of CNS inhibition of deep tendon reflexes (DTRs), is consistent with a UMNL and hyporeflexia with an LMNL. Reflexes are graded from 0 to +4 (Table 8.2). Clonus, or rapid involuntary alternating movements, may also be present with a UMNL.

Paralysis/Paresis/Muscle Tone

Spastic paralysis and/or hypertonicity is suggestive of a UMNL, while flaccid paralysis and/or hypotonicity is consistent with an LMNL. Spastic paralysis is hallmarked by an inability to move an extremity, both voluntarily and involuntarily. Muscle rigidity prevents, or at least restricts, passive motion and may even result in the so-called "cogwheel" response. This response appears as a jerky motion when the extremity is passively moved. Table 8.3 outlines the innervation of the more commonly tested extremity muscles.

Table 8.1 Upper versus Lower Motor Neuron Lesions

Test/Sign	UMNL	LMNL
Paralysis	**Spastic**	**Flaccid**
Muscle tone	+	−
Atrophy	+/−	+
Pathologic reflexes	+	−
Clonus	+	−
DTRs	+	−
Fasciculations	−	+

Note: + = present/increased; − = absent/decreased.

Fasciculations or Fibrillations

Fasciculations are palpable involuntary muscle contractions and fibrillations are invisible muscle contractions. These contractions are seen with an LMNL.

Pathologic Reflexes

A Babinski response (dorsiflexion of the great toe with spreading of the lateral four toes upon stroking the plantar surface of the foot) is diagnostic of a UMNL.

Table 8.2 Deep Tendon Reflex Grading

Grade	Findings
0	no reflex
1	hypoactive (diminished) reflex
2	normal
3	hyperactive (accentuated) reflex
4	hyperactive with clonus

Table 8.3 Neurologic Innervation of Extremity Muscles

Spinal Nerve Root	Muscles
C4	Levator scapulae (dorsal scapular nerve)
C5–6	Deltoid (C5) (axillary nerve) Biceps (C6) (musculocutaneous nerve) Brachioradialis (C6) (radial nerve) Supinator (C6) (radial nerve)
C6–7	Pronator teres (C7) (median nerve)
C6–8	Triceps (C7) (radial nerve) Extensor carpi ulnaris (C7) (radial nerve) Flexor carpi ulnaris (C8) (median/ulnar nerves)
C7–8	Digital extensors (C7) (radial nerve)
C8–T1	Thenar muscles (C8) (median nerve) Hypothenar muscles (T1) (ulnar nerve) Interossei (T1) (ulnar nerve)
L2–4	Quadriceps (L3,4) (femoral nerve) Iliopsoas (L2) (femoral nerve) Adductors (L3) (obturator nerve)
L4–5	Tibialis anterior (L4) (peroneal nerve) Hamstrings (L5) (sciatic nerve) Toe extensors (L5) (peroneal nerve)
L5–S2	Extensor hallucis longus (L5) (peroneal nerve) Peronei (peroneal nerve) Tibialis posterior (L5) (tibial nerve) Toe flexors (S1,2) (tibial nerve) Gastrocnemius/soleus (S1) (tibial nerve) Gluteus maximus (S1,2) (inferior gluteal nerve)

It should be remembered that children under the age of 12 to 18 months will have a positive Babinski response under normal circumstances.

Other common pathologic reflexes include the Hoffman's Reflex (opposition/flexion of the thumb when the middle finger is flicked), Kleist's Hooking Sign (with gentle elevation the patient's fingers cause reactive flexion and hooking onto the examiner's fingers), Gordon's Reflex (a Babinski response when the calf is squeezed/compressed), and Oppenheim's Sign (a Babinski response when the tibia is stroked firmly by the examiner).

If the lesion is determined to be an LMNL, it must then be decided if the defect is at the nerve root or in the peripheral nerve. (Table 8.4) Nerve root lesions are suggested by positive orthopedic tests for nerve root tension. Pain in a root lesion will also be noted from the spine to below the elbow or knee in a dermatomal pattern, whereas the pain and numbness of a peripheral lesion begins at the site of entrapment and does not follow a dermatomal pattern. Pain is less often seen with peripheral lesions. Dermatomes are illustrated in Figure 8–1.

If the lesion is determined to involve the CNS, it must then be decided whether the spinal cord or brain is the primary site of the lesion. (Table 8.5)

Spinal Cord Lesions

The spinal cord is divided into three basic columns—anterior, posterior, and lateral. The anterior column is primarily responsible for motor function, the posterior column is primarily responsible for sensory (proprioception) function, and the lateral column has an ascending sensory tract (pain and temperature) and a descending motor tract.

Lesions involving the anterolateral portion of the spinal cord will typically present with UMNL findings, often with a dermatomal defect and dissociation of sensory function in the extremities. Dissociation is the separation of sensory losses to opposite sides of the body. For example, if pain and temperature sensation are lost on one side of the body and proprioception on the contralateral side,

Table 8.4 **Nerve Root versus Peripheral Nerve Lesions**

Test/Sign	Root	Peripheral Nerve
Dermatomal dysesthesia	+	–
Root tension signs	+	–
Spinal nerve weakness distribution	+	–

Figure 8–1 Dermatomes

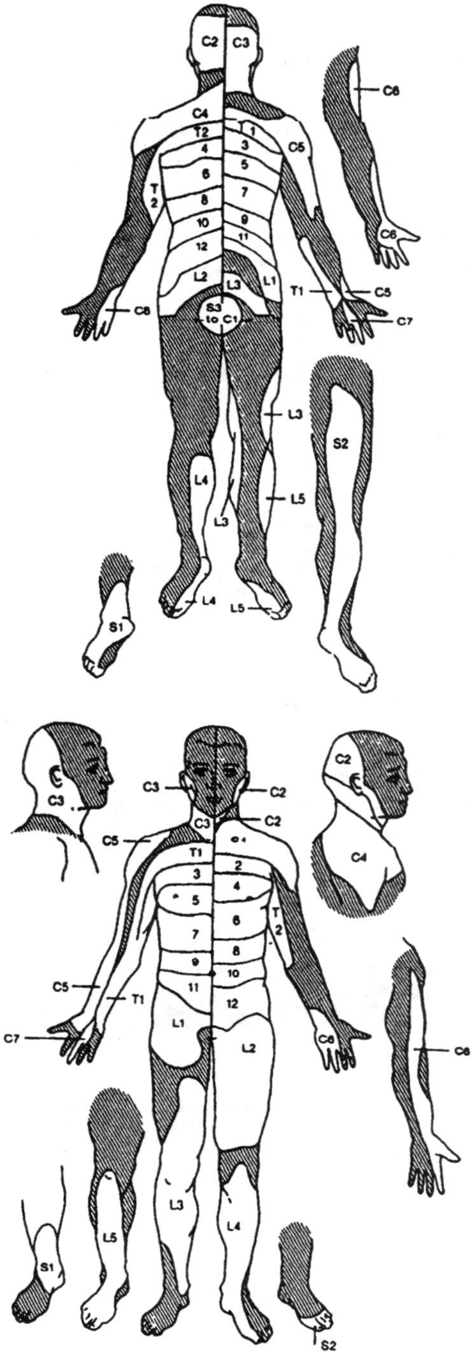

Table 8.5 Brain Versus Spinal Cord Lesions

Brain Lesion	Spinal Cord Lesion
UMNL	+/− UMNL
Cranial nerve deficit(s)	No cranial nerve deficit(s)
No dermatomal deficit(s)	+/− Dermatomal deficit(s)
Homolateral sensory loss	Dissociated sensory function
Altered consciousness	Normal consciousness
Changes in affect/mentation	No changes in affect/mentation
Aphasia	No aphasia
Posturing	No posturing

Note: "+/−" equals may or may not be present

the patient must have a spinal cord or brainstem lesion. Table 8.6 outlines the more common spinal cord syndromes and the clinical presentations.

Brain Lesions

Most cranial nerves originate in the brainstem because their nucleus resides there. It should be noted that their supranuclear tract descends from the cortex, however. Generally speaking, CN III and IV are located in the midbrain, CN V–VII are in the pons, and CN VIII–XII are in the medulla. If there is cranial nerve deficit, then the lesion must be above the foramen magnum or in one of the peripheral cranial nerves. A lesion in the cerebral cortex will cause a contralateral deficit of a cranial nerve, while an infranuclear lesion will cause an ipsilateral deficit. The lesion must be above the foramen magnum if there is ipsilateral loss of pain and temperature and proprioception along with a hemiplegia.

A word about "posturing" is important. There are two major postures that are important to note in patients with intracranial lesions: decorticate and decerebrate. Decorticate posturing (extension of the lower extremities and flexion of the upper extremities) suggests a supratentorial pathology, whereas decerebrate

Table 8.6 Spinal Cord Syndromes

Syndrome	Signs/Symptoms
Anterior cord syndrome	variable loss of motor/sensory/temperature function preservation of proprioception
Central cord syndrome	weakness more pronounced in upper extremities weakness of distal muscles predominates variable sensory loss more likely to lose pain and temperature sacral sensory sparing
Posterior cord syndrome	ataxia dysmetria loss of proprioception symptoms increase when closing eyes
Brown-Sequard's syndrome	ipsilateral loss of motor function/proprioception contralateral loss of pain and temperature
Conus medullaris syndrome	sudden onset of severe low back pain bilateral buttock and lower extremity pain loss of ankle jerk DTRs preservation of knee jerk DTRs loss of bowel and bladder control (early urinary retention) impotence (males) dissociation of lower extremity sensations
Cauda equina syndrome	loss of bowel/bladder control saddle anesthesia paresis/paralysis of both lower extremities loss of morning erections

posturing (extension and internal rotation of all extremities) indicates an infratentorial pathology. Because the lesion goes deeper in the brainstem, decerebrate posturing has a worse prognosis.

After the lesion is isolated to above the foramen magnum, it must further be located either above or below the tentorium cerebelli. (Table 8.7) Infratentorial lesions involve the cerebellum, pons, or brain stem, and supratentorial lesions involve the cerebral cortex and subcortical regions.

Table 8.7 **Supratentorial versus Infratentorial Lesions**

Cerebral Cortex Lesions (Supratentorial)
- contralateral loss of light touch, graphesthesia, two-point discrimination, and stereognosis (parietal lobe (post-central gyrus) involvement))
- contralateral loss of motor function (arm>leg=MCA territory, leg>arm=ACA territory)
- altered mentation
- aphasia (frontal lobe (expressive) and/or temporal lobe (receptive))
- personality changes (frontal lobes)
- ipsilateral facial and extremity involvement suggests a lesion above the brainstem
- conjungate gaze palsy (frontal lobes lesion) (eyes deviate toward lesion side)
- presence of seizures

Subcortical Lesions (Supratentorial)
- visual field defects (e.g., homonymous hemianopsia)
- dystonic postures (chorea, athetosis, hemiballismus) (basal ganglia lesion)
- equal facial, arm, and leg involvement (internal capsule lesion)
- loss of facial and extremity pain and sensory loss (thalamus lesion)

Infratentorial Lesions
- crossed hemiplegia (ipsilateral face, contralateral extremities) (brainstem lesion)
- lower cranial nerve findings (hearing loss, vertigo, dysarthria, dysphagia, tongue deviation) (brainstem lesion)
- nystagmus (medial longitudinal fasciculus) (brainstem)
- cerebellar findings (ipsilateral ataxia, dysmetria)

[ACA-anterior cerebral artery, MCA-middle cerebral artery]

If a cranial nerve deficit is contralateral to the side of hemiparesis or hemiplegia, then the brain stem must be involved. Lesions of the cerebral cortex will cause both of these deficits on the same side of the body and in many cases will not cause cranial nerve palsies because of crossover of their nerve fibers.

Cortical lesions are also hallmarked by altered mental status, such as loss of recent memory, personality changes, aphasia, inability to speak, and complete inability to perform normal motor tasks.

Extrapyramidal system lesions (e.g., parkinsonism) will produce bradykinesia with slowness of movement, tremor, shuffling walking with small steps, slow movements, resting tremor, and slowing of mentation as well as initiating movements.

Cerebellar lesions produce decomposition of movement, inability to perform movements smoothly (dysdiadochokinesia), hypertonia, rebound phenomenon, and intention tremor.

Radiculopathy

Compression of a nerve root, typically in the neural foramen, produces a dermatomal pattern of pain and paresthesias, hypoactive DTRs associated with the level of the lesion, weakness, hypotonia and atrophy of muscles associated with the spinal nerve root involved, and muscle fibrillations.

Peripheral Neuropathy

Fibrillations, weakness, typically normal DTRs, nondermatomal pain and paresthesias in the distribution of the peripheral nerve affected, and hypotonia and atrophy of involved muscles are suggestive of a peripheral nerve lesion.

Etiology of the Lesion

Now that the lesion has been located, the cause of the problem needs to be isolated. The list of etiologies responsible for neurologic disease is far too extensive to be covered in this text. Instead, this section will cover the causes of neurologic lesions most commonly seen in chiropractic general practice.

Peripheral Lesions

The most common peripheral nerve lesions are listed in Table 8.8. Diabetes mellitus often can cause peripheral polyneuropathy, especially affecting the hands and feet, the so-called "glove and stocking" paresthesias. Historical confirmation is made by affirming the presence of excessive thirst, hunger, and urination. Sustained serum hyperglycemia is the premiere indicator of diabetes mellitus. Confirmatory tests for hyperglycemia include glycosylated hemoglobin.

Peripheral nerve compression syndromes are common in clinical practice. Diseases such as carpal tunnel syndrome and thoracic outlet syndrome are diagnosed by orthopedic and neurologic testing

Nerve Root Lesions

Common nerve root lesions are listed in Table 8.9. The most often seen lesion is compression by a herniated disc with signs and symptoms of a radiculopathy. Classic symptoms of radiculopathy are outlined in Table 8.10. Encroachment of

Table 8.8 Common Peripheral Nerve Lesions

Diabetic neuropathy
- "glove-and-stocking" paresthesias
- polyneuropathy
- kidney disease
- cardiovascular disease
- diabetic retinopathy
- poor healing
- polydipsia, polyuria, polyphagia

Thoracic outlet syndrome
- brachial plexus/vascular compression
- nondermatomal upper extremity pain/paresthesias
- reduced upper extremity pulses/Raynaud's phenomenon
- orthopedic testing reproduces patients' complaints

Carpal tunnel syndrome
- median nerve compression
- thenar muscle atrophy
- thenar pain/paresthesias
- history of repetitive microtrauma
- positive Tinel's sign over carpal tunnel

Tarsal tunnel syndrome
- tibial nerve compression
- medial foot pain/paresthesias
- intrinsic foot muscle atrophy
- pain worse with eversion/dorsiflexion
- positive Tinel's sign over tarsal tunnel

an intervertebral foramen by either fibrosis or osteophytes causes a similar picture. Herpes zoster (shingles) and tabes dorsalis (neurosyphilis) can also result in nerve root involvement. Each nerve root lesion has typical signs and symptoms associated with it. These classic syndromes are outlined in Table 8.11.

Spinal Cord Lesions

There are a number of lesions that affect the spinal cord (Table 8.12) that can present with the signs and symptoms noted above. These include the Brown-Séquard's syndrome (hemisection of the cord); central disc herniations and

Table 8.9 Common Nerve Root Lesions

Herniated nucleus pulposus
Disc bulge
Dural sleeve adhesions
Dural root sleeve cyst
Conjoined nerve roots
Osseous foraminal encroachment
Lateral recess stenosis

Table 8.10 Signs and Symptoms of Radiculopathy

Dermatomal pain/paresthesia (past elbow/knee)
Muscle atrophy
Hypotonia/paresis/paralysis of muscles supplied by affected nerve root
Decreased DTRs
Fasciculations/fibrillations

Table 8.11 Common Nerve Root Syndromes

Spinal Level	Muscles	DTR	Sensation
C5	Deltoid, biceps	Biceps	C5 dermatome
C6	Biceps, brachioradialis	Brachioradialis	C6 dermatome
C7	Triceps	Triceps	C7 dermatome
C8	Finger flexors	None	C8 dermatome
L4	Quadriceps	Knee jerk	L4 dermatome
L5	Foot extensors (foot drop)	Hamstring	L5 dermatome
S1	Triceps surae	Achilles	S1 dermatome

Table 8.12 Common Lesions Affecting the Spinal Cord

Central HNP
Metastasis
Syringomyelia
Brown-Séquard's Syndrome
Spinal Canal Stenosis
Hematoma
Arteriovenous malformation
Ependymoma

tumors, which can result in the cauda equina syndrome; transection of the cord; and diseases intrinsic to the spinal cord, such as metastasis and syringomyelia.

Brain Stem Lesions

Lesions of the brain stem (medulla, pons, and mid-brain) are usually from either vascular disease or tumor. Common tumors of the brain stem include gliomas, acoustic neuromas, and meningiomas (Table 8.13)

Table 8.13 Common Brain Stem Lesions

Vascular
- Cerebrovacular ischemia/accident
- Arteriovenous malformation
- Vertebrobasilar system aneurysm

Neoplasm
- Gliomas
- Acoustic neuroma
- Meningioma

Osseous
- Basilar invagination (e.g., rheumatoid arthritis)
- Platybasia

Table 8.14 Common Cerebral Lesions

Vascular/Hemorrhagic
- Arteriovenous malformation
- Cerebrovascular ischemia/accident
- Subarachnoid hemorrhage
- Cerebral aneurysm
- Hematomas (epidural/subdural)

Neoplasm
- Glioma
- Astrocytoma
- Glioblastoma multiform

Infection
- Meningitis
- Cerebral abscess

Cerebral Lesions

Vascular diseases (such as ischemia, hemorrhage, and aneurysms) along with tumors (especially gliomas) are the most common cerebral lesions. (Table 8.14)

Treatment of the Lesion and Contraindications to Treatment

Most often, the treatment of a true neurologic lesion with acute paralysis, atrophy, and other ominous signs will be undertaken by a neurologist or neurosurgeon.

One of the main thrusts of diagnosis by the chiropractic clinician is to rule out the possibility of CNS lesions, surgical cases, and contraindications to manipulation. For example, the chiropractic physician will most often treat patients' nonsurgical neurologic lesions, such as disc herniations. (2,3,4) However, if a herniation causes a cauda equina syndrome or the patient has fasciculations or paralysis, the patient should be referred for neurosurgical consultation.

Challenges to the carotid and vertebrobasilar artery systems for patency have been performed on patients undergoing cervical spine manipulation with a great deal of regularity in past years. When those systems are compromised, aggressive dynamic manipulation of the patient's neck is contraindicated, and referral to a vascular or neurologic surgeon for more extensive investigation is required. Recent evidence suggests that the diagnostic yield of these tests is low with large numbers of false-positive and false-negative results. (5) In light of this new evidence, it is suggested that these tests not be used as a part of the standard diagnostic work-up of patients with neck pain and/or headache. Further information regarding this topic is included in the chapter on spinal manipulation.

There are many neuromusculoskeletal diseases and conditions with neuromusculoskeletal side effects that chiropractors treat frequently and with much success. The reader is referred to other chapters in this book and other texts for the investigation and treatment of these conditions.

The Neurologic Examination

- *Visual Inspection*
  - Abnormal movements (tremors, chorea, tics, athetosis, ballismus)
  - Personal hygiene (clothing appropriate for season)
  - Body habitus (cachexia, atrophy, plegia)
  - Speech pattern (dysarthria, receptive aphasia, expressive aphasia)
- *Mental Status Examination*
  - Serial reverse sevens–counting backwards from 100 by sevens (dyscalculia)
  - Orientation/level of consciousness–person, place, time, and situation
  - Object recall at five minutes
- *Cranial Nerve Examination*
  - I–Smell
  - II–Near/far visual acuity, visual fields
  - III, IV, VI–Cardinal ranges of motion of the eyes, pupillary response
  - V–Light touch on the face, corneal reflex
  - VII–Smile/frown
  - VIII–Finger rubbing, Weber/Rinne tests
  - IX, X–Gag reflex
  - XI–Shoulder elevation
  - XII–Protrude the tongue

- *Reflexes*
  - Deep tendon reflexes (DTRs)
    - Biceps (C5–6)
    - Brachioradialis (C6)
    - Triceps (C7)
    - Quadriceps (L4)
    - Hamstrings (L5)
    - Achilles (S1)
  - Pathologic reflexes (UMNL)
    - Babinski
    - Hoffman
    - Clonus
- *Sensory Examination*
  - Pain pinprick (lateral spinothalamic, thalamus)
  - Temperature (lateral spinothalamic, thalamus)
  - Vibration sense (posterior columns, thalamus)
  - Light touch (posterior columns, thalamus)
  - Kinesthesia (position sense) (posterior columns, somatosensory cortex)
  - Stereognosis (size and shape of objects) (posterior columns, somatosensory cortex)

Table 8.15 Muscle Strength Grading System

Grade	Explanation
0	No muscle contraction
+1	Visible muscle twitching/fasciculations
+2	Slight muscle contraction
+3	Movement with no gravity
+4	Movement against slight resistance
+5	Movement against full resistance

- graphesthesia (tactile sensation of written patterns on the skin (posterior columns, somatosensory cortex)
- *Motor Examination*
  - Muscle strength is graded in the affected region(s) (Table 8.15).
  - Pronator drift (UMNL)
- *Cerebellum*
  - Romberg test
  - Finger to nose
  - Finger to physician's moving finger

Peripheral Neuropathy

Lesions involving the peripheral nerves are relatively common, with diabetic neuropathy likely being the most common cause. There are myriad causes of peripheral neuropathy, and the more common ones are outlined in Table 8.16.

Signs and symptoms of peripheral neuropathy are those of an LMNL without any dermatomal deficits and instead, the sensory deficits are in the distribution of the peripheral nerve that is involved (e.g., peroneal nerve). These findings include decreased DTRs (where applicable), paresthesias, muscular hypotonia, decreased sensation, fasciculations, and fibrillations. Table 8.8 outlines the clinical findings of the more common peripheral nerve lesions.

Abnormal Gait

Ataxia–the patient spreads the legs apart to provide a wider base of support to compensate for an imbalance while standing or walking. In more severe cases, patients stagger as they walk.

Festinating gait–in some patients, the steps and pace may vary with a tendency for the patient to accelerate as he or she walks. Associated with extrapyramidal lesions such as Parkinson's disease.

Hemiparesis–the shoulder is adducted, the elbow is flexed, the forearm is pronated, and the wrist and fingers are flexed. In severe cases, the hand may be clenched; the knee is held in extension and the ankle is plantar flexed, making the paralyzed leg functionally longer than the other. The patient therefore has to circumduct the affected leg to ambulate. Associated with UMNLs, typically contralateral to the side of hemiparesis.

Table 8.16 Common Causes of Peripheral Neuropathies

Hereditary disorders
Charcot-Marie-Tooth disease
Friedreich's ataxia
Systemic or metabolic disorders
diabetes mellitus
vitamin B12 deficiency
alcoholic neuropathy
uremia
malignancy
Infectious or inflammatory conditions
AIDS
hepatitis
botulism
Colorado tick fever
diphtheria
Guillain-Barré syndrome
HIV infection without development of AIDS
Lyme disease
polyarteritis nodosa
rheumatoid arthritis
sarcoidosis
syphilis
systemic lupus erythematosus
amyloid
Toxic exposure
sniffing glue or other toxic compounds
nitrous oxide
industrial agents—especially solvents
heavy metals (lead, arsenic, mercury, etc.)
neuropathy secondary to drugs
Miscellaneous causes
ischemia
hypothermia/frostbite

Scissor (Spastic) gait–the legs are held in adduction at the hip and the thighs rub against each other as the patient walks; spasm of the inner thigh muscles also occurs. If the spasm is severe, with each advancing step the knees tend to slide over each other like the blades of a pair of scissors.

Shuffling gait–the individual takes very short steps almost to the point of not moving forward. In other words, the patient appears to shuffle his legs rather than put them forward. Associated with extrapyramidal lesions such as Parkinson's disease.

Steppage gait–the individual takes high steps as if climbing a flight of stairs while walking on a level surface. As the patient puts the feet down one by one, they slap the ground; hence the description of a foot-slapping gait. Associated with peripheral neuropathies or L5 radiculopathy.

Abnormal Involuntary Movements

Asterixis–this movement is elicited by having the patient extend both arms with the palms facing forward and the wrists dorsiflexed with the eyes closed. Transient jerky downward movements of the wrist are considered a positive sign.

Athetosis–slow writhing limb movements that occur along the long axis of the limb(s) or the body itself. These patients often assume different and often peculiar postures.

Chorea–quasi-purposeful movements that affect multiple joints with a distal preponderance. Associated with Huntington's chorea and other similar conditions.

Dystonias–muscle contractions that are more prolonged than myoclonus and result in spasms. Examples include blepharospasm, spasmodic torticollis, and writer's cramp.

Fasciculations–seen under the skin as quivering of the muscle. Fasciculations are typically benign, particularly when they occur in the calf muscles. They may also be seen with LMNLs and, when widespread, they can be associated with neuromuscular diseases such as amyotrophic lateral sclerosis (ALS).

Hemiballismus–violent flinging movement of one-half of the body. It is associated with lesions of the subthalamic nucleus.

Myoclonus–a brief (< one fourth second), generalized body-jerk, which at times is asymmetric.

Seizures–orofacial or appendicular automatisms, repeated eye blinks, or tonic or clonic motor activity are the most typical type seizures.

Tics–involuntary contractions of single muscles or groups of muscles that result in stereotyped movements. They can be familial or even associated with diseases such as Tourette's syndrome where patients have multiple tics and elaborate, complex movements and vocalizations (swearing, braking, nonsensical noises).

Differential Diagnosis of Common Signs and Symptoms

Anisocoria

Anisocoria is defined as pupillary inequality. Normal variant, Horner's syndrome, cranial nerve III palsy, iris damage, drug ingestion, brain tumor, and cerebral ischemia are just a few of the common causes. Cerebral magnetic resonance imaging (MRI) and computed tomography (CT) with contrast, along with laboratory investigation for ingested drugs and a chest film to rule out a Pancoast's tumor in the lung apex, are some of the common diagnostic modalities.

Bitemporal Hemianopsia

Pituitary tumors, optic chiasm tumors (such as meningiomas), hypothalamic masses, and a chordoma of the clivus are some of the more common causes for this finding.

Advanced imaging with CT if a bone lesion is suspected or MRI if a soft tissue lesion is suspected are helpful modalities.

Dementia

Alzheimer's disease (presenile dementia, Alzheimer's type), other forms of senility, brain tumors, hepatic disease, and vitamin deficiency are familiar etiologies.

Investigation is typically done by MRI although specialized forms of CT are also available.

Diplopia

Cranial nerve III, IV, VI palsies, meningitis, tumors, multiple sclerosis (MS), myasthenia gravis.

Evaluation of diplopia is typically performed with brain MRI with contrast.

Dizziness

Dizziness is a very nonspecific finding indicative of a list of diseases too detailed for this manuscript. Suffice it to say that orthostatic hypotension, cardiac arrhythmias, anemia, cerebellar disease, drug ingestion, endocrine diseases (such as Addison's disease), carotid sinus hypersensitivity, and inner ear disease are a few of the more traditional causes.

Evaluation of dizziness is directed at the more specific cause gleaned from the history and physical examination.

Headache

Muscle tension is by far the most common cause of headaches. Increased intracranial pressure, vascular spasm and dilatation (migraine), cluster headaches, ocular disease, dental disease, trauma, ischemic vascular disease, hemorrhage, and tumors have also been implicated.

Study of the cause for a patient's headache is again directed at evaluating possible causes elicited from the history and physical examination. Magnetic resonance imaging of the brain, CT of the brain, and other neurodiagnostic studies are helpful in this investigation. Table 8.17 outlines the diagnostic evaluation of headache.

Table 8.17 Evaluation of Headache

Cause	Diagnostic Procedure
Muscle tension	Orthopedic testing, history
Increased intracranial pressure	Magnetic resonance imaging Fundoscopic examination
Ocular disease	Eye examination Magnetic resonance imaging
Migraine	History
Cerebral ischemia	Magnetic resonance imaging Angiography
Cerebral hemorrhage	Computerized tomography Magnetic resonance imaging

Hyperreflexia

Brain and spinal cord tumors, trauma with hemorrhage, and demyelinating diseases (such as MS and cerebral ischemia) are the most common causes of increased DTRs.

Evaluation of hyperreflexia is most often undertaken with MRI although CT will be helpful in cases of suspected bone disease.

Hyporeflexia

Neuropathies, whether diabetic or otherwise, radiculopathy from foraminal encroachment by osteophytes, trauma with or without syringomyelia, spinal cord tumors, and tabes dorsalis can all result in diminished DTRs.

If an osseous cause is suspected, CT is helpful; soft tissue lesions are best investigated with MRI.

Ophthalmoplegia

Loss of the cardinal ranges of motion of the eye can result from a myriad of causes. Cranial nerve palsies, orbital diseases (such as infection and masses), myasthenia gravis, MS, brain tumors, and cerebral ischemia are a few of the more common causes.

Cranial and orbital imaging with CT and/or MRI are beneficial in the investigation of this disorder.

Polyneuropathy

Diabetes mellitus is probably the most common cause of peripheral polyneuropathy. Other causes include MS, hepatic cirrhosis, Charcot-Marie-Tooth disease, infectious mononucleosis, ingestion of toxins (such as lead, arsenic, and drugs), and the Guillain-Barré syndrome.

Evaluation of a polyneuropathy is best achieved with neurodiagnostic evaluation, including electromyography, somatosensory evoked potentials, nerve conduction velocities, and advanced imaging studies such as CT and MRI.

Syncope

Orthostatic hypotension, a vasovagal response of the physiologic type; autonomic neuropathies (such as diabetes mellitus); and cardiac diseases (such as arrhythmias, ischemic vascular disease, hyperventilation, and hypoglycemia) are

Table 8.18 Evaluation of Syncope

Suspected Cause	Diagnostic Procedure
Orthostatic hypotension	Blood pressures, standing and supine History
Diabetes/hypoglycemia	Serum glucose
Cardiac arrhythmias	Electrocardiogram
Cerebral ischemia	Magnetic resonance imaging Angiography

just a few of the more common etiologies for fainting. Table 8.18 outlines the diagnostic work-up for patients with syncope.

Tremors

The two most common causes for tremors are inherited physiologic tremors and Parkinsonism.

These lesions are best investigated with neurodiagnostic modalities (as outlined above) and cerebral MRI.

Vertigo

Vestibulopathy (inner ear disease), alcohol and drug intoxication, Meniere's disease, and benign paroxysmal positional vertigo should be the primary choices when investigating this complaint.

The caloric test, laboratory investigation for intoxication, and cerebral advanced imaging are the most helpful modalities when evaluating this complaint.

Weakness (Muscular)

The complaint of muscular weakness can be relatively nonspecific. Conditions that present with this disorder include myasthenia gravis, MS, drug ingestion, dystonias, brain tumors, spinal cord lesions, and peripheral nerve lesions.

Laboratory investigation for drug ingestion, MRI, and neurodiagnostic evaluation are traditionally used for evaluation of weakness.

Specialized Neurologic Testing

Evoked Responses

Evoked responses measure the electrophysiological responses of the nervous system to a variety of different stimuli. Almost any sensory modality can be tested, but in clinical practice only a select few are used on a routine basis. The ones most often encountered are the visual evoked potentials (VEP), somatosensory evoked potentials (SSEP), and brainstem auditory evoked responses (BAER).

The clinical use of evoked potentials (EP) has changed over time. Advances in imaging technology, particularly MRI, have limited the frequency of use of EP studies in clinical practice. Magnetic resonance imaging is an anatomical study, while the EP explains the functionality of certain pathways of the nervous system. In other words, the MRI scan gives more accurate information about structural pathology, while the EP provides information about the physiology of a certain anatomical pathway. Under many circumstances they may be complementary, but most clinical queries are answered better by MRI of relevant neurological structures.

Visual evoked potentials measure the function of the visual pathway from the retina to the occipital cortex. They measures the conduction of the visual pathways from the optic nerve, optic chiasm, and optic radiations to the occipital cortex. An important concept to remember is that, although the axons from the medial half of the retina decussate at the optic chiasm, the later axons do not. Lesions posterior to the optic chiasm may not be detected by some VEPs. This study is most useful in testing optic nerve function, whereas MRI is more useful for retrochiasmal lesions. The other important concept to appreciate about VEP is that the etiology of the lesion is not disclosed, and further study is necessary to evaluate the cause of the visual difficulty.

These studies are used in the evaluation of optic neuropathy, suspected toxic amblyopia, glaucoma, retrobulbar neuritis, ischemic optic neuropathy, multiple sclerosis, and tumors compressing the optic nerve, such as optic nerve gliomas, meningiomas, craniopharyngiomas, aneurysms, and pituitary tumors. A normal VEP virtually excludes an optic nerve or anterior chiasmatic lesion.

Cost is less for VEP when compared to MRI, and VEP is a more sensitive test for pre-chiasmatic lesions as well.

Brainstem auditory evoked responses measure the function of the auditory nerve and auditory pathways in the brainstem and are therefore useful in evaluating hearing loss. The test can be performed under sedation or under general anesthesia. These tests are very resistant to alteration by anything other than structural pathology in the brainstem auditory tracts, so medications do not generally affect the responses.

Cerebellopontine angle tumors, dymelinating diseases like MS, brainstem tumors, and brainstem vascular accidents are conditions that are amenable to investigation with BAER. In infants who have suspected hearing loss, BAER can be helpful. It is also helpful in determining brain death after trauma.

Electrical stimulation of predominantly large-diameter group Ia fibers and group II cutaneous afferents are responsible for the waveforms produced in SSEPs. This study evaluates the peripheral nerves, posterior columns, and lemniscal and thalamocortical pathways in the brain.

Any lesion that affects these pathways can be evaluated by SSEP. Multiple sclerosis (sensitivity similar to MRI), disc herniations, spondylosis, diabetic polyneuropathy, vitamin B-12 deficiency, intracranial tumors, and syringomyelia are classic examples. Intraoperative SSEPs are used to evaluate the success of decompressive procedures and to prevent neurosurgical complications. In addition, SSEP has a relatively high sensitivity in differentiating a brachial plexus lesion from cervical radiculopathy.

Motor Evoked Potentials (MEP)

With the advent of transcranial magnetic stimulation, the use of MEP has been making a comeback. This study is useful in the evaluation of MS, not only for diagnosis but as a tool for documentation of corticospinal tract dysfunction. Cervical myelopathy also appears to be a condition that is well-evaluated with MEP, as are spinal cord injuries, motor neuron diseases (ALS), and for prognosis for recovery from a cardiovascular accident.

This study is not without contraindications. The presence of epilepsy is a relative contraindication. Implanted stimulators (pacemaker, nerve stimulator), metallic foreign bodies, or a history of craniotomy are also contraindications.

Electromyography (EMG)

Electromyography is the recording of motor unit potentials. A needle electrode is inserted through the skin into the muscle. The electrical activity detected by this electrode is displayed on an oscilloscope and may be heard through a speaker as well.

A single needle electrode is inserted into several areas of a skeletal muscle's motor point region. The electromyographer then assigns an average of the muscle motor unit sample. This average varies according to the examiner's skill and clinical judgment.

After placement of the electrode(s), the patient may be asked to contract the muscle. The presence, size, and shape of the waveform produced on the oscilloscope provide information about the ability of the muscle to respond when the nerves are stimulated. Each motor unit (collection of muscle fibers associated with one nerve fiber and its collateral sprouts to individual muscle fibers) produces a multiphasic motor unit potential. The size of the muscle fiber affects the frequency and amplitude of the action potentials.

Normal muscles are electrically quiet at rest. Once the muscle activity caused by the needle insertion disappears, there should be no potentials on the oscilloscope. When the muscle is voluntarily contracted, motor unit potentials begin to appear. As contraction is increased, more and more muscle fibers produce motor unit potentials until a group of motor unit potentials of varying rates and amplitudes appears with full contraction.

The most common use of EMG is in the evaluation of weakness, most often associated with compressive neuropathy. Muscle fibrillations (electrical activity as rest), suggestive of a LMNL, are particularly well-evaluated with EMG. It is also helpful in distinguishing primary muscle disease from weakness associated with neurologic disorders.

Nerve compression syndromes such as radiculopathy and peripheral nerve entrapment (e.g., carpal tunnel syndrome), myasthenia gravis, inflammatory polyneuropathies (e.g., Guillain-Barré syndrome), and ALS are conditions commonly evaluated by EMG.

Special precautions may need to be taken in patients with coagulopathies and those on anti-coagulation therapy as well as those patients with HIV and hepatitis.

Nerve Conduction Velocity (NCV)

Often performed along with an EMG, an NCV study measures the speed of conduction of nerve impulses. It is a noninvasive procedure where surface electrodes are placed on a muscle belly in motor nerve conduction studies and over a sensory nerve in sensory nerve conduction studies. A stimulating electrode applies an external current at various sites along the peripheral nerve. The current is directed to the distal surface recording electrodes to determine segmental motor and sensory NCVs along a peripheral nerve. The distance between the stimulation sites and the time it takes to reach them are used to calculate the velocity of nerve conduction.

The amount of myelination of a nerve and the diameter of the nerve are both factors that affect conduction velocity. For example, in infants whose nervous systems are not completely myelinated, conduction velocities are much slower than adults.

Demyelinating diseases, neuropathy, and conditions that cause a conduction block will all demonstrate abnormal NCV values. Conditions commonly evaluated include diabetic neuropathy, disc herniations with probable radiculopathy, Guillan-Barré Syndrome, peripheral neuropathies (e.g., thoracic outlet syndrome), myasthenia gravis, and alcoholic neuropathy.

An example of the use of NCV is a combined evaluation with MRI to determine which disc protrusion/extrusion is causing the patient's signs and symptoms when multilevel herniations are present. Distal and proximal lesions, creating the "Double-Crush Syndrome," are best evaluated with this type of modality.

Electroencephalogram (EEG)

The electroencephalogram is a noninvasive procedure that provides information about the electrical activity of the brain. Recent advances in technology have made the use of ambulatory EEG available and clinically useful. With the ambulatory study, the patient is monitored for up to 72 hours while at home. This type of EEG is particularly helpful for finding small electrical discharges in the brain from small clinically undetectable epileptiform activity.

Electrodes are applied to key locations on the patient's head. The EEG instrument then picks up electrical impulses from the brain and records them. During the test, various procedures may be used to activate certain brain waves and make wave patterns clearer. For example, hyperventilation is often used, as is photic stimulation, where bright lights flash over the patient's closed eyes. Care should be taken in cases of suspected or known seizures as this photic stimulation can induce seizure activity. An electrocardiogram is recorded throughout the study to monitor cardiac function.

The EEG can help diagnose various conditions such as seizure disorders, cerebrovascular accidents, brain tumors, and CNS infections. It also can help the physician find the cause of other complaints such as headaches, syncope, and dizziness.

Lumbar Puncture (LP)

Lumbar puncture, also known as a spinal tap, involves collection of cerebrospinal fluid (CSF) from the subarachnoid space with analysis of the fluid contents.

Normal CSF is clear and colorless. Measurement of the levels of glucose, protein, including gamma globulin, white blood cells, and chloride are made. There should be no red blood cells in CSF. The opening pressure is also measured as the needle is inserted.

Conditions that are commonly evaluated with an LP include MS, encephalitis, meningitis, subarachnoid hemorrhage, Guillan-Barré Syndrome, and spinal tumors.

Suspicion of increased intracranial pressure is a contraindication for LP, as herniation of the brain may occur from pressure changes during the procedure.

Glossary of Neurologic Signs, Symptoms, and Diseases

abulia – Loss of will power or ability to make decisions.

acataphasia – Inability to formulate a statement or expression in an organized manner.

acoria (akoria) – Inability to feel satiated, regardless of how much is eaten.

Adie's tonic pupil – Dilated pupil that reacts poorly to light but better to accommodation. Indicates ciliary ganglion involvement.

ageusia – Absence of taste sensation. Suggests tongue lesions or cranial nerve VII and/or IX lesion.

agnosia – A general term for a loss of ability to recognize objects, people, sounds, shapes, or smells. This term is usually used when the primary sense organ itself is not impaired.

agraphesthesia – Inability to identify a letter or number being written on some part of the body.

agraphia (dysgraphia) – Inability to express thought in written language not due to mechanical dysfunction (aka dysgraphia).

akathisia – Motor restlessness, or the inability to sit still. Most often caused by defects in the extrapyramidal system.

akinesia (dyskinesia) – Unresponsiveness, with extreme reluctance to perform elementary motor activities. It is a form of apraxia.

alalia – Loss of the ability to speak.

alexia – Loss of the ability to understand written language. It is a subcategory of dyslexia.

allesthesia – Perception of a stimulus in the limb opposite to the one that was stimulated.

amblyopia – A unilateral or bilateral decrease in vision for which no cause can be found on physical examination. Usually requires a two-line difference in acuity from one eye to the other.

amelodia (aprosodia) – Absence of normal variations of pitch, rhythm, and stress in speech. Monotonous speech.

amentia – Extreme mental retardation.

amnesia (dysmnesia) – Total or partial loss of memory.

amusia – Inability to produce and/or appreciate musical sounds.

anacusia – Deafness.

analgesia – Absence of a normal sense of pain.

anhedonia – Inability to experience pleasure.

anisocoria – Pupillary inequality.

anomia (dysnomia) – General term for the inability to name objects.

anopsia – Blindness (e.g., hemianopsia).

anorexia – Loss of appetite or a clinical syndrome where there is a pathological fear of eating, in order to avoid weight gain.

anosmia – Loss of the sense of smell.

anosognosia – Unawareness of, denial of, or failure to recognize one's own neurological deficit. For example, someone paralyzed on his left side may claim he can move his left arm normally.

apastia – Refusal to eat.

aphasia (dysphasia) – Any impairment of the ability to use and/or understand words. Subcategories include: **Broca's (expressive) aphasia,** in which one can comprehend speech, but not produce it; and, **Wernicke's (receptive) aphasia,** in which one can produce speech but not comprehend speech.

aphemia – Inability to speak words, but able to make other sounds.

aphonia (dysphonia) – Loss of ability to speak; inability to produce speech sounds.

apraxia (dyspraxia) – Difficulty in performing a learned movement or coordinated motor task even though understanding, motor function, coordination, and sensation are intact.

aprosodia (amelodia) – Absence of normal variations of pitch, rhythm, and stress in speech.

Argyll Robertson pupil – Small, irregular pupil that does not react to light but does react to accommodation. Suggests neurosyphilis of the midbrain.

Arnold-Chiari malformation – Herniation of a portion of the contents of the posterior cerebral fossa through the foramen magnum. Three grades are recognized varying from simple partial herniation of the cerebellar tonsils with or without symptoms (Type I), herniation of the cerebellar vermis and hemispheres with kinking of the medulla and dysgenesis of the corpus callosum, most often associated with a meningiomyelocele (Type II) and herniation of the entire cerebellum, which is essentially incompatible with life.

asemia – Loss or inability to express or understand symbols or signs of thought.

asitia – Loathing of food.

astasia – Inability to stand due to lack of motor coordination in the presence of normal strength.

astereognosis – Inability to identify palpated objects.

asterixis – A clinical sign indicating a lapse of posture. It is usually manifest by a bilateral flapping tremor at the wrist, metacarpophalangeal, and hip joints.

asthenia – General weakness or debilitation.

asynergia – Loss of coordination of motor movement.

ataxia – Poor coordination and unsteadiness due to failure to regulate the body's posture, and strength and direction of limb movements. Typically cerebellar in etiology.

atonia – Lack of muscle tension or tone.

bulbar palsy – Results from bilateral impairment of function of CN IX, X, and XII motor nuclei. Results in dysarthria, dysphagia, dysphonia, and poor cough. It is distinguished from pseudobulbar palsy by the presence of lower motor neuron signs. Seen with MS, ALS, and stroke.

cauda equina syndrome – Compression of the cauda equina with a typical set of signs and symptoms including low back pain, saddle (bilateral buttock) paresthesias and/or anesthesia (may be gradual and unilateral in some cases), loss of bowel/bladder control, including urinary retention, hyporeflexia/areflexia of both L4 and S1 DTRs, loss of morning erections in males, clitoral/vulvar paresthesias in females. Paraplegia may also be seen. Requires emergent surgical decompression.

circumlocution – Evasive speech or use of unusual definitional terms.

confabulation – Answering of questions by an inappropriate, made-up attempt to explain.

conus medullaris syndrome – Compression of the conus medullaris with sudden onset of severe low back pain, bilateral buttock and lower extremity pain and paresthesias, loss of ankle DTRs with preservation of knee jerk DTRs, dissociation of senses in the lower extremities, loss of bowel and bladder control, including early urinary retention, impotence in males, and perianal paresthesias in both males and females.

dementia – General term for loss of intellectual or cognitive abilities.

diastematomyelia – Fibrous or osseous vertical bar projecting from the posterior aspect of the vertebral body and splitting the spinal cord into two sections.

The cord becomes tethered, and often nondescript neurologic symptoms begin in early adulthood. MRI is confirmatory. Treatment is surgical excision of the bar.

diplopia – Double vision.

dysacusis – Distortion of sound frequency or intensity, often painful.

dysantigraphia – Inability to copy writing or printed letters.

dysarthria – Imperfect articulation of speech due to disturbances of muscular control. This should be distinguished from *aphonia.*

dysbasia (abasia) – Difficulty walking, usually taking steps that are too big or too small.

dyscalculia (anarithmetria) – Inability to use mathematics.

dyschiria – Inability to tell which side of the body has been touched.

dyschronation – Lack of a sense of relativity in the conscious perception of time.

dysdiadochokinesia – Inability to perform rapidly alternating movements.

dysesthesia – Abnormal sensations of the skin.

dyslexia – A condition in which an individual with normal vision is unable to properly interpret or produce written language. Patients can see and recognize letters but have difficulty spelling and writing words.

dyslogia – Difficulty in expressing ideas.

dysmetria – Uncoordinated movement that misses its target.

dysmimia – Inability to express oneself by gestures or signs or the inability to physically imitate the actions of the clinician.

dysmorphophobia – Obsession that a normal body part is malformed or defective in appearance.

dysphagia – Difficulty in swallowing.

dysreflexia – Abnormal reflex in response to a stimulus.

dyssynergia – Disorganized muscle movement.

dystonia – Abnormal maintenance of a persistant posture or position.

echolalia – Imitation of sounds without comprehension of their meaning. This is a normal developmental stage in children, but an abnormality in adults.

hemiplegia – Weakness on one side of the body.

hyperpathia – Increased reaction to a stimulus, especially a repetitive stimulus, as well as an increased threshold. This sensation is inappropriately painful to the patient.

hypoacusis – Difficulty hearing.

internuclear ophthalmoplegia – Loss of adduction by the medial rectus muscle with conjugate eye movement, but with sparing during convergence. Associated with a lesion affecting the medial longitudinal fasciculus (ipsilateral to the affected eye) that connects the cranial nerve VI nuclei to the contralateral CN III nucleus. Often seen with MS and stroke.

lateral recess stenosis – Narrowing of the lateral recess of the spinal canal with attendant radiculopathy signs and symptoms.

myelopathy – Compression of the spinal cord with attendant upper motor neuron signs and symptoms.

paragraphia – Miswriting when responding to a spoken word or number.

paraphasia – Misreading of a written word or number.

paraplegia – Weakness/paralysis of the lower extremities.

parapnasia – Use of incorrect words or word combinations.

paresis – Partial or incomplete paralysis.

phantom limb – Sensation of a missing limb still being present.

piriformis syndrome – Compression of a portion of the sciatic nerve by the piriformis muscle. Typically caused by a portion of the sciatic nerve piercing the piriformis muscle. Results in peripheral neuropathy signs and symptoms in a nondermatomal pattern.

prosopagnosia – Inability to recognize faces, including one's own.

pseudobulbar palsy – Results from degeneration of the corticobulbar pathways to V, VII, X, XI, and XII cranial nerve nuclei. Cranial nerve III, IV, and VI nuclei are spared. Symptoms include weakness of the muscles of mastication, weakness of the muscles of facial expression, dysphagia, poor coughing, immobile atrophied tongue, exaggerated gag reflex, dysarthria, emotional liability, and absence of lower motor neuron signs involving these nerves. Most common in stroke patients, ALS, and MS.

quadriplegia – Weakness/paralysis in all four extremities.

radiculopathy – Compression of a nerve root with attendant signs and symptoms including decreased DTR, muscle weakness, and dermatomal sensory loss attributable to the level of the affected nerve root. Fasciculations and fibrillation potentials are also possible.

spinal canal stenosis – Narrowing of the spinal canal, oftentimes causing myelopathy or compression of the cauda equina or nerve roots. It may present with UMNL signs, LMNL signs, or a combination of both.

spondylotic myelopathy – Cervical spinal canal stenosis caused by degenerative joint disease.

supranuclear ophthalmoplegia – Condition most commonly seen with progressive supranuclear palsy, where control (above the nuclei) of eye movement results in vertical gaze impairment; downward gaze is affected before upward gaze.

synesthesia – An inappropriate sensory perception, such as perceiving a color in response to a particular odor.

syringomyelia – Dilatation of the central canal of the spinal cord secondary to trauma or congenital in etiology, with signs and symptoms including paresthesias/loss of pain and temperature sensation over the shoulders and upper arms, motor weakness, and atrophic neuropathic arthropathy, typically of the shoulder joints. Symptoms may also be seen in the lower extremities.

tinnitus – Ringing in the ears.

topagnosis – Inability to localize the site of tactile stimulation.

verbal dysdecorum – Inability to self-monitor the appropriateness of speech in social settings.

References

1. Haldeman, S., Kohlbeck, F.J., & McGregor, M. Stroke, cerebral artery dissection, and cervical spine manipulation therapy. *J Neurol.* 2002 Aug;249(8):1098–1104.
2. BenEliyahu, D.J. Magnetic resonance imaging and clinical follow-up: study of 27 patients receiving chiropractic care for cervical and lumbar disc herniations. *J Manipulative Physiol Ther.* 1996 Nov–Dec;19(9):597–606.
3. Floman, Y., Liram, N., & Gilai, A.N. Spinal manipulation results in immediate H-reflex changes in patients with unilateral disc herniation. *Eur Spine J.* 1997;6(6):398–401.
4. Quon, J.A., Cassidy, J.D., O'Connor, S.M., & Kirkaldy-Willis, W.H. Lumbar intervertebral disc herniation: treatment by rotational manipulation. *J Manipulative Physiol Ther.* 1989 Jun;12(3):220–227.
5. Licht, P.B., Christensen, H.W., & Hoilund-Carlsen, P.F. Carotid artery blood flow during premanipulative testing. *J Manipulative Physiol Ther.* 2002 Nov–Dec;25(9):568–572.

Chapter 9

Clinical Laboratory Diagnosis

Lawrence H. Wyatt, DC, DACBR, FICC

Introduction

Laboratory diagnosis is essential in evaluating patient complaints. Clinical laboratory tests can be vital tools for arriving at a final diagnosis, excluding pathology, and performing screening tests.

This chapter outlines clinical laboratory diagnosis by defining tests that are useful in chiropractic practice. If a decreased or increased value is not clinically useful (i.e., it has a low sensitivity and specificity), it has been excluded from this text.

Many facilities offer a panel of tests (e.g., SMA 12, CHEM 23) that are performed on a single sample. Physicians should investigate their facilities to learn the standard protocols.

The values listed in this chapter are for general use. Specific ranges are usually included on the reports from each institution. Unless otherwise specified, the listed values are for the adult patient. A list of helpful shorthand figures for laboratory values can be found in Figure 9–1.

Complete Blood Count (CBC)

The complete blood count includes the red blood cell (RBC) count, white blood cell (WBC) count, hemoglobin (Hgb), hematocrit (Hct), mean cellular volume (MCV), mean corpuscular hemoglobin, mean corpuscular hemoglobin concentration, and a platelet count. The breakdown of different types of WBCs

Figure 9–1 Laboratory Shorthand

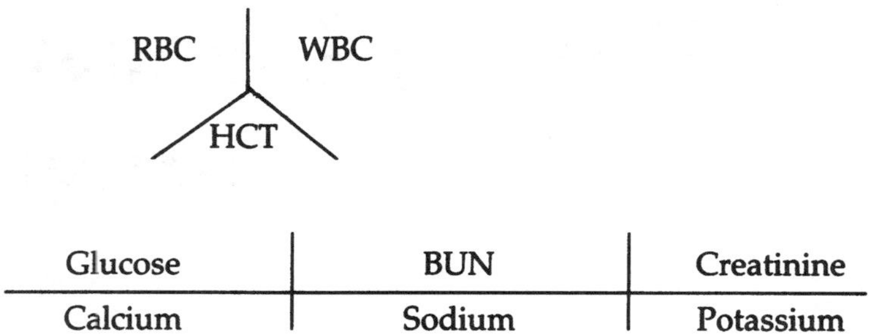

(differential) may be included or may have to be ordered separately. Reference ranges for CBC values are listed in Table 9.1.

Interpreting the CBC (common reference ranges in parentheses)

Red Blood Cell Count (male = 3.9–5.2 million/mm3)

Decrease: Anemias*

Increase: Polycythemias, high altitudes

*Note: The most common form of anemia is caused by iron deficiency. Any anemia in a patient over 40 should be considered to be caused by a gastrointestinal malignancy until proven otherwise. Follow up with rectal exam, testing for occult blood in the stool and serum iron.

Red Blood Cell Morphology

Anisocytosis: Irregular size of red blood cells. Anemias can present as normocytic, microcytic (iron deficiency), and macrocytic (megaloblastic anemia). This parameter is measured as MCV.

Poikilocytosis: Irregular shape of red blood cells. Examples include:

Sickling—sickle cell anemia

Nucleated—marrow replacement, hemorrhage, extramedullary hematopoiesis

Acanthocytes (burr cells)—liver disease

Target cells—any hypochromic anemia

Table 9.1 CBC Normal Values

Blood Component	Value
Red blood cells	3.9–5.2 million/mm3
White blood cells	3,800–10,000/mm3
Neutrophils	40–75%
Lymphocytes	18–47%
Eosinophils	0–6%
Basophils	0–2%
Monocytes	0–10%
Hemoglobin	12–16 gm/dL (female) 14–18 gm/dL (male)
Hematocrit	35–47% (female) 40–55% (male)
Platelets	130,000–400,000 mm3

Cellular inclusions

Basophilic stippling—heavy metal poisoning

Howell-Jolly bodies—postsplenectomy

Mean Corpuscular Hemoglobin (27–33 picograms)

Decrease: Hypochromic anemias (iron deficiency)

Increase: Hyperchromic anemias (megaloblastic)

White Blood Cell Count (3,800–10,000/mm3)

Decrease: Chronic infections

Increase*: Infections, tumors, arthritides

*Note: Mild to moderate elevations are most consistent with tumors, arthritides, systemic illness, and viral infection. High elevations are most consistent with bacterial infections, leukemia, and lymphoma.

White Blood Cell Differential

Segmented neutrophils = 40%–75%

Lymphocytes = 18%–47%

Eosinophils = 0%–6%

Basophils = 0%–2%

Monocytes = 0%–10%

Hemoglobin (male = 14–18 gm/dL; female 12–16 gm/dL)

Decrease: Anemias

Increase: Not usually seen, although may be temporarily increased with dehydration

Hematocrit (male = 40%–55%; female = 35%–47%)

Decrease: Anemias, hemorrhage

Increase: Hemoconcentration, polycythemias

Platelets (130,000–400,000/mm3)

Decrease: Thrombocytopenia syndromes, leukemias, chemotherapy, autoimmune disorders, medications

Increase: Myeloproliferative disorders, oral contraceptive use

Urinalysis

Normal adult values are noted parenthetically. Abnormal findings and their clinical significance are noted below each test. Table 9.2 summarizes the tests and their normal values.

Appearance (straw/clear)

Blue (or green)—beets

Brown—bile, hemoglobin, blood, food dyes

Cloudy (turbid)—phosphated, urates, WBCs

Dark (black)—porphyrins, melanin pigmentation

Foamy—protein, bile acids

Red—blood

Table 9.2 **Normal Urinalysis Values**

Characteristic	Value
Appearance	straw/clear
Specific gravity	1.01–1.03
Ph	4.5–8.0
Glucose	negative
Ketones	negative
Blood	negative
Nitrites	negative
Bilirubin	negative
Urobilinogen	negative

Specific Gravity (1.01–1.03)

The specific gravity of the urine is an indirect reflection of the kidney's ability to concentrate urine. If the first morning specimen has specific gravity of 1.025 or better, it is a good indication of adequate concentration by the kidneys.

Decrease: Intrinsic renal disease, diabetes insipidus

Increase: Diabetes mellitus, congestive heart failure (CHF), nephrosis (proteinuria)

Ph (4.5–8.0)

Acid urine: Ketoacidosis, chronic obstructive pulmonary disease, high protein diet, medications

Alkaline urine: Urinary tract infection (UTI), renal tubular acidosis, vomiting, high vegetable diet

Glucose (negative)

Normal urine never contains glucose, as the renal threshold before the glucose "spills over" into the urine is 180 mg%. If glucose is found in the urine, a diagnosis of diabetes mellitus should be entertained.

Positive: Diabetes mellitus, Cushing's syndrome, steroids, hyperthyroidism, pancreatic disease, renal tubular disease

Ketones (negative)

Positive: Diabetic ketoacidosis, vomiting, diarrhea, pregnancy, hyperthyroidism, starvation, high fat diet

Blood (negative)

If the dipstick is positive for blood but no cells are seen, there may be hemoglobin in the urine. Causes such as trauma should be sought.

Positive: Infection, stones, trauma, tumors. False positive in athletes from repetitive microtrauma.

Nitrites (negative)

Positive: Urinary tract infection (except when organism does not produce nitrites; therefore, a negative test does not rule out infection)

Bilirubin (negative)

Positive: Multiple myeloma, UTI, genitourinary malignancy, CHF, preeclampsia, malignant hypertension

Table 9.3 Urine Casts

Cast	Significance
Waxy	Advanced renal failure
Hyaline	Nonspecific/oliguria
RBC	Glomerulonephritis
WBC	Glomerulonephritis
Epithelial	Nephrotic syndrome, acute tubular injury
Fatty	Nephrotic syndrome
Granular	Tubular injury
Bacteria	Infection
Crystals	Metabolic diseases

Urobilinogen (0.1–1.0 mg/dL)

Increase: Cirrhosis, right-sided CHF, hepatitis, antibiotic therapy

All of the above tests, except the appearance of the urine, can be performed by the dipstick method with a freshly voided specimen. After the dipstick analysis is performed, the urine must be examined microscopically for the presence of cells, casts, and bacteria. Table 9.3 lists the casts found in urine and the clinical significance of each.

Culture and sensitivity to antibiotics may be in order for a patient with a suspected UTI. Gram staining of bacteria may also be performed. A urinalysis with gram staining and culture should be performed on all patients with a fever of unknown origin.

Serum Chemistries

Analysis of serum encompasses a large group of tests that are far beyond the scope of this text. The tests noted below are those that are most relevant to chiropractic practice. Some tests, although not a part of everyday general practice, have been included so that an overall picture of the patient's health can be formed.

The tests in this section are listed alphabetically. Normal values are noted parenthetically and the clinical significance of deviations from normal are also included. Table 9.4 lists the normal values of common serum chemistry tets.

Acid Phosphatase (<3 ng/mL or <0.8 IU/L)

This is a radioimmunoassay used in the evaluation of disease of the prostate gland.

Increase: (Metastatic) prostate cancer, prostatitis, benign prostatic hypertrophy

Alanine Aminotransaminase (ALT) (8–20 U/L)

See serum glutamic-pyruvic transaminase (SGPT).

Albumin (3.2–5.5 g/DL)

Albumin is protein measured for the evaluation of the kidneys and reticuloendothelial system as well as some connective tissue and gastrointestinal disorders. It is a relatively nonspecific test.

Table 9.4 Common Serum Chemistry Values

Test	Normal Value
Acid Phosphatase	<3 ng/mL or <0.8 IU/L
Alanine Aminotransaminase (ALT)	8–20 U/L
Albumin	3.2–5.5 g/DL
Albumin/Globulin Ratio (A/G Ratio)	1.0–2.2
Alkaline Phosphatase	20–70 U/L (child = 20–40 IU/L)
Alpha-fetoprotein (AFP)	<25 ng/mL
Amylase	25–125 U/L
Antistreptolysin-o Titre (ASO)	<165 units
Bicarbonate	22–28 mEq/L
Bilirubin	Total = <0.2–1.2 mg/dL
Indirect	<1.1 mg/dL
Direct	<0.3 mg/dL
Blood Urea Nitrogen (BUN)	7–25 mg/dL
Calcium	8.5–10.6 mg/dL
Chloride	95–110 mEq/L
Cholesterol	120–200 mg/dL
Creatine Phosphokinase (CPK)	25–150 IU/L
Creatinine	0.7–1.4 mg/dL
Gamma-glutamyl Transpeptidase (GGT)	0–45 U/L
Globulin	1.5–3.8 g/dL
Glucose	70–120 mg/dL
Hemoglobin A1C (Glycosylated Hemoglobin)	2.2–4.8%
High-density lipoprotein (HDL) cholesterol	>60
Human Chorionic Gonadotropin (HCG)	<3.0 mU/mL
Iron	40–155 mg/dL
Iron Binding Capacity (Total) (TIBC)	250–410 µg/dL
Lactate Dehydrogenase (LDH)	0–250 U/L
Lipase	0.0–2.0 U/mL
Low-density lipoprotein (LDL) Cholesterol	<160 mg/dL

Table 9.4 Common Serum Chemistry Values *(continued)*

Test	Normal Value
Parathyroid Hormone (LPTH)	100–600 pg/mL
Phosphorus	2.5–4.5 mg/dL
Potassium	3.5–5.3 mEq/L
Protein, Serum	6.0–8.5 g/dL
Rheumatoid Factor (RA Latex)	<1:40
Serum Glutamic-oxaloacetic Transaminase	0–50 U/L
Serum Glutamic-pyruvic Transaminase	0–55 U/L
Sodium	135–148 mEq/L
Thyroid Stimulating Hormone (TSH)	0.5–5.0 μg/mL
Thyroxine (T4 Total)	5–12 μg/dL
Triglycerides	20–150 mg/dL
Triiodothyronine (T3 RIA)	125–200 mg/dL
Troponin I	0.0–0.4
Uric Acid	2.5–7.5 mg/dL

Decrease: Multiple myeloma, Hodgkin's disease, leukemia, renal disease (nephrotic syndrome), inflammatory bowel diseases, hepatic disease, collagen-vascular diseases

Albumin/Globulin Ratio (A/G Ratio) (1.0–2.2)

This is another relatively nonspecific test used in the evaluation of bone, liver, and renal diseases.

Decrease: Multiple myeloma, nephrotic syndrome, cirrhosis, and other hepatic disease

Alkaline Phosphatase (20–70 U/L) (child = 20–40 IU/L)

This is an enzyme produced by both bone and liver tissue. Mildly elevated levels of this enzyme may be seen in children during adolescence and should not be mistaken for an abnormality. It may be necessary in some cases to fractionate the alkaline phosphatase to ascertain which organ system is causing the overproduction. Gamma-glutamyl transpeptidase determination is also helpful in making the distinction.

Increase: Bone malignancy, Paget's disease of bone, rickets/osteomalacia, hyperparathyroidism, hepatic disease, hyperthyroidism

Decrease: Excess vitamin D intake, malnutrition

Alpha fetoprotein (AFP) (<25 ng/mL)

This is a serum study used in the evaluation of cancer and in the prenatal evaluation of the mother's serum for predicting spina befida.

Increase: Hepatic carcinoma, testicular carcinoma, spina bifida

Amylase (25–125 U/L)

Amylase is an enzyme produced by the pancreas that causes the breakdown of complex sugars. Elevation is most often associated with disease of the pancreas.

Increase: Acute pancreatic disease, cholecystitis, peptic ulcer disease, mumps, renal disease, alcohol ingestion

Decrease: Pancreatic destruction, hepatic disease

Anti-double stranded DNA Antibody (Anti-dsDNA) (Negative)

This test is highly specific for lupus erythematosus, particularly lupus nephritis.

Antinuclear Antibody (ANA) (negative)

The presence of antibodies against nuclei is a good indicator of collagen-vascular disorders.

Positive: Systemic lupus erythematosus, scleroderma (progressive systemic sclerosis), rheumatoid arthritis, lupus syndromes (drug-induced)

Antistreptolysin-O Titre (ASO) (<165 units)

Increase: Infections (group-A hemolytic streptococcus), collagen-vascular disease (rheumatoid arthritis)

Aspartate Aminotransferase (AST)

See serum glutamic oxaloacetic transaminase (SGOT).

Bicarbonate (22–28 mEq/L)

This base acts as a buffer in the acid-base balance system.

Increase:	Respiratory acidosis, as compensation for metabolic acidosis, chronic obstructive pulmonary disease
Decrease:	Respiratory alkalosis, as compensation for metabolic alkalosis, diabetic ketoacidosis, severe diarrhea, salicylates

Bilirubin (Total = <0.2–1.2 mg/dL, indirect = <1.1 mg/DL, direct = <0.3 mg/dL)

This is the bile pigment formed mainly by the breakdown of red blood cells. The direct form is conjugated with glucuronide and the indirect form is unconjugated.

Increase (total):	Hemolysis, hepatobiliary disease, fasting
Increase (direct):	Hepatitis, biliary obstruction, drug-induced cholestasis (estrogen), hepatic cancer
Increase (indirect):	Gilbert's syndrome, hemolysis

Blood Urea Nitrogen (BUN) (7–25 mg/dL)

This chemistry is used in conjunction with creatinine in determining normal renal function.

Increase:	Renal failure, pre/postrenal azotemia, gastrointestinal hemorrhage, drugs (aminoglycosides)
Decrease:	Hepatic failure, pregnancy, nephrotic syndrome

Calcium (8.5–10.6 mg/dL)

Increase:	Bone tumors, osteoporosis, Paget's disease, sarcoidosis, hyperparathyroidism, immobilization, hyperthyroidism, excess vitamin D
Decrease:	Osteomalacia, rickets, renal failure, hypoparathyroidism

Chloride (95–110 mEq/L)

Increase: Diarrhea, renal disease

Decrease: Vomiting, diabetic ketoacidosis, renal disease

Cholesterol (120–200 mg/dL)

Increase: Hypercholesterolemia, diabetes mellitus, hyperlipoproteinemia, pregnancy

Decrease: Hepatic disease, steroid therapy, malnutrition, chronic anemia

Creatine Phosphokinase (CPK) (25–150 IU/L)

This enzyme has classically been used for the determination of myocardial damage. It is also elevated in a number of other diseases. Myocardial band (CPK-MB), muscle band (CPK-MM), and brain band (CPK-BB) have been identified and can be fractionated in order to determine which organ has been damaged.

Increase: Muscle damage (myocardial infarction, muscle trauma, rhabdomyolysis, polymyositis), cerebrovascular accident

Creatinine (0.7–1.4 mg/dL)

This test is the best serum determination of normal renal function. It is used in combination with blood urea nitrogen.

Increase: Renal failure, acromegaly, muscle disease

Decrease: Pregnancy

Fluorescent Treponemal Antibody Absorbed (FTA-ABS) (nonreactive)

Positive: Syphilis or other treponemal diseases

Gamma-glutamyl Transpeptidase (GGT) (0–45 U/L)

Increase: Hepatic disease, pancreatic disease

Globulin (1.5–3.8 g/dL)

Increase: Infection, leukemia, multiple myeloma, hepatic disease

Decrease: Renal disease, hypogammaglobulinemia

Glucose (70–120 mg/dL)

This test should be performed after the patient has fasted for 12 hours.

Increase: Diabetes mellitus, acromegaly, Cushing's syndrome, acute pancreatitis

Decrease: Pancreatic disease, hepatic disease, hypoglycemia, oral hypoglycemic drugs

Glycosylated Hemoglobin

See Hemoglobin A1C.

Hemoglobin A1C (Glycosylated Hemoglobin) (2.2–4.8%)

This test is used to monitor long-term serum glucose control, typically in diabetics.

Increase: diabetes mellitus, higher risk of complications from diabetes mellitus (retinal, renal, cardiovascular)

High-density lipoprotein (HDL) cholesterol (>60)

Increase: Lower risk of cardiovascular disease

Decrease (<35): Higher risk of cardiovascular disease

Human Chorionic Gonadotropin (HCG) (<3.0 mU/mL)

The beta subunit of HCG is used in the determination of pregnancy. Urine HCG can also be measured.

Increase: Pregnancy, testicular cancer, choriocarcinoma, molar pregnancy

Human Immunodeficiency Virus (HIV)

See human T-lymphocyte virus.

Human T-Lymphocyte Virus (HTLV) (negative)

Positive: Acquired immune deficiency syndrome

Iron (40–155 mg/dL)

Increase: Hemochromatosis, hemosiderosis, hemolysis

Decrease: Iron deficiency anemia, chronic disease, chronic infection

Iron Binding Capacity (Total) (TIBC) (250–410 μg/dL)

Increase: Hemorrhage, iron deficiency anemia, oral contraceptive agents, hepatic disease

Decrease: Chronic disease, chronic infection, hepatic cirrhosis, renal disease, hemochromatosis

Lactate Dehydrogenase (LDH) (0–250 U/L)

This enzyme is a nonspecific indicator of inflammation. Isoenzymes can also be fractionated.

Increase: Myocardial infarction, hepatic disease, malignant tumors, hemolysis, pulmonary and renal embolism/infarction

Lipase (0.0–2.0 U/mL)

This enzyme, which breaks down fats, is an indicator of pancreatic disease.

Increase: Acute pancreatitis, pancreatic duct obstruction

Low-density lipoprotein (LDL) Cholesterol (<160 mg/dL)

Increase: Higher risk of cardiovascular disease

Decrease: Lower risk of cardiovascular disease

Lupus Erythematosus Cell Preparation (LE Prep) (none seen)

This test is becoming less useful than previously thought.

Positive: Systemic lupus erythematosus, rheumatoid arthritis, scleroderma, drug-induced lupus-like syndromes (procainamide)

Monospot (negative)

This quick test is a useful tool in the diagnosis of infectious mononucleosis.

Positive: Infectious mononucleosis, viral hepatitis, rheumatoid arthritis (false positive), leukemias, lymphomas

Parathyroid Hormone (PTH) (100–600 pg/mL)

Increase: Primary and secondary hyperparathyroidism

Decrease: Idiopathic hypercalcemia, other nonparathyroid causes of hypercalcemia

Phosphorus (2.5–4.5 mg/dL)

Increase: Hypoparathyroidism, secondary hyperparathyroidism, bone diseases, renal failure

Decrease: Hyperparathyroidism, alcoholism, diabetes mellitus, gout, diuretic therapy, vitamin D deficiency

Potassium (3.5–5.3 mEq/L)

Increase: Renal failure, Addison's disease, hemolysis, potassium-containing drugs

Decrease: Diuretic therapy, vomiting, diarrhea, renal disease

Protein Electrophoresis (Serum) (SPE) (variable)

Serum proteins are fractionated into five groups: albumin, alpha-1 globulin, alpha-2 globulin, beta globulin, and the gamma globulins (IgA, IgG, IgM, IgD, IgE). The classic "M" spike (elevated albumin and gamma globulins) (Figure 9–2) is seen with multiple myeloma. Gamma globulin elevation is seen with collagen-vascular diseases, infections, and leukemia.

Figure 9–2 **Serum Protein Electrophoresis Patterns**

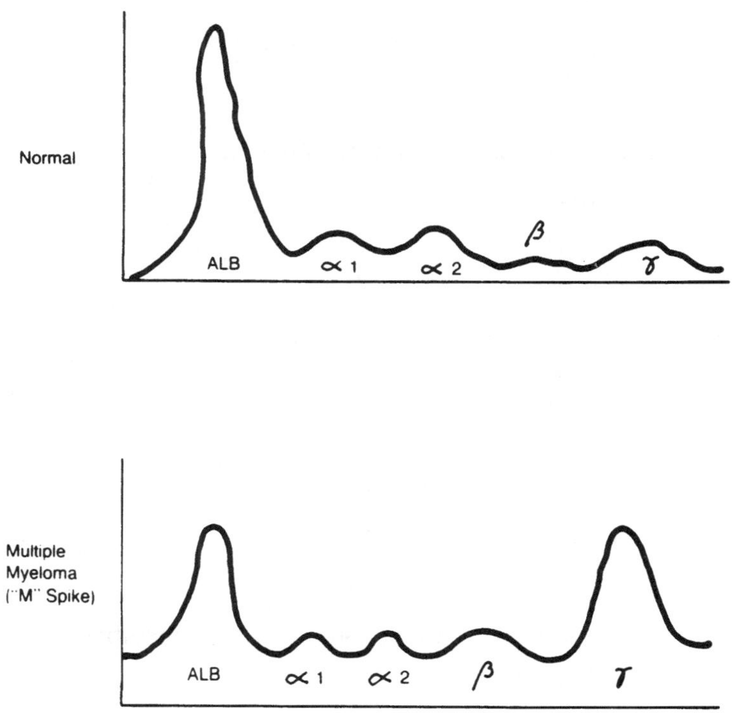

Protein, Serum (6.0–8.5 g/dL)

Increase: Multiple myeloma, sarcoidosis, acute inflammation

Decrease: Malnutrition, Hodgkin's disease, leukemia, inflammatory bowel disorders

Rheumatoid Factor (RA Latex) (<1:40)

The RA latex titer can be used as an indicator of the activity of the disease.

Increase: Rheumatoid arthritis, systemic lupus erythematosus, syphilis

Schilling's Test

Following an overnight fast, the patient is first injected intramuscularly with nonlabeled vitamin B12, sufficient to saturate the body's stores. This is followed by oral doses of vitamin B12 labeled with cobalt-58, and a second dose labeled with cobalt-57 bound to intrinsic factor. Prior saturation body stores ensures that the radio-labeled vitamin B12 is absorbed and rapidly excreted in the urine. Malabsorption is indicated if less than 10% is excreted in 24 hours.

Serum Glutamic-oxaloacetic Transaminase (SGOT) (0–50 U/L)

Increase: Hepatic disease, myocardial infarction, brain damage, renal disease, muscle disease

Serum Glutamic-pyruvic Transaminase (SGPT) (0–55 U/L)

Increase: Hepatobiliary disease, pancreatitis

Sodium (135–148 mEq/L)

Increase: Cushing's syndrome, diabetes insipidus

Decrease: CHF, hepatic cirrhosis, renal failure, multiple myeloma, vomiting, diarrhea

Thyroid Stimulating Hormone (TSH) (0.5–5.0 mU/L)

This test is good for screening for hypothyroidism.

Increase: Primary hypothyroidism

Decrease: Primary hyperthyroidism, pituitary insufficiency with secondary hypothyroidism

Thyroxine (T4 Total) (5–12 μg/dL)

This is an excellent screening test for hyperthyroidism.

Increase: Primary hypothyroidism

Decrease: Primary hyperthyroidism, pituitary insufficiency with secondary hypothyroidism

Triglycerides (20–150 mg/dL)

Increase: Hyperlipoproteinemia, hepatic disease, alcoholism, renal disease, pancreatitis, myocardial infarction

Triiodothyronine (T3 RIA) (125–200 mg/dL)

Increase: Hyperthyroidism, pregnancy, estrogen therapy
Decrease: Hypothyroidism

Troponin I (0.0–0.4)

This is a highly sensitive test for the investigation of suspected myocardial disease. Levels may stay elevated for up to 14 days after an infarction.

Increase: Myocardial ischemia/infarction

Uric Acid (2.5–7.5 mg/dL)

Increase: Gout, renal failure, leukemia

Venereal Disease Research Laboratory (VDRL) (nonreactive)

This is a good screening test for syphilis that, if reactive, can be confirmed with FTA-ABS testing.

Positive: Syphilis, systemic lupus erythematosus (false positive), pregnancy (false positive)

Special Studies

- *C-Reactive Protein*—Positive test is a nonspecific indicator of inflammation. Recent evidence has implicated elevated CRP levels in patients with cardiovascular disease.

- *Erythrocyte Sedimentation Rate*—Elevation is a nonspecific indicator of inflammation somewhere in the body. It is best used to gauge effectiveness of therapy than to diagnose disease.
- *Fecal Occult Blood (FOB)*—Used to diagnose occult blood in the stool. For this test to be positive it must reveal occult blood on at least three separate occasions. Approximately 1–4% false-positive rate results from ingestion of high doses of NSAIDs, vegetables, and red meat.

Specific Laboratory Panels

The investigation of specific organ system disease is augmented by the use of groups of laboratory tests specific to an organ or system. Table 9.5 lists some of the more common panels useful to the chiropractic clinician.

Table 9.5 Commonly Used Laboratory Profiles

Bone tumor profile	**Cardiac ischemia profile**
Calcium	CPK-MB
Phosphorus	SGOT
Alkaline phosphatase	LDH
Acid phosphatase (if blastic)	Troponin I
Arthritis profile	**Hepatic profile**
RA latex	SGPT
Uric acid	SGOT
HLA-B27	LDH
ESR	Bilirubin
Kidney profile	Albumin
BUN	Globulin
Creatinine	**Pancreatic Profile**
Albumin	Amylase
Globulin	Lipase
A/G ratio	Bilirubin
Cardiac risk profile	
Cholesterol (including HDL and LDL)	
Triglycerides	
Serum glucose	

Chapter 10

Diagnostic Imaging

Lawrence H. Wyatt, DC, DACBR, FICC

Introduction

Since its discovery, imaging of the human body has been a mainstay in the investigation of patient complaints. However, ionizing radiation is not without hazard. Its most deleterious effects are on body systems with the highest cell turnover such as the reproductive organs, the retinal and hematopoietic systems, and the gastrointestinal (GI) tract. It is for this reason that radiation in any form must be justified before use.

This chapter outlines the proper application of diagnostic imaging in a chiropractic general practice. Imaging protocols for common conditions are also delineated.

Ten Rules of Radiology

There are ten basic rules of radiology that, when followed meticulously, will lead the clinician to the proper imaging study and an accurate diagnosis.

1. Consult often with a radiologist. As a specialty consultant, the radiologist can supply the physician with written reports to aid in the diagnostic work-up of a patient. If there is ever a question regarding a radiographic finding or which study should be performed next, the radiologist is very helpful.
2. Perform only those studies that are clinically justified. (1,2,3,4) Ask this simple question: "Will the treatment or the prognosis for the patient

change if this study is performed?" If the answer is yes, then the study should be performed, barring any contraindications. If the answer is no, then serious thought should be given to other diagnostic studies that might be more helpful. Often, the patient regards the use of radiography as more important than it has been demonstrated to be by scientific evaluation. (5) Table 10.1 lists common indications for musculoskeletal radiography.

3. Choose the correct imaging procedure. For example, while magnetic resonance imaging (MRI) is an excellent diagnostic procedure in well-selected patient populations, its helpfulness has been called into question in a typical low back pain patient. (6) In these instances, plain film

Table 10.1 Common Indications for Musculoskeletal Radiography

Age >40
Alcohol abuse
Failure to improve with appropriate therapy
Fever
History of cancer
IV drug use
Loss of bowel and/or bladder control
Macrotrauma
Myelopathy
Night pain
Pain at rest or unchanged by patient position
Progressive neurologic abnormalities
Prolonged oral corticosteroid use
Radiculopathy
Repetitive microtrauma
Saddle anesthesia
Suspicion of inflammatory arthritis
Suspicion of osteoporosis
Unexplained weight loss

radiography had a similar impact on patient outcomes. Selection of the procedure with the highest diagnostic yield and therapeutic impact gives the clinician the most valuable information possible.

4. Always perform a complete series. This includes a minimum of 90-degree views of the area of chief complaint. If there is clinical suspicion that a patient may have true radiculopathy from cervical foraminal encroachment, then oblique views of the cervical spine are in order. (7)
5. Establish a standard protocol for working in the radiography suite. This ensures that a marker is never left off, for example.
6. Accept only good quality radiographs. It is a disservice to both the clinician and the patient to accept anything less. Poor quality films serve no useful purpose and even may result in litigation.
7. Develop a pattern approach to radiographic interpretation. If a pattern is established while viewing radiographs, the pattern soon becomes a routine and it becomes less likely that subtle but ominous radiographic signs will be missed. (8)
8. Compare with previous films, if at all possible. Serial radiography in patients with biomechanical spine pain is most often not helpful, (9,10) although progression of arthropathy, fracture healing, and other conditions can be followed. For example, a blastic lesion in the hip that appears benign that remains unchanged after two years is almost certainly benign. Without comparison films, the patient may have to undergo painful and expensive procedures to rule out a malignant lesion. Some authors claim that sagittal posture and changes toward a more "normal" sagittal posture are important (11,12), but to date the clinical utility of these procedures has not been demonstrated.
9. Understand the basic tenets of radiographic interpretation. There are several rules, germane to all radiographic studies, that should be followed. Utilization of these rules, which are presented in the next section, will help prevent oversight of any serious pathology.
10. Always have a written report in the patient's chart. Maintenance of a written report along with the views performed and the factors used to expose the patient are an integral part of any patient file. (13)

Basic Rules of Radiographic Interpretation

There are a number of basic rules in radiology that should be memorized, understood, and utilized any time the clinician interprets a radiographic study. The following are only guidelines; there are exceptions to these rules but, in most instances, the rules will be helpful.

General Bone Radiology

1. Osteopenia is a radiographic description of loss of bone density; osteoporosis is a disease. The diagnosis of osteoporosis can seldom be made from a radiograph. Clinical signs and symptoms should be consistent with the diagnosis.
2. Hyperemia causes osteopenia; avascular necrosis causes osteosclerosis.
3. Painful lesions are usually aggressive; nonpainful lesions are usually benign.
4. Slow growing lesions are usually not aggressive.
5. A benign painless lesion that becomes painful is suspicious for malignant degeneration.

Bone Tumors

1. A solitary lytic/blastic lesion in a patient over 40 is malignant until proven otherwise; consider metastasis and multiple myeloma.
2. A solitary diaphyseal lucency in any patient is malignant until proven otherwise; consider leukemia and metastatic neuroblastoma in children and reticuloendothelial malignancies in adults.
3. The most common skeletal malignancy is lytic metastasis.
4. Bilateral symmetry suggests a normal variant.
5. Patients over 40 years of age have malignancies; patients under 40 have benign lesions.
6. Diffuse osteopenia in a male may be the only sign of multiple myeloma.
7. Calcified lesions are usually benign (except chondrosarcoma).
8. Thick sclerosis around the edge of a lesion suggests benignancy; consider fibrous lesions.
9. Thirty to fifty percent bone destruction is required before any plain film radiographic findings become evident.
10. Metastasis favors the pedicles; multiple myeloma spares the pedicles.
11. Long lesions in long bones usually have a fibrous matrix.

Arthritides

1. Older patients have degenerative arthritides; younger patients have inflammatory arthritides.
2. Always rule out atlantoaxial instability in any patient with inflammatory arthritis; consider transverse ligament rupture.
3. Bilateral symmetry suggests rheumatoid arthritis.
4. Inflammatory arthritis in young males is most often due to a seronegative spondyloarthropathy; consider ankylosing spondylitis.
5. A monarticular arthritis is infectious until proven otherwise.
6. Pure bone erosion without bone production suggests rheumatoid arthritis; bone erosion with bone production suggests a seronegative spondyloarthropathy.
7. Degenerative joint disease is, by far, the most common form of arthritis.
8. Degenerative joint disease in an articulation that does not normally develop degenerative joint disease is most likely secondary to crystal deposition or trauma.

Trauma

1. Compression fractures where both the anterior and posterior vertebral body heights are lost are pathologic until proven otherwise.
2. Transverse fractures are pathologic until proven otherwise.
3. Avulsion of the lesser trochanter is pathologic until proven otherwise.
4. Multiple injuries at different stages of healing indicate battered child syndrome (child abuse) until proven otherwise.
5. Spiral fractures in children are suspicious for child abuse.
6. Metaphyseal beak fractures are almost pathognomonic for child abuse.
7. Symmetry suggests a normal variant; consider nonfusion of a secondary growth center. Do comparison views when necessary.
8. Distraction and rotation of fracture fragments are ominous prognostic indicators.
9. A healed fracture is a clinical decision, not a radiographic one.
10. If there is a greater than 25% compression of vertebral body height, order a computerized tomography (CT) or MRI scan to rule out retropulsion of bone fragments into the spinal canal.

Infection

1. Rapid progression of a lesion, days to weeks, usually suggests an infectious etiology.
2. Infections invade and blur fascial planes; tumors deflect fascial planes.
3. Joints are especially vulnerable to tuberculosis.
4. Multifocal infections are found in infants and geriatric patients.
5. Infection, along with infarction and avascular necrosis, suggests sickle cell anemia.

Congenital Lesions

1. If there is one anomaly, look for another.
2. Lumbar spine anomalies are often associated with genitourinary anomalies.
3. Thoracic spine anomalies are often associated with cardiopulmonary anomalies.

Soft Tissues

Abdomen

Although most chiropractic practices concentrate on bone and joint radiology, there are many times when evaluation of soft tissues with radiography becomes necessary, as noted below.

1. The maximum normal anteroposterior diameter of the abdominal aorta is 3.5 centimeters. Anything larger suggests an abdominal aortic aneurysm.
2. The most common abdominal calcification is a calcified mesenteric lymph node.
3. The most common pelvic calcification occurs in the pelvic veins (phlebolith).
4. Absence or haziness of a fascial plane suggests inflammation (peritonitis).
5. The maximum normal diameters of the small and large intestines are 3.0 and 5.0 centimeters, respectively. Significant enlargement suggests obstruction or adynamic ileus.

Chest

1. The cardiac silhouette should be no larger than one-half the largest lateral measurement of the thoracic cage.

2. The first diagnostic step after finding a pulmonary mass is to compare the most recent film with previous films. Growth of the lesion during a 2-year period should be looked upon with suspicion for malignancy, while stability for 2 years suggests benignancy.
3. Chest films with a less than full inspiration give the false appearance of congestive heart failure.
4. Deviation of the trachea suggests that either something is pushing it away (mass) or pulling it toward (atelectasis) the side of the lesion.
5. Calcification within a pulmonary lesion, especially when centrally located, suggests benignancy.

Differential Diagnosis and Follow-up Imaging

One of the most challenging aspects of radiology is to determine, once the lesion is located, what the next step is for the diagnostic work-up. Table 10.2 outlines the differential diagnosis of common radiographic lesions.

Table 10.3 delineates the traumatic spine lesions that might be seen in a chiropractic practice. Table 10.4 outlines the traumatic upper extremity skeletal lesions and Table 10.5 the lower extremity skeletal lesions.

Table 10.6 outlines the more common radiographic signs and the diseases and conditions associated with them.

Aggressive Lesion Characteristics

Many times it becomes prudent for patients with aggressive lesions to be referred to another physician for diagnosis or treatment. To determine if such referral is necessary, characterize the lesion using the information in Tables 10.7, 10.8, 10.9 and 10.10.

Common Causes of Common Lesions

Table 10.11 lists the most common causes of common lesions seen in a chiropractic general practice.

Radiographic Evaluation in the Abdomen and Chest

[Def=definition, DDx=differential diagnosis,
Investig=diagnostic investigation]

Table 10.2 Differential Diagnosis of Common Radiographic Skeletal Lesions

Radiographic Sign	Differential Diagnosis
Blastic lesion (solitary)	Metastasis Bone island Osteoid osteoma Stress fracture
Blastic lesions (multiple)	Metastasis Osteopoikilosis
Chondrocalcinosis	Idiopathic Degenerative joint disease Calcium pyrophosphate crystal deposition Gouty arthritis

Lucent lesion (solitary)	Metastasis
	Malignant tumor
	  Multiple myeloma
	  Ewing's sarcoma
	  Fibrosarcoma
	  Telangiectatic osteosarcoma
	  Giant cell tumor
	  Chondrosarcoma
	  Benign tumor
	  Aneurysmal bone cyst
	  Enchondroma
	  Giant cell tumor (quasi-malignant)
	  Solitary bone cyst
	  Osteochondroma
	  Hemangioma
	  Chondroblastoma
	  Fibrous cortical defect
	  Nonossifying fibroma
	  Chondromyxoid fibroma

Lucent lesions	Metastasis Multiple myeloma
Missing pedicle	Metastasis Agenesis

Table 10.2 **Differential Diagnosis of Common Radiographic Skeletal Lesions *(continued)***

Radiographic Sign	Differential Diagnosis
Multi-loculated lucent lesion	Aneurysmal bone cyst Chondroblastoma Enchondroma Fibrous dysplasia Giant cell tumor Hemangioma Nonossifying fibroma Osteoblastoma Plasmacytoma Solitary bone cyst
Osteopenia in a male	Multiple myeloma Metastasis Osteoporosis Chronic corticosteroid use
Painful scoliosis	Trauma Aneurysmal bone cyst Chondroblastoma Giant cell tumor Osteoid osteoma Osteoblastoma
Sacroiliitis	Ankylosing spondylitis Reiter's syndrome Psoriatic arthritis Enteropathic arthritis Infectious arthritis
Sclerotic (Ivory) vertebra	Metastasis Paget's disease Lymphoma Idiopathic

Table 10.3 Traumatic Spine Lesions

C1 fractures
Solitary ring fracture-post. arch, hyperextension, stable
Jefferson-four fracture sites, unstable, axial compression
C2 fractures
Type I-tip of odontoid, stable, hyperflexion
Type II-base of odontoid, unstable, mc dens fracture, hyperflexion
Type III-body of C2, least common, stable/unstable, hyperflexion
Hangman's-traumatic spondylolisthesis, unstable, hyperextension
Lower cervical fractures
Pillar fx-compression of facet, mc cervical fx, stable, seen on pillar view
Wedge compression-stable (unless retropulsion of fragments), hyperflexion
Pathologic compression-unstable, underlying bone pathology
Teardrop-avulsion of vertebral corner, unstable, hyperflexion/hyperextension
Clay shoveler's-spinous process of C6, 7, T1, stable, rotation-flexion
Cervical dislocations
Unilateral facet-stable, <50% subluxation, flexion-rotation
Bilateral facet-unstable, >50% subluxation, hyperflexion, severe ST injury
Thoracic fractures
Wedge compression-stable without retropulsion of fragments, hyperflexion, osteoporosis
Pathologic compression-unstable, underlying bone pathology
End plate infractions-"fish" vertebra(e), osteoporosis, often multiple, stable
Lumbar fractures
Wedge compression-stable without retropulsion of fragments, hyperflexion, osteoporosis
Pathologic compression-unstable, underlying bone pathology
End plate infractions-"fish" vertebra(e), osteoporosis, often multiple, stable
Chance-separation of vertebra into superior and inferior fragments, unstable
Pelvic fractures
Pubis-stress fx seen in osteoporosis mc, can be macrotraumatic
Rider's bone-fx of ischial tuberosity in kids with bone overgrowth
ASIS-avulsion fx seen in athletes (e.g., soccer)
Sacrum-direct blow/fall on buttocks, oblique, unstable if "through and through"
Coccyx-stable, direct blow/fall on buttocks

Note: mc = most common

Table 10.4 Traumatic Upper Extremity Skeletal Lesions

Shoulder fractures
- Clavicle-stable, check for neurovascular compromise
- Surgical neck of the humerus-rule out neurovascular compromise
- Bankart lesion-inferior labrum tear with/without fx

Shoulder dislocations
- Anteroinferior-mc, can have Bankart lesion also
- Posterosuperior-seen in electrocution, tonic-clonic seizures

Elbow fractures
- Supracondylar-many fracture planes possible, can be comminuted
- Condylar-capitellum, trochlea, medial condyle, lateral condyle
- Radial head-look for fat pad changes, can be very subtle, step-defect

Elbow dislocations
- Posterior-radius/ulna dislocates posteriorly, can be associated with fx
- Nursemaid's elbow-radial head dislocation in child, easily reducible

Forearm fractures
- Colles'-distal radius fx with post. dorsal displacement of the carpus, silver-fork deformity, can have associated ulnar styloid fx
- Smith's-distal radius fx with post. palmar displacement of the carpus, can have associated ulnar styloid fx
- Barton's-intra-articular radius fx with wrist subluxation
- Galeazzi's-distal radius fx with ulnar disloc. at the elbow
- Monteggia's-proximal ulnar fx with radial head dislocation
- Nightstick-mid-shaft ulna fx, often a defensive injury

Wrist fractures
- Scaphoid-waist is mc, AVN is common sequela, fall on outstretched wrist
- Hook of the hamate-direct trauma to hamate (e.g., golfers)

Wrist dislocations
- Lunate-moves anteriorly, fall on outstretched wrist
- Scapholunate dissociation-scaphoid and lunate separate in coronal plane, Terry Thomas sign

Finger fractures
- Bennett's- intra-articular fx/dislocation at base of 1st carpometacarpal joint
- Boxer/barroom-4th/5th metacarpal head fx

Table 10.5 Traumatic Lower Extremity Skeletal Lesions

Hip fractures

Femoral neck-subcapital, mid-cervical, basocervical, intertrochanteric, sub-trochanteric; first three are intracapsular and slow-healing

Acetabular-posterosuperior acetabulum mc, often seen with dislocations

Hip dislocations

Posterosuperior-mc, dashboard impact injury, often with fx

Anteroinferior-uncommon injury

Knee fractures

Condylar-medial, lateral, supracondylar

Tibial plateau-valgus or varus stress resulting in plateau compression fx

Ankle fractures

Medial malleolus-inversion/shear, eversion/avulsion

Lateral malleolus-eversion/shear, inversion/avulsion

Pott's-malleolar fx(s) with dislocation, usually laterally

Foot fractures

Dancer's-spiral fx of 5th metatarsal neck, inversion

Jones'-transverse through base of the 5th metatarsal, avulsion

Lisfranc- fx/dislocation between metatarsals cuneiforms and cuboid, trauma, neuropathic foot without significant trauma

Bedroom-distal phalanx, slow-healing

* - diseases noted with an asterisk may need to be placed at the top of the differential diagnosis list under appropriate clinical circumstances, as they carry a generally poor prognosis if not discovered early.

Abdomen

Adrenal Calcification

Def: calcification of the adrenal gland

DDx: usually occurs secondarily to some form of inflammatory disease. Birth trauma is by far the most common cause for adrenal calcification, followed by cancer* and infection of the adrenal gland.

Investig: CT, MRI

Table 10.6 **Common Named Radiographic Signs**

Sign	Disease/Condition
Bamboo spine	Anklylosing spondylitis
Blade of grass sign	Paget's disease
Blister of bone	Aneurysmal bone cyst
Bone in bone sign	Osteopetrosis
Boutonniere sign	Rheumatoid arthritis
Button sequestrum	Eosinophilic granuloma
Corduroy vertebra	Hemangioma
Cotton wool sign	Paget's disease in the skull
Crescent sign	Avascular necrosis
Elbow fat pad sign	Joint effusion
Fallen fragment sign	Simple (unicameral) bone cyst
Fat-blood interface	Lipohemarthrosis
Fish vertebrae	Osteopenic diseases
'H' vertebrae	Sickle cell anemia
Hair-on-end sign	Hemolytic anemia (skull)
Heel pad sign	Acromegaly
Intradiscal vacuum cleft	Disc injury (at disc-vertebra junction)
Intravertebral vacuum cleft	Avascular necrosis (e.g., radiation)
Inverted Napoleon hat sign	Sponlylolisthesis in AP lumbar radiograph
Ivory Phalanx	Psoriasis
Ivory vertebra	Blastic metastasis, Paget's disease, lymphoma
Sail sign	Elbow joint effusion
Sausage digit	Psoriasis
Scotty dog sign	Spondylolysis
Swan neck deformity	Rheumatoid arthritis
Terry Thomas sign	Scapholunate dissociation
Trolley-track sign	Ankylosing spondylitis
Vacuum phenomenon	Degenerative disc disease

Table 10.7 Benign Lesions of Bone

Signs of Benignancy
Small size
Thick rim of sclerosis
Thick or no periosteal reaction
Cortical expansion without destruction
No soft tissue mass
Geographic pattern of bone destruction
Calcification (except for chondrosarcoma)
Negative bone scan

Types of Benign Bone Lesions
Cartilaginous
- Enchondroma
- Osteochondroma
- Chondroblastoma

Osseous
- Enostoma (bone island)
- Osteoma
- Osteoblastoma

Fibrous
- Fibroxanthoma
- Fibrous dysplasia

Miscellaneous
- Aneurysmal bone cyst
- Chondromyxoid fibroma
- Giant cell tumor
- Osteoid osteoma
- Simple bone cyst

Dysphagia

Def: inability to swallow objects without difficulty. It usually begins with difficulty with liquids and progresses to solids.

DDx: cancer*, whether intrinsic esophageal or extrinsic from some other regional organ, primary achalasia, reflux esophagitis with stricture, hypertrophic spinal diseases (such as diffuse idiopathic skeletal hyperostosis

Table 10.8 Aggressive Lesions of Bone

Signs of Aggressiveness
Large size
Absence of sclerotic rim
Laminated or spiculated periosteal reaction
Cortical destruction
Soft tissue mass
Moth-eaten or permeative bone destruction
No calcification (except for chondrosarcoma)
Positive bone scan

Types of Aggressive Bone Lesions
Osteomyelitis
- Pyogenic
- Fungal

Cartilaginous
- Chondrosarcoma

Osseous
- Osteosarcoma

Fibrous
- Fibrosarcoma
- Malignant fibrous histiocytoma

Miscellaneous
- Multiple myeloma
- Chordoma
- Giant cell tumor
- Ewing's sarcoma
- Lymphoma
- Leukemia

and degenerative disc disease), globus hystericus (no true esophageal luminal stricture but a sensation of dysphagia (diagnosis by exclusion of other causes).

Investig: barium swallow, upper GI series, esophagogastroduodenoscopy (EGD)

Table 10.9 Unstable Spinal Lesions

Signs of Instability

Vertebral body compression of more than 50%

Vertebral anterolisthesis of more than 25% of vertebra below

Intersegmental vertebral sagittal rotation (flexion) of more than 11 degrees

Atlantodental interspace of greater than

- 5 mm in children
- 3 mm in adults

Retropulsion of bone fragments into spinal canal

Types of Unstable Bone Lesions

Cervical spine

- Odontoid fractures (Types II and possibly III)
- Flexion teardrop fracture
- Extension teardrop fracture
- Burst fracture
- Bilateral facet dislocation

Thoracolumbar spine

- Burst fracture
- Bilateral facet dislocation
- Chance fracture

Table 10.10 Patterns of Bone Destruction

Pattern	Description	Typical Significance
Geographic	Large, well defined	Benign
Moth-eaten	Mid-sized, ill defined	Aggressive
Permeative	Pinpoint, ill defined	Aggressive

Table 10.11 Common Causes/Locations of Common Lesions

	Lesion	Cause/Location
Tumors		
	Skeletal malignancy	Lytic metastasis/thoracolumbar
	Primary skeletal malignancy	Multiple myeloma/thoracolumbar
	Tumor w/skeletal mets	Bronchogenic carcinoma/thoracolumbar
	Benign tumor of skeleton	Enostoma (bone island) (pelvis/hips)
	Benign tumor of spine	Hemangioma/thoracic
	Diffuse osteopenia	Multiple myeloma/thoracolumbar
Arthritides		
	Arthritis	Degenerative joint disease (DJD)/lumbar
	Destructive arthritis	Rheumatoid arthritis/hands
	Lumpy and bumpy joints	DJD/knees
Trauma		
	Fracture plane in adults	Oblique/clavicle
	Fractured bone in body	Clavicle/oblique
	Fracture of spine	Simple compression fracture/thoracolumbar
	Fractured bone in wrist	Scaphoid
	Fracture of elbow	Radial head
	Fracture of hip	Subcapital
	Dislocation of shoulder	Anteroinferior
	Dislocated bone in wrist	Lunate
	Dislocation of hip	Posterior
Metabolic/endocrine		
	Cause of osteopenia	Osteoporosis
	Cause of osteomalacia	Renal osteodystrophy
Congenital		
	Spinal congenital lesion	Spina bifida occulta/lumbosacral
	Transitional segment	Lumbosacral
	Hemivertebra	Thoracic spine
	Block vertebra	Cervical spine
Vascular		
	Osteochondritis dissecans	Lateral aspect of medial femoral condyle
	Bone infarction	Sickle cell anemia/knee

Hematemesis

Def: vomiting of blood

DDx: malignancy*, peptic ulcer disease, gastritis, esophageal varices (alcoholics)

Investig: EGD, upper GI series

Hematochezia

Def: passage of bright red blood per rectum

DDx: hemorrhoids (mc), inflammatory bowel disease (ulcerative colitis, irritable bowel syndrome, Crohn's disease), cancer of the rectum*, intestinal polyps

Investig: barium enema (BE), upper GI series, EGD

Hepatomegaly

Def: enlargement of the liver

DDx: cirrhosis, hepatitis, cancer*, congestive heart failure

Investig: MRI, ultrasound (US), endoscopic retrograde cholangiopancreatography (ERCP), magnetic resonance cholangiopancreatography (MRCP), biopsy

Abdominal Mass (Adult)

Def: abnormal mass within the abdominal cavity

DDx: Saccular abdominal aortic aneurysms*, pregnancy, ovarian cysts and tumors, renal masses, gallbladder disease, colon cancer*

Investig: plain film radiograph, US, CT, MRI

Melena

Def: black tarry stools

DDx: GI bleeding proximal to the mid-transverse colon, proximal GI malignancy*, inflammatory bowel disease, peptic ulcer disease

Investig: BE, upper GI series, colonoscopy

Pancreatic Calcification

Def: opacities in the pancreas

DDx: chronic pancreatitis, pancreatic pseudocyst and cancer of the pancreas*

Investig: CT, MRI, ERCP, MRCP, US

Pneumoperitoneum

Def: air in the peritoneal cavity

DDx: post-operative abdomen, perforation of a hollow viscus (peptic ulcer, colon diverticulitis), douching, sexual intercourse, idiopathic

Investig: plain film radiographic examination in the upright and lateral decubitus postures, laparoscopy, CT, MRI

Renal Calcification

Def: opacities in the kidneys or renal arteries

DDx: renal calculus, infection, cancer*, renal papillary necrosis, renal artery aneurysm

Investig: US, CT, MRI

Splenic Calcification

Def: opacities in the spleen or renal artery

DDx: splenic artery atherosclerosis and/or aneurysm, splenic cysts, healed hematoma, infarction (sickle cell anemia)

Investig: US, CT, MRI

Splenomegaly

Def: enlargement of the spleen, often in concert with an enlarged liver

DDx: leukemia and lymphomas,* infections, portal hypertension

Investig: US, CT, MRI

Vas Deferens Calcification

Def: opacification of the walls of the vas deferens

DDx: diabetes mellitus, idiopathic, infection

Investig: US

Chest

Consolidation

Def: filling of the alveoli with a substance, usually blood, pus, water, protein or cells (aka pulmonary infiltrate)

DDx: pulmonary edema (congestive heart failure (CHF)), pneumonia, pulmonary contusion, lymphoma and alveolar cell carcinoma*, pulmonary alveolar proteinosis

Investig: plain film radiography, biopsy, bronchial lavage

Effusion (Pleural)

Def: fluid (water, blood) in the pleural space

DDx: CHF, infection, and cancer (lymphangitic metastasis)*

Investig: plain film radiography, thoracocentesis

Extrapleural Sign

Def: non-parenchymal pleural-based, tapered-bordered lesion projecting into the chest

DDx: rib metastasis, rib fracture, loculated pleural effusion, mesothelioma

Investig: plain film radiography, CT

Hilar Enlargement (Bilateral)

Def: enlargement of the lymph nodes of the hila

DDx: lymphoma (especially Hodgkin's disease), sarcoidosis, lymphangitic metastasis, tuberculosis

Investig: plain film radiography, CT, MRI, biopsy

Hilar Enlargement (Unilateral)

Def: unilateral enlargement of a hilum

DDx: bronchogenic carcinoma*, vascular disease, sarcoidosis, lymphoma, tuberculosis

Investig: plain film radiography, CT, MRI, angiography, biopsy

Mediastinal Mass (Anterior)

Def: mass in the retrosternal space

DDx: thymoma, teratoma, thyroid (substernal), aortic aneurysm, lymphoma

Investig: plain film radiography, CT, MRI, biopsy

Mediastinal Mass (Middle)

Def: mass in the middle mediastinum

DDx: lymphoma, bronchogenic carcinoma, bronchogenic cyst, aortic

Investig: CT, MRI, biopsy

Mediastinal Mass (Posterior)

Def: mass in the retrocardiac/paraspinal region of the thorax

DDx: neurogenic tumors, aortic aneurysm, hiatal hernia, neurenteric cyst

Investig: CT, MRI, biopsy

Multiple Pulmonary Nodules

Def: multiple masses in the lung parenchyma

DDx: metastasis, old infections (tuberculosis, fungal) especially when calcified

Investig: plain film radiography, CT, biopsy

Unresolving Pneumonia

Def: pneumonia that is slow to resolve or fails to resolve with therapy

DDx: malignancy until proven otherwise, improper therapy, benign bronchial obstruction

Investig: plain film radiography, CT

Solitary Pulmonary Nodule

Def: single parenchymal lung mass

DDx: bronchogenic carcinoma, infectious or noninfectious granuloma, metastasis, benign tumors

Investig: evaluation begins with a comparison of the most recent chest radiographs with any taken in the past. If there has been an increase in the size of the lesion, especially if the volume of the lesion has doubled within 1 to 18 months, then malignancy is the prime concern. If the lesion has remained stable for two years or more, it can be considered benign. Advanced imaging with CT is helpful in finding calcifications within the lesion, which most often signify a benign etiology.

Radiation Physics Made Easy

Basic Rules

The following basic rules help make radiation physics more easily understood, especially as far as applying physics to everyday clinical practice.

1. Milliampere-seconds (mAs) control density (blackness) of the radiograph. The relationship of this setting to density is generally linear, i.e., doubling

the mAs will cause a doubling of film blackness. Use mAs and not kilovoltage potential to control density. There must be at least a 30% change in mAs for a change to be seen on the radiograph. Change the mAs by changing the time, not the mA.

2. Kilovoltage potential (kVp) controls contrast (number of shades of gray). Its relationship to film density is logarithmic. Do not use kVp to control density. The only time to vary kVp from standard protocols (depicted in Figure 10–1) is with obese patients. Use lower kVp to reduce scatter radiation and thus reduce film fog. If the patient measures over 30 centimeters, a general rule is to increase kVp by two for each centimeter over 30. If the outlines of the bones can be seen, enough kVp has been used. Film density can now be controlled with mAs.
3. Any body part measuring over 13 centimeters should be X-rayed with a grid to reduce scatter radiation.
4. Always err on the side of too much density. An underexposed film is useless, unless of course a foreign body in the soft tissues is being sought.
5. Always use the shortest time and longest patient-to-film distance possible to reduce magnification, distortion, and patient motion.
6. The inverse square law is useful if the clinician moves the tube (e.g., from 40 inches to 72 inches for a lateral lumbar spine film).

Radiography Procedure

Definition: Using ionizing radiation and plain film examination to investigate pathology.

Materials

- X-ray unit
- X-ray film
- Positioning aids (if necessary)
- X-ray technique calculator
- Film processor
- Right/left side markers
- Filters
- Gonad shields
- Lead gloves/apron
- Measuring calipers

Figure 10–1 Standard kVp for Different Body Regions

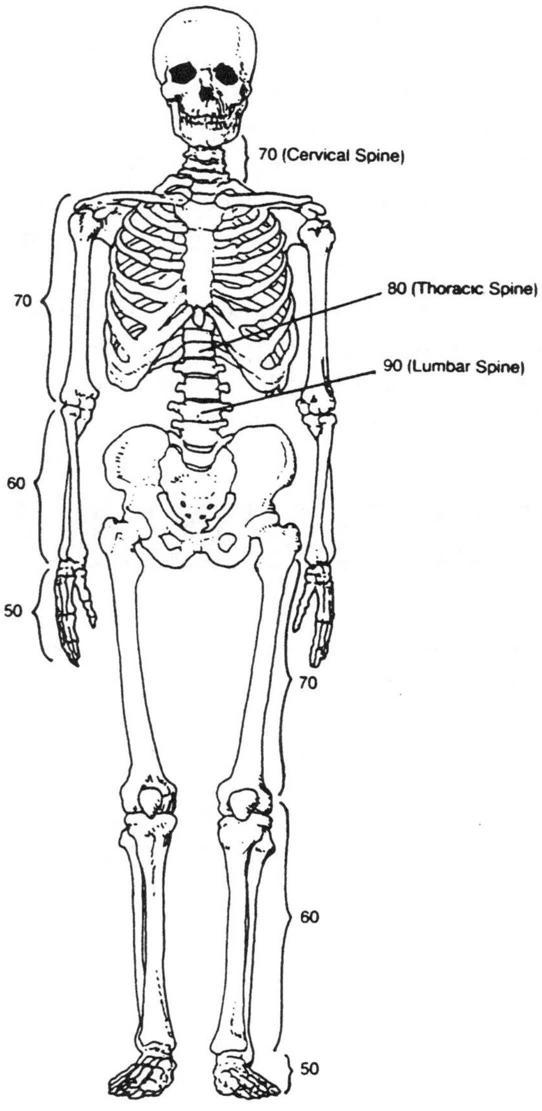

Procedure: Although X-ray units and positioning for each radiographic view differ, the same procedure can be used on all patients to ensure excellent radiographs in all cases. (These procedures are also summarized in Table 10.12.)

1. Explain the procedure, including the benefits and risks, to the patient. If the patient is a female, ensure that the procedure is being performed within 10 days after the onset of her last menstrual period. This rule applies unless the health of the mother is in imminent danger.
2. Obtain the informed consent of the patient for the X-ray procedures to be performed. Have a witness sign the form.
3. Have the patient undress and don a gown. Make certain the patient has removed any clothing or jewelry that may contain metal (earrings, brassieres, etc.).
4. Measure the body part to be examined with calipers.
5. Input the measurement into the technique chart or the technique calculator and figure the proper radiographic exposure factors. Always remember to use the shortest time possible.

Table 10.12 Radiography Procedures

Radiography Procedures
Explain procedure to patient
Ensure the 10-day rule applies
Obtain informed consent
Have patient undress and don gown
Remove jewelry
Measure part to be X-rayed
Input technique factors
Insert cassette with marker
Position the patient
Check focal film distance
Tilt tube
Position central ray
Recheck positioning
Give breathing instructions
Make the exposure

6. Input the technique factors into the X-ray machine.
7. Place the X-ray cassette with the side marker attached into the tray or on the tabletop, whichever is necessary for the view being performed. Ensure the film tray is pushed all the way into the Bucky.
8. Position the patient properly, including any rotation or tilting necessary.
9. Tilt the X-ray tube as necessary. Remember that tube tilt must be compensated for by decreasing the tube film distance one inch for every five degrees of tube tilt.
10. Place the central ray in the proper position, making sure it is centered with the film in the holder or on the tabletop.
11. Recheck all positioning and ensure the proper factors have been programmed into the machine.
12. Give the patient the proper breathing instructions.
13. Expose the patient, ensuring that the button(s) is (are) depressed until the "beep" is heard.

Table 10.13 outlines the standard techniques for the more common radiographic projections of the spine and pelvis, Table 10.14 the upper extremity, and Table 10.15 the lower extremity.

Standard Radiographic Views

Standard radiographic views of the skeleton, chest, and abdomen are outlined in Table 10.16.

Radiology Reports

Radiology reports should adhere to the following format:

- name, age, and sex of the patient
- studies performed
- date of the study and report
- body of the report (paragraph form)
- impressions (conclusions from the body)
- comments (recommendations for further investigation)
- signature

Table 10.13 Select Spine Radiographic Techniques

View	Film Size	TFD	Tube Angulation	CR*	Specials
Cerv-AP	8 × 10	40″	15° ceph	C4	Collimate eyes
Cerv-APOM	8 × 10	40″	0°	C1	Tight coll.
Cerv-Lat	10 × 12	72″	0°	C4	Air gap
Cerv-Obl	8 × 10	72″	15°	C4	Post obl better
Cerv-Flex	8 × 10	72″	0°	C4	Tuck chin first
Cerv-Ext	8 × 10	72″	0°	C4	
Cerv-Pillar	8 × 10	40″	40° caud	C4	Chin turned
Thor-AP	14 × 17, 7 × 17	40″	0°	T6	Susp. Respir.
Thor-Lat	14 × 17, 7 × 17	40″	0°	T6	Susp. Respir.
Swimmers	10 × 12	40″	0°	T1	
Lumb-AP	14 × 17, 7 × 17	40″	0°	L3	Susp. Exhale
Lumb-Lat	14 × 17, 7 × 17	40″	0°	L3	Susp. Exhale
Lumb-Obl (45°)	10 × 12	40″	0°	L3	Susp. Exhale
Lumb-AP Spot	12 × 10	40″	25° ceph	L5-S1	
Lumb-Lat Spot	8 × 10	40″	0°	L5-S1	
Full Spine-AP	14 × 36	72″	0°	T6	Filter Cerv
Full Spine-Lat	14 × 36	72″	0°	T6	Filter Cerv
Pelvis-AP	17 × 14	40″	0°		
Sacrum-AP	8 × 10	40″	15° ceph		
Sacrum-Lat	8 × 10	40″	0°		
Sacroiliac Joint	8 × 10	40″	0°		25° obl
Coccyx-AP	8 × 10	40″	10° caud		
Coccyx-Lat	8 × 10	40″	0°		

[CR-Central ray, Cerv-Cervical spine, Thor-Thoracic spine, Lumb-Lumbar spine, AP-anteroposterior, Lat-Lateral, Obl-Oblique, Flex-Flexion, Ext-Extension, Ceph-Cephalad, Caud-Caudal, Coll-Collimation, Susp-Suspend, Respir-Respiration]

*Unless otherwise noted, the central ray should be in the center of the body part to be imaged.

To increase clarity and readability, follow these guidelines in writing reports.

1. Be brief without forsaking completeness. Include only the pertinent positives and pertinent negatives.
2. Write in a narrative format and use short, complete sentences.
3. Use the present tense when referring to what is seen on the film. Use the past tense only when referring to previous studies.
4. Avoid using phrases like "there is" at the beginning of sentences. It becomes monotonous to the reader.

Table 10.14 **Select Upper Extremity Radiographic Techniques**

View	Film Size	TFD	Tube Angulation	CR*	Specials
Shoulder-AP	10 × 12	40″	0°		
Shoulder-Int Rot	8 × 10	40″	0°		
Shoulder-Ext Rot	8 × 10	40″	0°		
Shoulder-Baby Arm	10 × 12	40″	0°		90° Abduct.**
Elbow-AP	8 × 10 (½)	40″	0°		
Elbow-Lat	8 × 10 (½)	40″	0°		
Elbow-Obl	8 × 10 (½)	40″	0°		
Elbow-Tang	8 × 10	40″	0°		Post hum flat
Wrist-PA	8 × 10 (¼)	40″	0°		
Wrist-Lat	8 × 10 (¼)	40″	0°		Lunate Disloc.
Wrist-Obl (45°)	8 × 10 (¼)	40″	0°		O.K. pos.***
Wrist-Ulnar Dev	8 × 10 (¼)	40″	0°		Scaphoid view
Hand-PA	8 × 10	40″	0°		
Hand-Lat	8 × 10	40″	0°		
Hand-Obl (45°)	8 × 10	40″	0°		
Hand-Ball Catcher	8 × 10	40″	0°		Catch pos****

[AP-anteroposterior, Lat-Lateral, Obl-Oblique, Int Rot-Internal Rotation, Ext Rot-External Rotation, Tang-tangential, Ulnar Dev-Ulnar Deviation of the wrist]

*CR-Central Ray; unless otherwise noted, the central ray should be in the center of the body part to be imaged.

** Shoulder is externally rotated to 90° and abducted to 90° similar to an infant during a startle reflex.

***Thumb and index finger in a circle with tips touching, lateral fingers spread, as if making the okay sign.

****Hand cupped and supinated as if ready to catch a ball; useful for finding small erosions associated with inflammatory arthritides.

5. If there is a specific question regarding, for example, trauma, explain that "no fractures are identified" in the report.
6. Vary the wording of reports. Using the same sentences consistently runs the risk of missing an important but subtle finding.
7. Note the most important findings first and save the incidentals for last.
8. Save diagnostic conclusions for the impressions section of the report.
9. Clearly express any clinical impressions and the confidence felt in each.

Table 10.15 Select Lower Extremity Radiographic Techniques

View	Film Size	TFD	Tube Angulation	CR*	Specials
Hip-AP	10 × 12	40″	0°		
Hip-Frog Leg Lat	10 × 12	40″	0°		Frog leg pos**
Femur-AP	7 × 17, 14 × 17	40″	0°		
Femur-Lat	7 × 17, 14 × 17	40″	0°		
Knee-AP	8x10	40″	0°		
Knee-Lat	8x10	40″	0°		
Knee-Tunnel	10 × 12	40″	***		
Knee-Tang	8 × 10	40″	0°		† prone, >90° flex
Lower Leg-AP	7 × 17	40″	0°		
Lower Leg-Lat	7 × 17	40″	0°		
Ankle-DP	8 × 10	40″	0°		
Ankle-Lat	8 × 10	40″	0°		
Ankle-Mortise (20°)+	8 × 10	40″	0°		
Ankle-Obl	8 × 10	40″	0°		
Foot-DP	8 × 10	40″	0°		
Foot-Lat	8 × 10	40″	0°		
Foot-Obl (45°)	8 × 10	40″	0°		

[AP-anteroposterior, DP-Dorsoplantar, Lat-Lateral, Obl-Oblique, Tang-tangential]
*CR-Central Ray; unless otherwise noted, the central ray should be in the center of the body part to be imaged.
**Hip externally rotated and knee flexed to 90°
***Patient prone with knee partially flexed, tube housing should be parallel to lower leg
†prone with knee flexed past 90°; CR through patellofemoral joint
+20° medial oblique

Table 10.16 Standard Radiographic Views

Body Region	Radiographic Views
Cervical spine	AP, APOM, Lat, Obl, Flex, Ext
Thoracic spine	AP, Lat
Lumbar spine	AP, Lat, Obl, AP Angulated L5-S1 spot
Pelvis	AP
Hip	AP, Frog leg Lat
Femur	AP, Lat
Knee	AP, Lat, Sunrise, Tunnel
Lower Leg	AP, Lat
Ankle	AP, Lat, Mortise (20° medial obl)
Foot	DP, Lat, Obl
Shoulder	AP, Int rot, Ext rot, Baby arm
Humerus	AP, Lat
Elbow	AP, Lat, Obl
Forearm	AP, Lat
Wrist	PA, Lat, Obl
Hand	PA, Lat, Obl
Skull	Lat (Rt and Lt), Towne's, Caldwell's
Chest	PA, Lat
Abdomen	AP (recumbent), AP (standing)

[AP-anteroposterior, Lat-lateral, Obl-Oblique, Int Rot-Internal rotation, Ext Rot-External rotation, DP-Dorsoplantar, Flex-Flexion, Ext-Extension]

Advanced Diagnostic Imaging

Use of advanced imaging has become common in the modern chiropractic practice.

These modalities can be helpful in the diagnostic, treatment, and prognostic decisions that must be made regarding patient care.

Computerized Tomography (CT)

Computerized axial tomography, while utilizing x-radiation as an imaging source, can be extremely helpful in diagnosing many osseous and soft tissue lesions.

Table 10.17 Common Indications for Computerized Tomography

Follow-up of unusual plain film findings
- Clinically significant subluxation
- Spinal canal/foraminal stenosis
- Fractures/dislocations
- Clinically significant congenital anomalies
- Infection
- Tumors

Abdominal masses (e.g., abdominal aortic aneurysm)
Herniated nucleus pulposus (CT discogram)
Intracanalicular space-occupying lesions (CT myelography)
Headache
Cauda equina syndrome
Cerebral space-occupying lesions
Postoperative pain
Cerebral ischemia
Intracranial bleeding

While much controversy exists regarding the utility of CT in the diagnosis of central nervous system (CNS) disease, especially with the advent of magnetic resonance imaging, it is still useful in a number of different instances (Table 10.17).

Patients who will require iodinated contrast agents during a CT examination should be queried regarding any allergy or adverse reaction to contrast agents and their component substances.

Magnetic Resonance Imaging (MRI)

MRI has become a staple in the investigation of CNS disorders in recent years. The use of MRI in the diagnosis of musculoskeletal disease is well-demonstrated. (14) Imaging of solid abdominal organ pathology is also easily accomplished. (15) Magnetic resonance angiography is a recent technology that is demonstrating promise in the investigation of aneurysms, coronary artery disease, and other vascular pathology. (16) MRI is a safe procedure as it does not require the use of ionizing radiation and has very few side effects. (17) Some patients may be claustrophobic and may require the use of anxiolytics/sedatives before the procedure can be performed. The use of contrast enhancement is typically reserved for investigation of abdominal and CNS disease as well as for post-operative spine pain. In addition, the differentiation of post-operative fibrosis from re-herniation of disc material is best accomplished with contrast enhancement. Table 10.18 outlines the indications and contraindications for using MRI.

Table 10.18 Common Indications and Contraindications for Magnetic Resonance Imaging

Indications

Arnold-Chiari malformation
Avascular necrosis (e.g., hip)
Basilar invagination
Bone tumors (with contrast)
Cauda equina/conus medullaris syndromes
Disc disease
Internal joint derangement

- glenoid labrum tears
- meniscus lesions
- ligament tears (e.g., knee, ankle)

Intracranial disease (with contrast)

- tumors
- hemorrhage
- cerebrovascular accident/ischemia
- demyelinating disease (multiple sclerosis)
- vascular lesions (arteriovenous malformation)

Post-operative spine (with contrast)
Rotator cuff disease
Solid organ visceral disease (liver, kidneys, spleen, pancreas) (with contrast)
Spinal canal stenosis
Spinal cord disease (with contrast)
Spinal trauma
Subchondral fractures
Syringomyelia (with contrast)
Tendinopathy

Contraindications

Cerebral aneurysm clips
Implanted ferromagnetic devices (e.g., cardiac pacemaker, stents)
Metallic foreign bodies (e.g., schrapnel)

Table 10.19 Common Indications for Radionuclide Bone Scanning

Skeletal metastasis
Primary bone tumors
Osteomyelitis
Stress/occult fracture

Radionuclide Bone Scanning

The chiropractic doctor is occasionally called upon to evaluate the possibility of malignancy in a patient. The intravenous injection of a radiopharmaceutical that has an affinity for bone (i.e., radionuclide bone scanning) is a helpful procedure. A gamma camera is used to detect any areas in the skeleton that take up an abnormal amount of the radiotracer. Table 10.19 outlines the more common indications for radionuclide bone scans.

Diagnostic Ultrasound (US)

The use of sound waves has become useful in the diagnosis of soft tissue diseases of the human body. US has become most popular in the evaluation of abdominal and pelvic organs. For the chiropractic physician, it may also be helpful in the investigation of suspected vascular disease. Table 10.20 demonstrates some of the indications for diagnostic US.

Table 10.20 Common Indications for Diagnostic Ultrasound

Abdominal aortic aneurysm
Carotid/vertebral artery disease
Ascites
Hepatobiliary disease
Ovarian disease
Pregnancy
Uterine disease

Plain Film Interpretation

Chest Radiographs

Evaluation of the chest radiograph is outlined in Table 10.21.

Abdomen Radiographs

Evaluation of abdomen radiographs is outlined in Table 10.22.

Table 10.21 Chest Radiograph* Interpretation and Positioning

Skeletal structures
- rib fractures
- spine
- clavicles (check for rotation)
- shoulders

Mediastinum
- widening (cardiomegaly, specific chamber enlargement)
- distinct heart border (silhouette sign-overlying lung consolidation/collapse)
- aortic knob (enlargement with atherosclerosis, hypertension, aneurysm)
- aorticopulmonary window (lymphadenopathy)
- hila (enlargement, nodes, masses)

Lung fields
- pneumothorax, pneumomediastinum, pneumoperitoneum
- masses
- fluid (blood, pus, protein, water, cells)
- effusions (check lateral film)
- apices (scarring, cephalization of blood flow)
- symmetry (nodules, loss of volume)
- thickened fissure lines (fluid)
- Kerley B lines (short lines laterally, interstitial edema)

Inflation - count number of ribs to diaphragm
- hyperinflation (chronic obstructive pulmonary disease)
- underinflation (atelectasis)

*Chest radiograph performed posterior-anterior at 72″ on a 14 × 17 cassette with the patient at full inspiration. High kVp should be used (>100) for long scale of contrast.

Table 10.22 Abdomen Radiograph* Interpretation and Positioning

Skeletal structures
- rib fractures
- spine
- pelvis
- hips

Abdominal organs
- hepatomegaly (convex inferior border)
- splenomegaly (inferomedial shift of magenblase)
- calcification (phleboliths most common)
    - pancreas (pancreatitis)
    - kidneys (infection)
    - vasculature (atherosclerosis, diabetes mellitus, hypertension, aneurysm)
    - lymph nodes (sign of previous infection)
    - liver/spleen (infections, cysts)
    - gallbladder (stones, cholecystitis, porcelain gallbladder (pre-malignant))

Ascites (cirrhosis)

Free Air (pneumoperitoneum (post-surgical, perforated viscus)

Bowel size/aeration (adynamic ileus, bowel obstruction)

*Abdomen radiographs performed anterior-posterior at 40″ on a 14 × 17 cassette with the patient in supine and upright positions.

Spine Radiographs

Evaluation of spine radiographs is outlined in Table 10.23.

Extremity Radiographs

Evaluation of extremity radiographs is outlined in Table 10.24.

Skull Radiographs

Evaluation of skull radiographs is outlined in Table 10.25.

Table 10.23 Spine Radiograph Interpretation

Soft tissues
- blurring of fascial planes
- organomegaly
- calcifications

Fracture
- fracture plane
- location
- simple/compound
- pathologic fractures
- associated deformity

Dislocation
- location
- named by superior vertebra
- associated deformity

Scoliosis

Overall bone density

Lytic/blastic lesions
- location(s) (examine pedicles closely)
- cortical destruction
- soft tissue mass

Joints
- degenerative joint disease
- inflammatory arthritis

Mensuration

Table 10.24 **Extremity Radiograph Interpretation**

Soft tissues
- blurring of fascial planes
- calcifications

Fracture
- fracture plane
- location
- simple/compound
- comminution
- pathologic fractures
- associated deformity
- healing stage

Dislocation
- location
- named by distal bone
- associated deformity

Overall bone density

Lytic/blastic lesions
- location(s)
- zone of transition
- cortical destruction
- soft tissue mass
- periosteal reaction
- bone expansion

Joints
- degenerative joint disease
- inflammatory arthritis

Mensuration

Table 10.25 Skull Radiograph* Interpretation and Positioning

Soft tissues
- hematoma formation
- calcifications

Fracture
- location
- simple/compound
- depression of fracture fragments
- comminution
- does the fracture line cross a vascular groove?

Sella turcica
- size (normal ~12 (S-I) × 16 (A-P) mm)
- shape (normal is ovoid)
- erosion of clinoid processes
- calcification (petroclinoid ligament, intrasellar)

Brain
- calcifications (amorphous, vascular, punctuate) (pineal gland normally calcified)
- intracranial air

Bone
- skull shape (normocephalic, brachycephaly (short AP dimension)), scaphocephaly (short coronal dimension)
- bone density (osteoporosis, myeloma, metastasis)
- thickened cranial vault (Paget's disease)

Sutures
- separation (diastasis)
- premature closure in pediatric patients

Sinuses (frontal, maxillary, ethmoid, sphenoid)
- fluid/air-fluid levels (sinusitis)
- thickened mucosal lining (sinusitis)

*Towne's View- patient seated/supine, anteroposterior position, 40″ TFD, 10 × 12 cassette, chin tucked to neck, 30° caudal tube tilt.
*Caldwell View- patient seated/supine, posteroanterior position, 40″ TFD, 10 × 12 cassette, canthomeateal line parallel to floor, 15° caudal tube tilt.
*Lateral View (bilateral)- patient seated/supine, side of skull flat against cassette with body rotated out of the way, 10 × 12 cassette, 0° tube tilt.

References

1. Wyatt, L., & Schultz, G. The diagnostic efficacy of lumbar spine radiography: a review of the literature. In Hodgsen, M. (ed). *Current Topics in Chiropractic.* Palmer College of Chiropractic-West, Sunnyvale, CA: 1987.
2. Frymoyer, J. Spine radiographs in patients with low back pain. *JBJS.* 1984; 66-A:7: 1048–1055.
3. Deyo, R., Diehl, A., & Rosenthal, M. Reducing roentgenography use: can patient expectations be altered? *Arch Internal Med.* 1987;147(1):141–145.
4. Kendrick, D., Fielding, K., Bentley, E., Kerslake, R., Miller, P., & Pringle, M. Cost-effectiveness of lumbar spine radiography in primary care patients with low back pain. *Spine.* 2002 Oct 15;27(20):2291–2297.
5. Espeland, A., Baerheim, A., Albrektsen, G., Korsbrekke, K., & Larsen, J.L. Patients' views on importance and usefulness of plain radiography for low back pain. *Spine.* 2001 Jun 15;26(12):1356–1363.
6. Jarvik, J.G., Hollingworth, W., Martin, B., Emerson, S.S., Gray, D.T., Overman, S., Robinson, D., Staiger, T., Wessbecher, F., Sullivan, S.D., Kreuter, W., & Deyo, R.A. Rapid magnetic resonance imaging vs radiographs for patients with low back pain: a randomized controlled trial. *JAMA.* 2003 Jun 4;289(21):2810–2818.
7. Schultz, G., Phillips, R., Howe, J., & Cherachanko, D. Oblique views: useful or useless. Proceedings of International Conference on Spinal Manipulation. May 1990:27–30.
8. Peterson, C. Factors associated with success or failure in radiological interpretation: diagnostic thinking approaches. *Med Educ.* 1999 Apr;33(4):251–259.
9. Plaugher, G., Cremata, E.E., & Phillips, R.B. A retrospective consecutive case analysis of pretreatment and comparative static radiological parameters following chiropractic adjustments. *J Manipulative Physiol Ther.* 1990 Nov–Dec;13(9):498–506.
10. Gautier, J., Morillon, P., & Marcelli, C. Does spinal morphology influence the occurrence of low back pain? A retrospective clinical, anthropometric, and radiological study. *Rev Rhum Engl Ed.* 1999 Jan;66(1):29–34.
11. Troyanovich, S.J., Harrison, S.O., Harrison, D.D., Harrison, D.E., Payne, M.R., Janik, T.J., & Holland, B. Chiropractic biophysics digitized radiographic mensuration analysis of the anteroposterior lumbopelvic view: a reliability study. *J Manipulative Physiol Ther.* 1999 Jun;22(5):309–315.
12. Harrison, D.E., Harrison, D.D., Betz, J.J., Janik, T.J., Holland, B., Colloca, C.J., & Haas, J.W. Increasing the cervical lordosis with chiropractic biophysics seated combined extension-compression and transverse load cervical traction with cervical manipulation: nonrandomized clinical control trial. *J Manipulative Physiol Ther.* 2003 Mar–Apr;26(3):139–151.
13. Taylor, J.A.M. Writing radiology reports in chiropractic. *J Can Chirop Assoc.* 1990; 34(1):30–34.

14. Stoller, D.W., Cannon, W.D., Jr., & Anderson, L.J. The knee. In: Stoller, D.W. *Magnetic Resonance Imaging in Orthopaedics and Sports Medicine.* 2nd ed. Philadelphia: Lippincott Williams & Wilkins, 1997:203–442.
15. Salmanzadeh, A., & Shirkhoda, A. Hepatic lesions that "fill in" on contrast-enhanced CT and MRI: imaging patterns and diagnostic pitfalls. *Radiologist.* 2000;7(1):1–12.
16. Grist, T.M. MRI of the abdominal aorta and lower extremities. *J Magn Reson Imaging.* 2000;11(1):32–43.
17. Shellock, F.G. *Pocket Guide to MR Procedures and Metallic Objects: Update 2000.* Lippincott Williams & Wilkins, 2003. (Contraindications Table)

Chapter 11

Specialized Procedures

Lawrence H. Wyatt, DC, DACBR, FICC

Introduction

This chapter outlines the many procedures that are used in chiropractic practice. No attempt has been made to justify the procedures or their rationale. Instead, the proper steps taken for each procedure are included.

Venipuncture (Phlebotomy)

Definition: The insertion of a needle into a peripheral vein so that venous blood can be withdrawn for analysis.

Materials

- Tourniquet
- Alcohol pad
- Specimen tubes (see Table 11.1)
- An 18–22 gauge needle (the smaller the gauge, the larger the needle)
- Vacutainer holder
- Gauze/cotton balls
- Bandaids

Table 11.1 Blood Specimen Tubes

Tube	Test(s)
Red top	Serum studies
Purple top	Complete blood count
Green top	HLA-B27
Grey top	Glucose tolerance test
Tiger top	Serum studies
Royal blue top	Heavy metals

Procedure

1. Have all the necessary materials close at hand and easily accessible.
2. Palpate the antecubital fossa for prominent veins (Figure 11–1) and select the one to be used. To make the veins more easily visible/palpable, have the patient pump the hand by opening and closing the fist; then gently but briskly tap on the fossa with your index and middle fingers.
3. Apply the tourniquet approximately 5 to 10 cms above the site of the puncture. Then have the patient make a fist and hold it. Relocate the vein to be used and follow its course for a short distance proximally.
4. Swab the area with the alcohol prep. Wipe off any excess alcohol with gauze or cotton.
5. Insert the needle and tube into the holder in their proper respective positions but do not puncture the rubber stopper on the tube yet.
6. Insert the needle with the bevel up (Figure 11–2) into the skin adjacent to the vein. After the needle is through the skin, stabilize the vein with your free hand to prevent it from rolling.
7. Enter the vein at approximately a 30° angle, being careful not to pierce through the opposite side of the vein.
8. Withdraw the sample by piercing the rubber stopper on the tube with the needle in the holder by advancing the tube forward. The vacuum inside the tube will automatically collect the sample.

Figure 11–1 Veins of the Right Antecubital Fossa

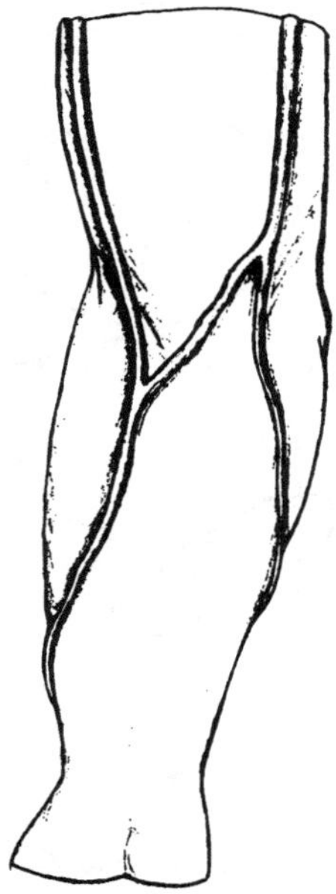

9. If another tube is to be drawn, gently remove the first tube from the holder, place it aside, and insert the new tube onto the needle. Repeat this same procedure for any other tubes that need to be drawn.
10. After the sample(s) has been drawn, remove the tourniquet, withdraw the needle, and apply firm pressure on the puncture site with a small piece of gauze folded into quarters. Elevating the extremity may be helpful.
11. Place tape over the folded gauze and ensure that the patient tolerated the procedure well.
12. Perform whatever procedures are necessary for preparation of the sample for study, such as centrifugation.

Urine Specimen Collection

Definition: Collection of a patient's urine so that urine can be analyzed for the presence of a number of different chemicals, cells, and crystals.

Figure 11–2 **Proper Needle Insertion for Venipuncture**

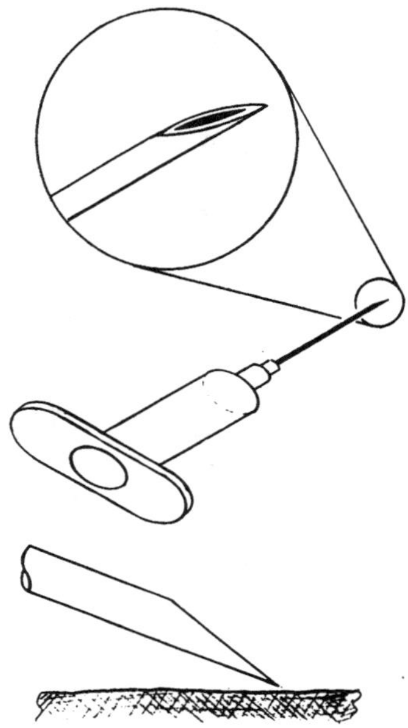

Note: The bevel of the needle is up.

Materials

- Urine collection cup and label

Procedure (for clean catch specimen)

1. Instruct the patient to go into the bathroom and to follow the procedures listed below.
    - Have the patient void a small amount of urine and then stop the stream. This purges the urethra of any residual sediment.
    - The patient should begin the stream again and urinate into the container provided until the cup is half full, and then void the remaining urine. If the patient cannot fill the cup half full, have him or her void until the bladder is almost empty and then stop the stream.
2. The specimen should be examined immediately, as urine degrades rather quickly in warm temperatures. If some time will elapse before the specimen will be examined, it should be refrigerated.

Electrocardiogram (ECG)

Definition: Measuring the electrical conducting system of the heart to diagnose disease of the heart and other organ systems.

Materials

- Electrocardiographic machine with electrodes
- Electrode gel or prefabricated electrode pads

(Machines used for ECGs vary with the institution. Some are even automated. Become familiar with the specific machine used in a specific institution.)

Procedure

1. Be certain the patient is comfortably positioned in the supine position.
2. Explain the procedure to the patient and assure him or her that there is no pain involved. Also ensure that the patient understands the importance of remaining motionless during the examination. This will prevent any artifacts that would obscure proper interpretation of the examination.
3. Plug in the ECG machine and turn it on.
4. Attach each of the electrodes as outlined below (also see Figure 11–3).
    - Most often the color coding system delineates the proper placement of the electrodes.
      White—right arm (RA)
      Black—left arm (LA)
      Green—right leg (RL)
      Red—left leg (LL)
      Brown—chest (V1, V2, V3, V4, V5, V6)
    - Each of the limb leads is attached along the distal ventral portion of the extremity. Apply electrode gel unless premoistened electrode pads are available.
    - The placement of the precordial leads is as follows:
      V1—Fourth ICS to the right of the sternum
      V2—Fourth ICS to the left of the sternum
      V3—Midway between leads V2 and V4
      V4—Midclavicular line above the left fifth ICS
      V5—Left fifth ICS at the anterior axillary line
      V6—Left fifth ICS at midaxillary line
5. Once the leads are in proper position and the machine is ready, follow the instructions for that particular machine and obtain the tracings.

Figure 11–3 Proper ECG Electrode Placement

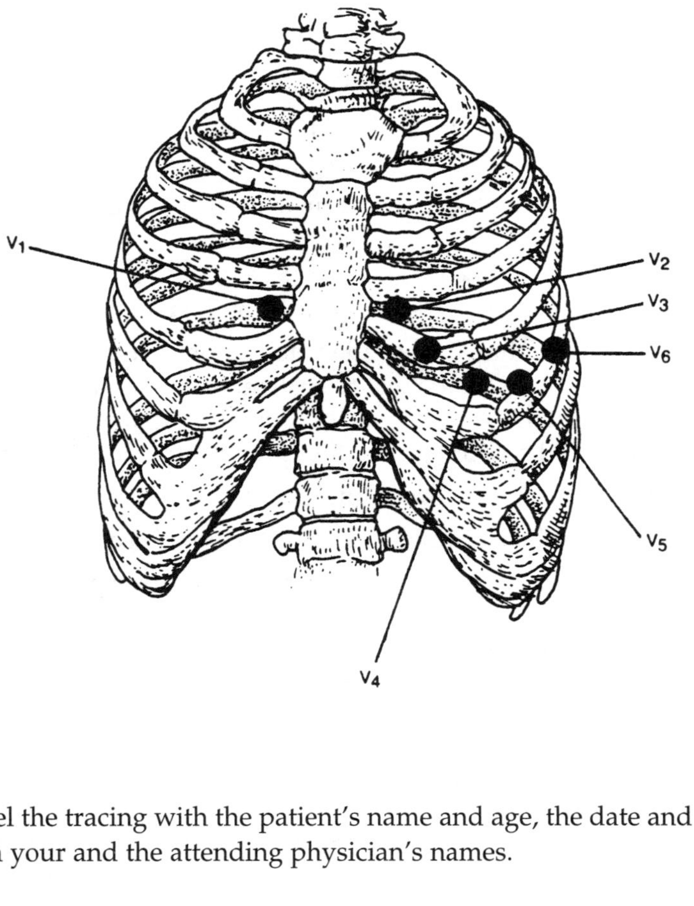

6. Label the tracing with the patient's name and age, the date and time, and both your and the attending physician's names.

Digital Rectal Examination

Definition: Digital examination of the rectum and prostate for any palpable signs of pathology. Many rectal polyps can be found with digital examination. Because of the frequency of colon carcinoma, digital examination of the rectum and testing for occult blood should be performed on patients over 40. It should be remembered that this procedure is uncomfortable and many times embarrassing for patients. Reassuring the patient and explaining the procedure as it is being performed will help allay some of those fears.

Materials

- Lubricating gel
- Examination glove or finger cot
- Occult blood testing materials

Procedure: There are a number of different positions that can be used for proper examination of the patient. Use the one that will be most comfortable for the patient and most useful for the physician. The positions are listed below:

- *Left lateral decubitus*—Best position when evaluating for rectal masses. The patient lies on the left side with the knees pulled up comfortably to the chest.
- *Knee-chest position*—Best position for palpating the prostate. The patient is placed on the table on his knees with his head and shoulders touching the examining table.
- *Dorsolithotomy position*—Particularly useful when examining female patients.
- *Bent over a table*—Useful for examining the prostate. The table should be waist high for patient comfort.

1. Position the patient.
2. The anal region should be inspected for signs of pathology such as hemorrhoids, fissures, fistulae, and skin lesions. Any pain or tenderness should be noted.
3. Place a small amount of lubricant on the index finger of the gloved hand.
4. Apply gentle but steady pressure on the anal sphincter while having the patient perform a Valsalva maneuver. This will facilitate entry.
5. Palpate the walls of the rectum for any signs of a mass or tenderness.
6. If the patient is a male, the finger is then rotated until the prostate gland is felt. It is then plapated for size, consistency, masses, and tenderness. Any masses are noted as to their size, tenderness, consistency, and contour. The normal prostate is a bi-lobed, nontender, smooth midline structure about the size of a walnut. Normal prostatic tissue feels similar to the feel of the tip of the nose.
7. Have the patient bear down again. This may make lesions that were beyond reach palpable.
8. The finger is gently withdrawn and the character of the stool on the gloved finger is noted. Black tarry stool is consistent with proximal gastrointestinal tract bleeding. This stool is then checked for occult blood. (Standard tests for occult blood are available in most laboratories.)

Cardiopulmonary Resuscitation (CPR)

Definition: The administration of external cardiac compressions and breathing to sustain a clinically dead patient until advanced cardiac life support can be initiated. The procedures used here are based on the American Heart Association Standards, 2000.

Materials: No special materials are necessary.

Procedures: CPR is most easily remembered by using the mnemonic ABC: airway, breathing, and circulation. It is assumed that the reader has been trained in CPR; the procedure noted here is in quick reference form. Remember that even with the best CPR technique, one is delivering only approximately one third of normal cardiac output.

Adult CPR

1. Assess the level of responsiveness of the patient by shaking and shouting at patient.
2. If the patient is unresponsive, call loudly for help.
3. Place the patient in the supine position on a flat firm surface. If the patient is in a bed or on an adjusting table, move him or her to the floor.
4. Ascertain whether the patient has spontaneous respirations. Tilt the patient's head using the head tilt-chin lift maneuver and look, listen, and feel for respirations. If respirations are nonexistent or agonal (less than 6/minute), then artificial respirations must be administered.
5. Begin artificial respirations. Administer two slow deep breaths while pinching the patient's nose. A mask may also be utilized.
6. Assess circulation by palpating the ipsilateral carotid pulse for 5 to 10 seconds.

One-Person CPR

8. If there is no pulse, begin external chest compressions in the cycle of 15 compressions and then two breaths at a rate of 80–100 compressions per minute (15 compressions/two breaths). The hand is placed on the lower half of the sternum and compressions are 1½ to 2 inches in depth. If patient has a pulse, continue artificial respirations at a rate of 12 breaths per minute (1 every 5 seconds).
9. Pause after one minute to check pulse and respirations. If they are still absent, continue the cycle and pause every five minutes to check pulse and respirations.

Two-Person CPR

10. Begin compressions with five compressions for each breath at a rate of 80 compressions per minute.
11. Pause at one minute to check for pulse and respirations. If still absent, continue the cycle and pause every five minutes to check pulse and respirations.

Child CPR
Same as the adult, except:

1. Use less force for respirations.
2. Use heel of one hand only for compressions and compress 1–1½ inches.

Infant CPR
Same as adult, except:

1. Palpate brachial instead of carotid pulse.
2. Use only two fingers to compress the sternum ½–1 inch.
3. Compress at a point one finger width below the inter-nipple line.
4. Use only puffs of air, not full breaths.

PART III

Differential Diagnosis

Chapter 12

Rheumatology

Lawrence H. Wyatt, DC, DACBR, FICC

Introduction

Certainly, arthritis and related disorders are the most commonly encountered diseases in clinical chiropractic practice. Degenerative joint disease (DJD) probably accounts for fully half of the complaints of chiropractic patients. The study of connective tissue disorders is extensive, and this chapter is by no means exhaustive.

It is the purpose of this chapter to outline the more common rheumatologic disorders, including their etiology, diagnosis, and treatment, both medical and chiropractic. Disease categories as well as precise history and physical examination procedures are also outlined.

Classification of Rheumatologic Diseases

There are myriad rheumatologic diseases, each of which can be grouped into one of many categories. Table 12.1 gives the classification of the major joint diseases.

History

The key to the diagnosis of any connective tissue disorder is meticulous historical analysis. It is not an understatement to say that most diagnoses in this disease category can be made by proper history taking.

There are a number of questions that must be asked of all patients suspected of having a rheumatologic disease. The proper questions are illustrated below;

Table 12.1 Classification of Arthritides

- Inflammatory arthritides
  - Rheumatoid arthritis (RA)
  - Seronegative spondyloarthropathies (SNSA)
  - Ankylosing spondylitis (AS)
  - Reiter's syndrome
  - Arthritis associated with enteropathy
  - Arthritis associated with psoriasis
  - *Cis*-retinoic acid arthropathy
- Crystal deposition arthropathy (CDA)
  - Gouty arthritis
  - Calcium pyrophosphate arthropathy (pseudogout)
  - Hydroxyapatite deposition disease (HADD)
- Infection
  - Suppurative
  - Nonsuppurative
- Degenerative joint disease (DJD)
  - Primary osteoarthritis (primary OA)
  - Secondary osteoarthritis (secondary OA)
  - Traumatically induced DJD
- Connective tissue arthropathies (CTA)
  - Systemic lupus erythematosus (SLE)
  - Progressive systemic sclerosis (PSS) (scleroderma)
  - Polymyalgia rheumatica
- Miscellaneous
  - Erosive osteoarthritis (EOA)
  - Juvenile chronic arthritis (JCA)
- Non-inflammatory arthropathies
  - Diffuse idiopathic skeletal hyperostosis (DISH)
  - Ossification of posterior longitudinal ligament
  - Neuropathic arthropathy
  - Nonarticular rheumatism
- Endocrine diseases (with musculoskeletal complaints)
  - Hyperthyroidism
  - Hypothyroidism
  - Hyperparathyroidism
  - Cushing's syndrome
  - Pituitary disorders
  - Diabetes mellitus
- Fibromyalgia syndrome

diseases indicated by positive responses are noted parenthetically. It must be remembered that the diseases mentioned are generalizations and that there are some exceptions to these rules.

1. Sex of the patient?
   Female? (RA, primary/erosive OA, DJD)
   Male? (SNSA, DJD)
2. Is the disease monarticular? (infection, acute trauma [synovitis], chronic trauma [DJD], CDA)
3. Is the disease polyarticular? (inflammatory arthropathy, DJD, CTA)
4. Is the disease symmetric? (RA, CTA)

Asymmetric? (DJD, SNSA, CDA, traumatic arthropathy)

Other questions that can lead to a more exact etiology of the patient's complaint include:

1. Has the patient had a recent surgery (including tooth extraction) or is there a history of tuberculosis? (infection)
2. Has the patient had Crohn's disease, ulcerative colitis, or irritable bowel syndrome? (enteropathic arthritis)
3. Has the patient had urethritis, conjunctivitis, balanitis, or a sexually transmitted disease? (Reiter's syndrome)
4. Is there a history of skin disease? Psoriasis? (arthritis associated with psoriasis) Malar rash? (SLE)
5. Is there dysphagia? (DISH, PSS)
6. Is the patient diabetic? (neuropathic arthropathy, DISH)
7. Is the patient an alcoholic? (neuropathic arthropathy)
8. Is there a family history of arthritis?

Physical Examination

Physical examination of the joints and other connective tissues can also be very helpful in establishing a diagnosis. The following physical examination procedures should be performed on all rheumatology patients. Suggested diseases are noted below examination procedures.

1. Is there soft tissue swelling around the affected joint? If so, is it concentric? (inflammatory arthritis, infection) Eccentric? (gouty arthritis, HADD, amyloidosis)

2. Are there firm bony nodules around the joint? (DJD)
3. Is there redness and heat at the affected joint(s)? (infection)
4. Is there a cutaneous fistula with drainage? (infection, RA)
5. Is the patient febrile? (infection)
6. Is there inflammatory ocular disease? (AS, Reiter's syndrome)
7. Is there inflammatory anal disease? (enteropathic arthritis)
8. Are there scaly red lesions in the external auditory canal? (arthritis associated with psoriasis)
9. Are there subcutaneous nodules? (RA, HADD)
10. Is the disease primarily confined to the feet? (Reiter's syndrome, RA, gouty arthritis)
11. Is the disease primarily confined to the hands? (RA, primary OA, erosive OA, psoriatic arthritis)
12. Does the disease primarily involve:
    large joints? (DJD)
    small joints? (RA)
    spine? (SNSA)

Laboratory Investigation

The use of the clinical laboratory in the investigation of arthritides is almost requisite. In addition to standard admission protocols of a complete blood count and urinalysis, the following investigations are helpful in the rheumatology patient.

- Erythrocyte Sedimentation Rate (ESR)—This test is a nonspecific indicator of inflammation anywhere in the body. It can be used to monitor the progress of the disease and effectiveness of therapy.
- Rheumatoid Factor (RF)—This test is positive in most RA patients. High titres are frequently associated with more severe disease.
- Anti-nuclear Antibodies—The presence of these antibodies is most often times seen in SLE; however, this is a relatively nonspecific test.
- Anti-DNA Antibodies—This is a relatively specific test for SLE.
- LE Cell Prep—This test is expensive but beneficial in the diagnosis of SLE.
- HLA-B27—This antigen test is most frequently positive with the seronegative SNSA.

- HLA-DR4—This antigen test is not uncommonly seen in RA.
- Serum Glucose—Many patients with DISH will also have diabetes mellitus.

Radiographic Investigation

The following radiographic findings are helpful in the diagnosis of arthropathy; their particular suggested diseases are listed parenthetically.

1. Is there periarticular osteopenia?
   Yes? (RA, SLE)
   No? (SNSA, CDA, DJD)
2. Is there bone erosion?
   Yes? (RA, SNSA, gouty arthritis [late in the disease])
   No? (DJD, CTA)
3. Is there bone production?
   Yes? (DJD, SNSA)
   No? (RA, CTA, CDA)
4. Are there calcified soft tissue masses?
   Yes? (CDA)
5. Is there joint space narrowing?
   Concentric? (inflammatory arthritis)
   Eccentric? (DJD)
6. Is there osseous ankylosis of joint?
   Yes? (SNSA, RA [carpus/tarsus only], JCA)

Rheumatologic Diseases

The following is a summary of the more common rheumatologic diseases seen in chiropractic practice. The reader is referred to more in-depth texts for further study. Each of the disease outlines contains the following information: incidence (Incid:), etiology (Etiol:), pathogenesis (Path:), history (Hx:), physical examination (PE:), laboratory (Lab:), radiology (Rad:), and treatment (Tx:).

Rheumatoid Arthritis

Incid: Middle-aged females
Etiol: Unknown
Path: Pannus formation leading to joint destruction

Hx/PE/Lab: Four of these for >6 weeks is diagnostic
- Morning stiffness > one hour
- Soft tissue swelling (3 or more joints)
- Swelling of wrist, MCP, PIP joints
- Bilaterally symmetric arthritis
- Subcutaneous nodules
- Positive RF (+ HLA-DR4)
- Radiographic evidence of RA in the hands/wrist

Rad: Fusiform (concentric) soft tissue swelling
Periarticular osteopenia
Erosions of periarticular bone
Concentric loss of joint space
Subchondral cyst formation
Atlantoaxial instability
Facet joint erosions (cervical spine)

Tx: nonsteroidal anti-inflammatory drugs (NSAIDS), corticosteroids, gold, penicillamine, methotrexate, physical therapy

Ankylosing Spondylitis

Incid: Young males
Etiol: Unknown
Path: Pannus formation with joint destruction (less agressive than RA)
Hx: Low back pain (sacroiliac and thoracolumbar)
Progressive stiffness
Inflammatory ocular disease
PE: Decreased lumbar range of motion
Thoracic kyphosis
Lumbar hypolordosis
Decreased chest expansion
Aortic regurgitation
Uveitis/iritis
Lab: Positive HLA-B27
Elevated ESR
Negative RF
Rad: Bilaterally symmetric sacroilitis/fusion
Erosions at corners of vertebral bodies
Sclerosis at corners of vertebral bodies
Thin vertical syndesmophyte formation
Bony fusion
Tx: NSAIDs, corticosteroids, manipulation, physical therapy

Arthritis Associated with Psoriasis

Incid: 30–50 males and females
Etiol: Unknown
Path: Similar to AS
Hx: Psoriasis (arthritis can precede psoriasis)
Pain and stiffness (hands and thoracolumbar spine)
Nail deformity (pitting)
Inflammatory ocular disease
PE: Classic psoriatic skin lesions
Uveitis/iritis/keratoconjunctivitis
Decreased range of motion (hands and spine)
Nail pitting
Lab: Positive HLA-B27
Elevated ESR
Negative RF
Rad: Asymmetrical sacroilitis/fusion
Thick parasyndesmophytes
Vertebral fusion
DIP erosions (PIP/MCP also)
Terminal phalangeal sclerosis
Entirety of single digit involved
Periosteal reaction along the metacarpal shafts
Tx: NSAIDs, corticosteroids, manipulation, physical therapy

Reiter's Syndrome

Incid: Young males
Etiol: Unknown, but may occur after a sexually transmitted disease (e.g., gonorrhea)
Path: Similar to AS
Hx: Classic triad (urethritis, conjunctivitis, arthritis) balanitis, keratoderma Blennorrhagicum
Low back pain
PE: Usually confined to spine and lower extremity
Swelling of fingers/toes/heels
Decreased range of motion
Lab: Positive HLA-B27
Elevated ESR
Negative RF
Rad: Erosions at calcaneus/MTPs

	Assymmetric sacroiliac erosions/fusion
	Thick parasyndesmophytes
	Spinal fusion
	Periosteal reaction along the metatarsal shafts
Tx:	NSAIDs, corticosteroids, manipulation, physical therapy

Arthritis Associated with Enteropathy

Other than a history of inflammatory bowel disease, enteropathic arthritis can resemble any of the SNSAs.

Gouty Arthritis

Incid:	Middle-aged males
Etiol:	Synovial deposition of monosodium urate crystals
Path:	Crystals induce an inflammatory arthropathy
Hx:	Sudden onset of excruciating monarticular arthralgia
	Affects great toe most commonly (podagra)
	Lumps and bumps around affected joint(s)
	Fever/chills
	Alcohol abuse
PE:	Acutely inflamed joint with redness and swelling
	Periarticular soft tissue masses
	Soft tissue masses in the pinna of the ear
Lab:	Strongly negative birefringent crystals from joint aspirate under polarized light microscope
	Elevated ESR
	Negative RF/HLA-B27
	+/− Hyperuricemia
Rad:	Nonmarginal erosions of bone with overhanging edges
	Eccentric soft tissue masses (+/− calcification)
	Severe joint destruction
	May be 10–12 years before any radiographic findings
Tx:	Colchicine, allopurinol, NSAIDs, increased fluid intake (prevents gouty nephropathy), avoidance of alcohol, purine containing foods, caffeinated beverages, chocolate/cocoa

Calcium Pyrophosphate Crystal Deposition Disease

Incid:	Adults
Etiol:	Deposition of calcium pyrophosphate dihydrate crystals in joints
Path:	Crystals incude a destructive synovitis

Hx: Usually an acute monarthritis
Can be chronic pseudo-DJD pattern
Occurs in joints not usually affected by DJD
Pain/swelling/stiffness
PE: Similar to any inflammatory arthritis
Lab: Positively birefringent crystals from joint aspirate under polarized microscopy
+/− Elevated ESR
Negative RF
Negative HLA-B27
Rad: Chondrocalcinosis
DJD in a joint that does not normally have DJD
Tx: Joint aspiration, NSAIDs, manipulation, physical therapy

Hydroxyapatite Deposition Disease

Incid: Adult males and females
Etiol: Hydroxyapatite crystal deposition
Path: Crystal deposition in inflamed tendons and ligaments
Hx: Chronic tendinitis/bursitis/enthesitis
Old/chronic trauma
PE: Tender ligaments and/or tendons
+/− Palpate soft tissue mass in painful area
Lab: +/− Elevated ESR
Rad: Calcification in a tendon, ligament, or bursa
Tx: NSAIDs, physical therapy (especially ultrasound)

Degenerative Joint Disease

Incid: Older males and females
Etiol: Chronic "wear and tear"
Path: Dehydration, fibrillation, and degeneration of articular cartilage
Hx: Chronic pain and stiffness
Most common in spine and large joints of lower extremities
May cause signs and symptoms of spinal canal stenosis
Single joint is suggestive of traumatic induction
PE: Decreased range of motion
Periarticular bony nodules
+/− Mild swelling
Lab: Noncontributory in most cases
Rad: Eccentric loss of joint space

	Subchondral sclerosis
	Subchondral cyst formation
	Osteophyte formation
	Erosions in hands with EOA
Tx:	Manipulation, physical therapy, NSAIDs, surgery (arthroplasty, laminectomy, foraminotomy)

Diffuse Idiopathic Skeletal Hyperostosis (DISH)

Incid:	Middle-aged males
Etiol:	Unknown
Path:	Ossifying diathesis
Hx:	Chronic spinal stiffness
	+/− Pain
PE:	Decreased range of motion
	Altered spinal contours
Lab:	+/− Hyperglycemia
Rad:	Flowing anterolateral thick syndesmophytes that bridge vertebral bodies
	Relative preservation of disc heights
	Sparring of the facet joints
	+/− Ossification of the posterior longitudinal ligament
Tx:	Manipulation
	Physical therapy
	Exercise

Fibromyalgia Syndrome

Incid:	Female of childbearing age
Etiol:	Unknown
Path:	Fibrous infiltration of muscles
Hx:	Emotional stress
	Chronic fatigue
	Diffuse stiffness/pain
	Sleep disturbance
PE:	Palpation of the following points will elicit tenderness bilaterally:
	• Nuchal line of occiput
	• Mid-upper trapezius
	• Scapular insertion of the rhomboids
	• Pectoralis major at second costosternal area
	• Bicipital groove

- Distal to lateral epicondyle at the elbow
- Gluteus maximus at lateral iliac crest
- One-inch posterior to greater trochanter
- L4/L5 interspinous ligament
- Pes anserine bursa
- Gastrocnemius/Achilles tendon junction

The following control points should not be tender:

- Mid-forehead
- Mid-ventral forearm
- Thumbnail
- Anterior thigh musculature

Lab: Negative RF
Negative ANA/LE cell prep
Negative HLA-B27
Rad: Noncontributory
Tx: Manipulation
Physical therapy
NSAIDs

Chapter 13

Clinical Oncology

Lawrence H. Wyatt, DC, DACBR, FICC

Introduction

The diagnosis of cancer has, in past years, been associated with terminal illness. With recent advances in chemotherapy and radiation therapy, the mortality rates with certain types of cancers have become amazingly low. One of the most beneficial aspects of cancer therapy is early diagnosis. This chapter will explain some of the most widely used methods of screening for cancer in various organ systems and also the best diagnostic methods for determining whether a patient has cancer.

Screening Methods

Screening examinations must yield a significant amount of information that will benefit the patient, even if the disease is found early in its course. Table 13.1 lists cancer screening methods. They must also be reasonably priced. After all, the primary focus is to find disease when it is clinically asymptomatic. All of the recommendations in this section are taken from a compilation of a number of references.

Lung Cancer

One of the most widely used screening examinations in health care circles was the routine chest radiograph. The use of this tool as a screening method has been abandoned in recent years. There are no clinically reliable methods of screening for lung cancer.

Table 13.1 Cancer Screening Methods

Type of Cancer	Screening Method
Central nervous system	None available
Lung cancer	None available
Colon cancer	Rectal examination Endoscopy Hemoccult
Breast cancer	Self-examination Physician examination Mammogram
Prostate cancer	Rectal examination Ultrasound
Genital cancer (female)	Pelvic examination Ultrasound Pap smear
Genital cancer (male)	Self-examination Physician examination

Colon Cancer

It has been said that many colon malignancies should be palpable on digital rectal examination. For this reason, this examination should be performed in all patients over 40 years of age on a yearly basis. Testing for occult blood in the stool (stool guaiac) is recommended every year for all persons older than the age of 50, and sigmoidoscopy should be performed every 3–5 years in patients older than 50.

Breast Cancer

Second only to lung cancer, cancer of the breast is a leading cause of mortality in American females. Three types of examinations are useful. Self-examination of the breasts is recommended every month in all females older than age 20. Examination by a physician is recommended every three years in females 20–40 years of age and every year thereafter. Mammography, especially with the advent of low kilovoltage techniques, is again becoming popular. A baseline study should be performed between the ages of 35 and 39 and every year in all females older than 50. Frequency of mammograms between the ages of 40 and 49 should be every 1–2 years.

Female Genital Cancer

Uterine and ovarian cancers account for many deaths in females each year. A Pap test should be performed every three years in patients who have had two successive negative yearly examinations, and more often in high-risk females. This examination should begin at age 18 or when the patient becomes sexually active, whichever is earlier. Pelvic examination in females aged 20–40 should be performed every three years and then yearly in females older than 40.

Prostate

Prostate cancer is a common cancer in older men. Digital rectal examination, ultrasound, and prostate specific antigen are screening methods commonly used in practice.

Clinical Examination

The clinical examination is the first line of defense in the investigation of a patient with suspected cancer. Symptoms and signs that are indicative of cancer in each organ system are outlined below. Weight loss, malaise, and anorexia symptoms are found in almost all forms of cancer.

Bladder

A history of chronic cystitis along with a palpable suprapubic mass, suprapubic pain, and urethral discharge traditionally are found with bladder cancer.

Brain

Changes in personality, usually recognized by family members, and headaches are common signs of intracranial space-occupying lesions. Seizures that are focal (i.e., involve one limb or a single body region) are also ominous signs of a cerebral tumor. Visual field defects signify an intracranial mass; this type of defect also helps localize the mass. Loss of motor, bowel, and bladder control, syncope, and altered deep tendon reflexes may also signify brain tumors. The presence of pathologic reflexes is a sign of an upper motor neuron lesion as well.

Spinal Cord

Dermatomal defects, loss of motor control, altered deep tendon reflexes, and the presence of pathologic reflexes should prompt suspicion of an intracanalicular space-occupying mass.

Bone

The signs and symptoms that are most suggestive of osseous malignancy include deep unrelenting bone pain unrelieved by position or salicylates, and acute focal pain after minimal trauma, which is suggestive of pathologic fracture and diffuse skeletal pain.

Breast

A hard, immovable, nontender mass, especially located in the upper outer quadrant of the breast, with or without skin dimpling, nipple retraction and/or nipple discharge, and skin ulceration, should be regarded as malignant until proven otherwise. The presence of a family history positive for breast cancer should make the female patient regard any changes in the breast with suspicion.

Lung

The most unfortunate aspect of lung cancer is that it is usually asymptomatic until metastasis has already occurred. By that time, the prognosis for cure is poor. Signs and symptoms that are common to lung cancer include hemoptysis, cough, hoarseness, chest pain, and persistent or recurrent pneumonia.

Genital (Female)

Dysmenorrhea, dyspareunia, abnormal menstruation, a pelvic mass, vaginal discharge, a cervical mass, and a positive family history of genital cancer are strong indicators of cancer, especially in patients older than the age of 40.

Genital (Male)

The presence of testicular pain, penile discharge, dysuria, difficulty starting the urinary stream, and a nontender, hard scrotal mass should prompt suspicion of malignancy.

Colon

Colon cancer is a leading cause of death in older persons in the United States. Signs and symptoms consistent with this diagnosis include abdominal pain with or without a mass, bloating, alternating diarrhea and constipation, hematochezia, and melena.

Liver

Most forms of hepatic carcinoma are invasive and, as such, do not cause signs and symptoms until late in the course of the disease. When they are present, abdominal pain, jaundice (especially when painless), and hepatomegaly are ominous signs.

Pancreas

The classic triad of abdominal pain, jaundice, and weight loss are the most common findings associated with pancreatic carcinoma. Signs of duodenal obstruction can also be present.

Kidney

An abdominal mass, flank pain, and hematuria, especially when painless, should prompt an investigation for renal carcinoma.

Stomach

Gastric cancer, although not as commonly found in the United States as in the Far East, carries with it a poor prognosis. The appearance of epigastric pain, melena, bloody vomitus, a gastric ulcer that does not heal, and dyspepsia should be regarded with suspicion for malignant change.

Leukemia

Leukemia most often affects young persons. Signs and symptoms include ecchymoses, hepatosplenomegaly, pallor, fever, and lymphadenopathy.

Lymphoma

A relatively young patient with a relapsing fever lymphadenopathy (which is often times painful with the ingestion of alcohol), hepatosplenomegaly, an abdominal mass, and/or a Virchow's node should be investigated for the possibility of lymphoma.

Laboratory Investigation of Cancer

Although laboratory investigation of patients with suspected cancer is often nonspecific, it can be useful and can lead the physician to other more sensitive and specific diagnostic tests. The following is a list of some diagnostic tests that are helpful. Specific reference values should be sought from your particular laboratory.

- *Hemoccult*—Tests the patient's stool for the presence of blood; three consecutive positive tests are necessary for definitive diagnosis; helpful in the diagnosis of gastrointestinal malignancy

- *Carcinoembryonic Antigen*—Nonspecific but useful in the diagnosis of carcinoma of the colon, pancreas, lung and stomach; also increased in smokers and with hepatic and inflammatory bowel diseases
- *Alpha fetoprotein*—Nonspecific but useful in the diagnosis of hepatic carcinoma and testicular carcinoma

Table 13.2 Tests for Specific Malignancies

Type of Malignancy	Suggested Test
Skeletal	Calcium Alkaline phosphatase Acid phosphatase Prostate-specific antigen Serum protein electrophoresis Computerized tomography (CT) with contrast Magnetic resonance imaging (MRI) with contrast Radionuclide bone scan
Prostate	Acid phosphatase Prostate specific antigen Ultrasound MRI with contrast
Kidney	Urinalysis Complete blood count MRI with contrast
Reticuloendothelial	Complete blood count MRI with contrast
Colon	Hemoccult Complete blood count CEA CT with contrast
Central nervous system	MRI with contrast
Breast	Mammography MRI with contrast
Thyroid	Thyroid function tests Ultrasound MRI with contrast

- *Human Chorionic Gonadotropin*—Useful in the diagnosis of testicular tumors and choriocarcinoma; also elevated with pregnancy
- *Prostate Specific Antigen*—Useful in the diagnosis of prostate cancer but also elevated with benign prostatic hypertrophy in some cases
- *Alkaline Phosphatase*—Elevated with bone malignancy, especially blastic forms
- *Acid Phosphatase*—Elevated with prostate malignancy but also with other prostate diseases and medullary replacement disorders
- *Protein Electrophoresis*—Elevated albumin and gamma globulins are suggestive of multiple myeloma
- *White Blood Cell Count*—Nonspecific but severe elevation is suggestive of leukemia; Auer rods are seen with acute myelogenous leukemia
- *Calcium*—Increased with metastatic bone tumors but highly nonspecific
- *Complete Blood Count*—Nonspecific but can be an indicator of anemia and demonstrate specific cell types seen with certain malignancies

Table 13.2 lists diagnostic studies that can be performed when certain types of malignancies are suspected.

Diagnostic Imaging of Cancer

Although the plain film radiograph is the pillar of general clinical practice, it is usually of little help in the diagnosis of malignancy, especially in the early stages. Advanced imaging procedures such as radionuclide bone scanning, CT, and MRI are much more sensitive and specific methods in the investigation of cancer. The following list gives the most effective procedures for certain types of malignancies.

- *Skeletal Malignancy*—See Figure 13–1.
- *Lung Cancer*—See Figure 13–2. Plain film radiographs are not often diagnostic in early bronchogenic carcinoma.
- *Central Nervous System Malignancy*—MRI with contrast.
- *Hepatic, Pancreatic, Bladder, Colon, and Stomach Cancers*—CT with oral and intravenous contrast, MRI with contrast. Ultrasound and angiography can also be of some benefit in many cases.
- *Lymphomas*—CT with contrast, MRI with contrast.
- *Leukemias*—Usually require a combination of techniques, including plain film radiography, radionuclide bone scanning, CT, and MRI.

Figure 13–1 Investigation of Skeletal Malignancy

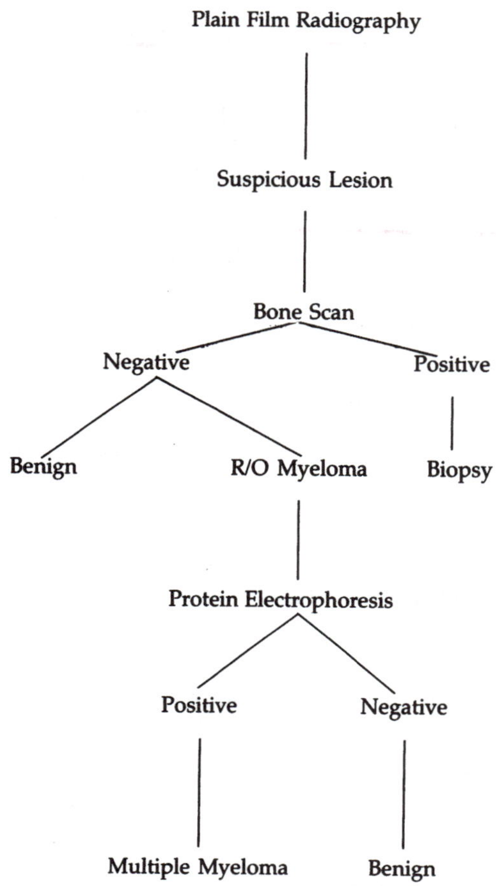

Selected Skeletal Tumors

Below are descriptions of selected skeletal tumors that may be seen in a chiropractic practice. Salient features of the tumors are italicized.

Malignant Bone Tumors

Multiple Myeloma

Incid: 45–75 years old, M:F 2:1, *especially African-American*

Path: bone marrow malignancy of plasmacytes

Figure 13–2 Investigation of Lung Cancer

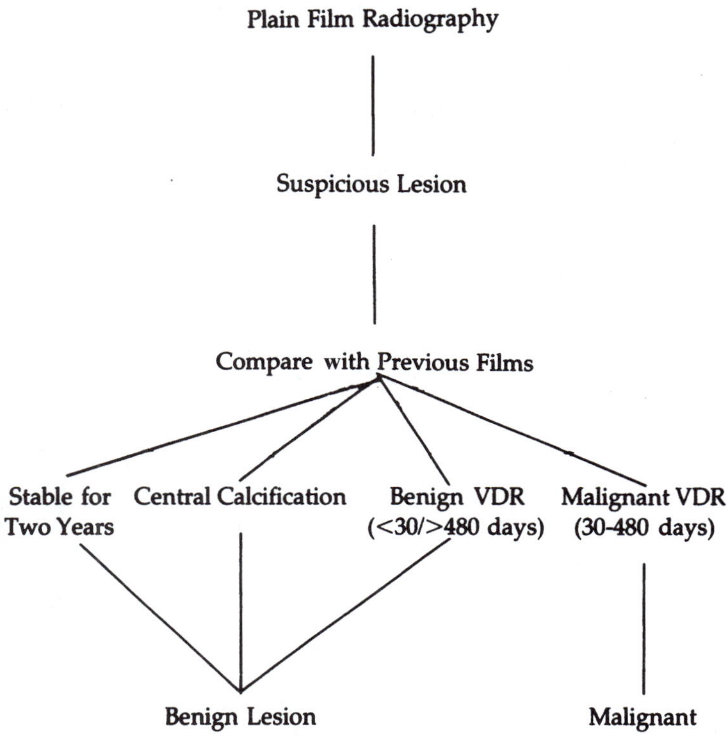

Note: **If the lesion is indeterminate but probably benign, re-x-ray at 1-, 3-, 6-, 9-, 12-, and 24-month intervals for changes suggestive of malignancy. (VDR = volume doubling rate)**

Hx: *insidious onset,* diffuse bone pain, spine pain, skull pain, pelvic pain, weight loss, fatigue, renal problems

PE: painful spine/skull/pelvis palpation, wasting, peripheral edema (renal disease), *may be very non-descript,* low-grade fever

Lab: *'M' spike on serum protein electrophoresis,* Bence Jones proteinuria, anemia

Loc: *spine,* skull, pelvis, long bones

X/R: *diffuse spinal osteopenia,* pathologic vertebral compression fractures, *spares pedicles in spine,* solitary bubbly lytic lesion, "punched-put" skull lesions, normal radiographs, metastatic calcifications to kidneys

Imag:	MRI (+C), CT (+C), bone scan (most often negative)
DDX:	lytic metastasis

Chordoma

Incid:	45–75 M
Path:	notochordal remnant malignant tumor
Hx:	*midline buttock pain,* headache, back pain, upper neck pain, *insidious onset*
PE:	+/− *palpable midline mass,* weight loss, fatigue
Lab:	N/A
Loc:	*sacrum,* cervicocranial region, clivus
X/R:	lytic lesion with large soft tissue mass, *may cross disc spaces,* +/− calcification
Imag:	MRI (+C), CT (+C)
DDX:	lytic/mixed metastasis, osteomyelitis, chondrosarcoma, giant cell tumor

Osteosarcoma

Incid:	dependent on cell type, osteogenic form is 10–25 years old, M>F
Path:	malignant osteocytes
Hx:	*Insidious onset* of pain around *knee,* hip, shoulder; may be a history of trauma but *pain out of proportion to trauma,* soft tissue mass, low-grade fever, chest pain, shortness of breath
PE:	localized pain, *soft tissue mass,* low-grade fever, *pulmonary findings*
Lab:	? alkaline phosphatase, +/− anemia
X/R:	large permeative lytic/blastic/mixed metaphyseal lesion with soft tissue mass, periosteal reaction (spiculated), *Codman's triangle*
Imag:	MRI (+C), CXR (metastasis), CT (+C+) chest (metastasis)
DDX:	*Ewing's sarcoma,* chondrosarcoma, lymphoma, leukemia, soft tissue sarcoma invading bone, *Paget's disease (older patient)*

Chondrosarcoma

Incid:	50–60, M:F 2:1
Path:	malignant chondrocytes, *low-grade tumors are most common primary type,* may occur in preexisting osteochondroma/enchondroma
Hx:	*insidious onset* of dull aching pain, +/− soft tissue mass, hip and pelvis most common, *pain in a preexisting enchondroma/osteochondroma*
PE:	localized pain, +/− soft tissue mass, low-grade fever
Lab:	N/A

X/R: permeative lytic lesion, *sometimes subtle;* hazy or speckled *calcification,* +/− soft tissue mass
Imag: CT (+C), MRI (+C)
DDX: osteosarcoma, osteochondroma, enchondroma, bone infarction

Fibrosarcoma

Incid: 15–30, M>F, may occur in much older patients as well (3-83)
Path: malignant fibrous tissue, low-grade and high-grade forms
Hx: *insidious onset* of pain around knee, ankle, hip, shoulder
PE: painful mass, may be diaphyseal, low-grade fever
Lab: N/A
X/R: permeative lytic/hazy metadiaphyseal lesion, +/− soft tissue mass, *fairly nondescript and can be subtle on plain films*
Imag: CT (+C), MRI (+C)
DDX: Ewing's sarcoma, osteosarcoma, lymphoma, leukemia

Ewing's Sarcoma

Incid: *5–20 year olds,* M>F; rare in African-Americans
Path: unknown etiology, thought to be reticulum marrow cells, *highly aggressive*
Hx: *mimics osteomyelitis,* high-grade fever, malaise, fatigue, weight loss, *insidious onset,* pain near *diaphysis of long bones*
Lab: elevated white blood cell count, anemia, erythrocyte sedimentation rate
X/R: permeative poorly-circumscribed diaphyseal long bone lesion with periosteal reaction
Imag: CT (+C), MRI (+C)
DDX: *osteomyelitis,* osteosarcoma

Giant Cell Tumor of Bone

Incid: 25–50 year olds, M>F
Path: quasi-malignant, locally aggressive, osteoclasts
Hx: *insidious onset,* localized pain around the knee, wrist, sacrum, ankle; +/− mass
Lab: N/A
X/R: expansible lytic *epiphyseal/subarticular* lesion, +/− periosteal reaction, +/− soft tissue mass
Imag: CT (+C), MRI (+C)
DDX: aneurysmal bone cyst, brown tumor of hyperparathyroidism

Lymphoma of Bone

Incid: 20–50, M>F
Path: metastasis/local invasion of soft tissue lymphoma
Hx: *insidious onset, lymphadenopathy,* splenomegaly, repeated infections; spine, knee, pelvis, rib pain
Lab: lymphocytosis, anemia, white blood cell count
X/R: *"ivory" vertebra(e),* permeative diaphyseal lesion in a long bone, +/− periosteal reaction, +/− soft tissue mass
Imag: CT (+C), MRI (+C)
DDX: fibrosarcoma, Ewing's sarcoma, Paget's disease, blastic metastasis

Benign Bone Tumors

Hemangioma

Incid: 40–70 year olds
Path: fatty/vascular lesion, *mc benign tumor of the spine*
Hx: asymptomatic unless expansile and puts pressure on other structures
Lab: N/A
X/R: *"corduroy cloth" appearance in spine,* uncommon in extremities
Imag: not usually necessary, radionuclide bone scan, CT (+C), MRI (+C)
DDX: osteoporosis, Paget's disease (when expansile)

Enostoma (Bone Island)

Incid: not age dependent
Path: hamartoma, no malignant potential; *osteopoikilosis* is the multiple form; also associated with *Maffucci's syndrome,* mc benign tumor of the skeleton
Hx: asymptomatic
Lab: N/A
X/R: well-circumscribed blastic lesion typically around hips, edges look like a rose thorn; *can be confused with blastic metastasis*
Imag: radionuclide bone scan to rule out metastasis
DDX: blastic metastasis

Osteochondroma (Exostosis)

Incid: 5–65
Path: osteoid base with a cartilaginous cap, minimal *malignant potential when closer to the axial skeleton* and when multiple lesions associated with hereditary multiple exostosis are present

Hx: asymptomatic unless fractured or putting pressure on another regional structure
Lab: N/A
X/R: sessile-broad-based expansile eccentric cortical metaphyseal expansion with calcifications; pedunculated-narrow-based eccentric cortical metaphyseal expansion with calcified cauliflower-like "cap"; any change over time should be suspicious for malignant transformation
Imag: usually not necessary, radionuclide bone scan, MRI (+C) used to find malignant degeneration
DDX: N/A

Enchondroma

Incid: 15–25 year olds
Path: benign chondrocytic tumor cells with fibrous matrix, associated with enchondromatosis (*Ollier's disease*)
Hx: *asymptomatic unless fractured or undergoing malignant transformation* (risk increases with locations closer to axial skeleton)
Lab: N/A
X/R: centrally located expansile lytic lesion *with calcification*
Imag: usually not necessary unless concerned with fracture or malignant degeneration, radionuclide bone scan, CT (+C), MRI (+C)
DDX: bone infarction, low-grade chondrosarcoma

Chondroblastoma

Incid: 10–30 year olds
Path: benign tumor of chondroblasts that *can invade and cross growth plates of epiphyses and apophyses,* mc tumor of the patella, said to be the adolescent form of giant cell tumor
Hx: *insidious onset* of pain near a joint or an apophysis
Lab: N/A
X/R: well-circumscribed lytic ovoid lesion near/crossing a growth plate, calcification is common
Imag: not usually necessary
DDX: giant cell tumor

Chondromyxoid Fibroma

Incid: 10–20 year olds
Path: benign myxoid and chondroid tumor with fibrous tissue intermingled; may invade growth plate
Hx: *insidious onset* of pain around a joint (knee), high recurrence rate

Lab: N/A
X/R: eccentric, sometimes-loculated, lytic lesion without calcification but with a sclerotic rim in the metaphysis of a long bone
Imag: usually not necessary
DDX: chondrosarcoma, chondroblastoma, aneurysmal bone cyst, fibroxanthoma

Osteoma

Incid: adolescents, rare tumor
Path: hamartoma, may be seen with multiple colonic polyps in Gardner's Syndrome
Hx: asymptomatic unless it obstructs ostium of a sinus
Lab: N/A
X/R: homogenous blastic lesion typically seen in the skull/sinuses
Imag: unsually not necessary, CT of sinuses to rule out obstruction
DDX: N/A

Osteoblastoma

Incid: any age group, mc in 15–25 year olds
Path: benign tumor of osteoblasts
Hx: *painful scoliosis,* long bone (femur) pain, *insidious onset,* +/− night pain
Lab: N/A
X/R: expansile lytic lesion mc in posterior vertebral arch, metaphyseal in long bones
Imag: CT (+C), MRI (+C)
DDX: aneurysmal bone cyst, osteoid osteoma

Osteoid Osteoma

Incid: 10–25 year olds, rare in patients older than 40
Path: central vascular nidus surrounded by sclerotic reactive bone, tumor will recur if nidus not removed, occasionally self-resolving
Hx: *painful scoliosis, insidious onset* of long bone (knee) pain, fever, *night pain, relieved by aspirin*
Lab: N/A
X/R: central lytic nidus (often obscured) surrounded by thick rim of sclerosis, *sclerotic pedicle*
Imag: radionuclide bone scan, CT (+C), MRI (+C)
DDX: osteoblastoma, Brodie's abscess

Simple Bone Cyst (Unicameral Bone Cyst)

Incid: 4–15 year olds
Path: epithelium-lined fluid filled cyst of bone, no malignant potential
Hx: asymptomatic unless fractured
Lab: N/A
X/R: lytic, centrally-located, metaphyseal lesion; may see a "fallen fragment" from a fracture in the dependent portion of the cyst that will move with patient position, migrates down shaft of bone as child reaches adulthood
Imag: N/A
DDX: aneurysmal bone cyst, enchondroma

Aneurysmal Bone Cyst

Incid: 10–20 year olds, uncommon after 30
Path: proliferation of vascular tissue that forms a lining around a blood-filled cystic lesion, can be associated with minor regional trauma, no malignant potential, *grows very rapidly*
Hx: rapid onset of pain around knee, hip or shoulder and sometimes in the spine, +/− palpable mass, *painful scoliosis*
X/R: highly expansile, rapidly growing, lytic metaphyseal lesion with very thin outer cortex, +/− periosteal reaction; expansile lytic posterior arch lesion in the spine
Imag: usually not necessary
DDX: giant cell tumor, osteoblastoma, chondroblastoma

Fibroxanthoma (Fibrous Cortical Defect, Nonossifying Fibroma)

Incid: 4–20 year olds
Path: benign fibrous tumor that eventually *ossifies with skeletal maturity*, very common childhood lesion
Hx: asymptomatic unless fractured, which is rare
X/R: eccentric hazy lesion with thick sclerotic rim, long axis of the lesion parallels long axis of the bone
Imag: not necessary
DDX: fibrous dysplasia, chondromyxoid fibroma

Fibrous Dysplasia

Incid: 10–40 year olds
Path: monostotic and polyostotic forms, misplaced dysplastic fibrous tissue that often causes bone deformity; polyostotic form associated with

precocious puberty and *café au lait* skin pigmentation in young girls (Albright's syndrome)

Hx: asymptomatic unless causing bone deformity or fracture occurs; occasionally painful

X/R: eccentric hazy long lesions that *parallel the long axis of long bones;* diaphyseal location, *shepherd's crook deformity* of proximal femur; also occurs in flat bones; *great imitator of bone disease*

Imag: radionuclide bone scan determines if lesions are active

DDX: fibrous bone tumors, Paget's disease, practically any bone lesion

Glossary of Oncology Terms

Adenocarcinoma: malignant tumor of glandular tissue

Adenoma: benign tumor of epithelial tissue

Anaplasia: lack of differentiation characteristic of a cancer cell

Angioma: a knot of atypically and irregularly arranged dilated vessels

Benign: a mass that does not metastasize and is cured by removal

Carcinoma: malignant tumor of epithelial cells

Carcinoma *in situ:* epithelial cancer confined to the site of origin without invading neighboring tissues

Chemotherapy: treatment of cancer by means of chemicals that selectively destroy rapidly developing and/or cancer cells

Cyst: epithelium-lined fluid-filled cavity

Dysplasia: preneoplastic abnormal cell growth, with disordered cellular orientation, atypical cellular morphology, increased cell proliferation, and reduced cellular maturation

Glioma: neuroectodermal tumor of neuroglial origin (e.g., astrocytoma) that invades adjacent neural tissue but does not metastasize

Hamartoma: tumor-like but nonneoplastic overgrowth of tissue that is disordered in structure

Hyperplasia: an increase in the number of normal cells in normal arrangement in a tissue

Hypertrophy: enlargement of a tissue secondary to an increase in the size of its cells

Leiomyoma: benign smooth muscle tumor, also known as a fibroid

Lipoma: benign tumor of adipose tissue

Malignant: a mass that spreads and invades other tissues, particularly those at a distance from the primary organ of origin

Metaplasia: change in the type of adult cells in a tissue to a form that is not normal for that tissue

Metastasis: the transfer of disease from one organ to another not directly connected with it

Neoplasia: abnormal new growth

Oncogene: mutated version of a normal gene that can convert a cell into a tumor cell

Papilloma: benign tumor of epithelial cells (e.g., wart)

Primary tumor: the mass of tumor cells at the original site of the neoplasm

Remission: complete or partial disappearance of the signs and symptoms of disease in response to treatment; not necessarily a cure

Sarcoma: malignant tumor of connective tissue cells

Secondary tumor: a tumor that is the result of metastasis

Tumor: an abnormal mass of tissue, which performs no useful function, that results from excessive cell division that is uncontrolled and progressive (aka, neoplasm)

Chapter 14

Spine Pain

Lawrence H. Wyatt, DC, DACBR, FICC

Introduction

One of the most important tasks for the chiropractic physician is to accurately diagnose the cause of a patient's neck or back pain. The list of diseases that can cause pain of this type is almost endless. This chapter describes the most common causes of spine pain, both within and outside the spinal column.

Structural Spinal Landmarks

Several landmarks are helpful in isolating which vertebral level is actually being palpated. The following is a list of those landmarks with the vertebral level noted parenthetically.

- First palpable spinous process (C2)
- Hyoid bone (C3)
- Thyroid cartilage (C4-5)
- Cricoid cartilage (C6)
- Spine of the scapula (T3)
- Inferior angle of the scapula (T7)
- Umbilicus (T10)
- Iliac crest (L4)
- Posterior superior iliac spine (S2)

Spinal Biomechanics

Facet Planar Motions

Motion through the facet joints is different dependent upon which spinal region one is evaluating. The following list delineates the various planes and motions of each spinal region based upon its facet morphology.

- Cervical spine–facets are oriented in the transverse plane allowing rotation
- Thoracic spine–facets are oriented in the coronal plane allowing lateral flexion
- Lumbar spine (L1-4)–facets are oriented in the sagittal plane allowing flexion and extension
- Lumbosacral (L5-S1)–facets are oriented in the coronal plane allowing lateral flexion

Coupled Motions

All motions of the spine are coupled to some degree. The following list outlines those coupled motions.

- lateral flexion is coupled with rotation
  –spinous processes rotate into the convexity in the cervical and upper thoracic spine
  –spinous processes rotate into the concavity in the lower thoracic and lumbar spine
- flexion is coupled with anterior translation
- extension is coupled with posterior translation
- rotation is coupled with lateral flexion

Vertebrogenic Spine Pain

The following is a list of intrinsic spine disorders that can result in pain in the spine or paraspinal regions. Table 14.1 lists common vertobrogenic causes of spine pain.

Arthritides

- *Ankylosing Spondylitis (AS)*—This disease begins by causing pain in the sacroiliac joints (sacroiliitis), usually bilaterally and symmetrically, and then progresses to the thoracolumbar spine, and then cephalically and

Table 14.1 Common Vertebrogenic Causes of Spine Pain

Arthritides	**Infectious**
AS	Brucellosis
DDD	Coccidioidomycosis
DISH	E. coli.
Aseptic diskitis	Pseudomonas
Enteropathic arthritis	Tuberculosis
Facet arthrosis	Facet arthrosis
Psoriatic arthritis	**Metabolic**
Reiter's syndrome	Hyperparathyroidism
RA	Osteoporosis
Biomechanical	**Miscellaneous**
Hypermobility	Paget's disease
Hypomobility	Trauma
Functional spinal lesion	Disc bulge/HNP
Developmental	Fracture/dislocation
Basilar invagination	Facet syndrome
Block vertebrae	Spondylolisthesis
Arnold-Chiari	Fibrous dysplasia
Dysplasias	Sprain/strain
Transitional segments	**Tumors**
Miscellaneous	Benign
	Malignant

caudally from that point forward eventually resulting in osseous spinal fusion with a classic forward flexed fixed posture and a short shuffling gait.

- *Degenerative Disc Disease (DDD)*—Chronic, dull, achy pain is the hallmark of DDD. Patients are most often stiff when first arising from recumbency but the stiffness subsides with movement. Pain can be radiating in cases when spinal canal/lateral recess/neural foramen stenosis has developed, but can improve with a flexed posture, such as when riding a bicycle.
- *Diffuse Idiopathic Skeletal Hyperostosis (DISH)*—The pain of this disease is mild and nonspecific in most cases. If ossification of the posterior longitudinal ligament (seen more commonly in diabetics) is also present, signs of spinal canal stenosis can prevail.

- *Diskitis (aseptic)*—Often found in young persons, this disease most often presents with moderate to severe focal thoracic spine pain. A calcified disc may be noted radiographically.
- *Enteropathic Arthritis*—The pain pattern of this disease is similar to AS, although lower extremity complaints are more common and the disease tends to be bilateral but asymmetrical.
- *Osteoarthritis of the Facet Articulations*—Local pain at the level(s) of degeneration along with radiating pain, usually not beyond the elbow or knee, are the common presentations. Extension aggravates the pain. It may eventually lead to foraminal stenosis with radiculopathy.
- *Psoriatic Arthritis*—Again, pain pattern is similar to AS, but concomitant hand pain is also seen. This disease also tends to be bilateral but asymmetrical. Skin psoriasis is seen in 85% of patients.
- *Reiter's Syndrome*—Pain in the heels and feet usually accompany low back and sacroiliac pain. The disease is bilateral but asymmetrical. Classic triad of symptoms is conjunctivitis/iritis ("can't see"), urethritis ("can't pee"), and arthritis in the foot ("can't dance with me").
- *Rheumatoid Arthritis (RA)*—Most often this disease involves chronic pain, with periodic acute exacerbations, in the cervical spine. Basilar invagination is a significant concern in these patients. It occasionally causes unilateral sacroiliitis. Fusion of the spine is fibrous, except in the juvenile form (Juvenile Chronic Arthritis) where bony fusion is the rule.

Biomechanical

- *Intervertebral Hypermobility*—Pain can be localized to a single level or may radiate, but not usually below mid-extremity. May result in instability.
- *Intervertebral Hypomobility*—Pain is similar to hypermobility except that stiffness accompanies the pain.
- *Myofascitis*—Muscle pain adjacent to the spine is common with many of the diseases in this category. The pain may radiate and simulate radiculopathy/visceral disease patterns when trigger points are present.
- *Spinal Joint Dysfunction*—This lesion can cause focal or diffuse spine pain, radiating pain not below the elbow or knee, and/or referred pain simulating visceral disease.

Developmental

- *Basilar Invagination*—The pain of this condition is usually suboccipital in nature, but there may be referral of the pain into the extremities and down the spine as well. It may also be seen secondary to trauma and inflammatory arthritis.

- *Block Vertebrae*—The hypermobility above and below a synostotic segment can cause pain, as other forms of hypermobility can.
- *Congenital Dysplasias*—(e.g., Marfan's syndrome). The pain seen with these diseases is dependent upon the disease present and its severity.
- *Lumbosacral Transitional Segments*—Although pain from this anomaly is no more common than in those without the anomaly, occasionally focal lumbosacral pain, with or without radiation, can occur. Patients with a unilateral pseudoarthrosis are at increased risk of developing a disc protrusion at L4-5. The pain from this anomaly can be very confusing, however.
- *Miscellaneous Vertebral Anomalies*—(e.g., hemivertebra). Pain patterns are dependent upon the anomaly present.
- *Occipitocervical Transitional Segments*—Just as with lumbosacral transitional segments, the pain pattern can be very confusing. It can cause focal spine pain, radiating pain, and even headaches.

Infectious

- *Coccidioidomycosis*—The pain of this fungus is usually localized to an apophysis. The lungs are the primary route of infections, and the spine becomes involved when there is dissemination.
- *E. coli.*—This infection can result from septicemia from another infection or in drug abusers.
- *Pseudomonas*—This is another infection seen in intravenous drug abusers. Pain is insidious in onset and chronic in nature.
- *Tuberculosis*—Tuberculosis of the spine can be very devastating, with severe destruction of the discs and vertebrae and a resultant gibbous deformity.

Metabolic

- *Hyperparathyroidism*—The pain from this condition is usually located in the sacroiliac joints; however, when there is bone resorption in the vertebral bodies, pain is felt there as well.
- *Osteoporosis*—Osteoporosis becomes especially painful when compression fractures occur, although infractions (microfractures) of the endplates are painful as well.

Miscellaneous

- *Fibrous Dysplasia*—This lesion is usually painless unless there has been a pathologic fracture. Polyostotic forms of the disease can be painful by themselves.
- *Paget's Disease*—The pain of Paget's disease is usually chronic and may become acute if there is a pathologic fracture.

Trauma

- *Disc Bulge*—Focal pain, many times with radiation to the extremities, is the hallmark presentation.
- *Disc Protrusion/Extrusion/Sequestration*—Focal back or neck pain without dermatomal radiation to the hands or feet is the most common presentation. Radiculopathy can result, although this is quite uncommon ($<5\%$ of cases). The cauda equina syndrome can be the result of a large central disc herniation.
- *Dislocation*—Acute focal pain, with myelopathy if there is instability, is the rule.
- *Facet Syndrome (synovitis)*—Focal pain at the level of involvement with radiation to the knee or elbow is common. There may also be a pseudovisceral referral pattern as well.
- *Fracture*—Pain is very similar to a dislocation. Pain also tends to be in the midline.
- *Spondylolisthesis*—The pain of this lesion is oftentimes an enigma. No specific pain pattern is extremely common, but bilateral buttock pain is not uncommon.
- *Sprain/Strain*—Focal muscular and vertebral pain is most common, although there can be some mild radiation of the pain.

Tumors

- *Benign Tumors*—The pain of benign spinal tumors is usually focal and unless the tumor is expansible and causes spinal canal stenosis, there is little or no radiation of pain. Types of benign tumors include aneurysmal bone cyst, giant cell tumor (quasimalignant), osteoblastoma, and osteoid osteoma, and hemangioma (most common/rarely painful).
- *Malignant Tumors*
  Chordoma—The pain from this tumor is usually localized to the sacrum, as this is the most common location in the spine.

Metastasis—The pain of this condition can be focal or diffuse depending upon the extent of the disease. In either event, the pain is chronic and unrelieved by changes in position.
Multiple Myeloma—The pain of this reticuloendothelial malignancy is very similar to the pain of metastasis.

Referred Spine Pain

There are a number of nonspinal disorders that may refer pain to the spine and paraspinal structures. This clinical presentation can be quite confusing. When the clinician is directed to a pattern of referred pain from the history and physical examination, the following list of differential diagnoses, grouped by the region to which each of them refers pain, will be helpful. (These are summarized in Table 14.1.)

Cervical Spine

- *Brain Lesions*—All of these lesions cause diffuse pain referred to the cervical spine. Spinal stiffness may accompany infection and hemorrhage, as well. Causes of brain lesions include arteriovenous malformations, aneurysm, cerebrovascular accident, infection, subarachnoid hemorrhage, subdural hematoma, and tumors.
- *Coronary Artery Disease* (CAD)—The pain of myocardial ischemia is usually referred to the left neck and jaw.
- *Dental Caries/Periodontal Abscess*—Pain is usually referred to the upper cervical spine.
- *Esophageal Disease*—The location of pain is dependent upon the location of the esophageal lesion.
- *Laryngeal/Pharyngeal Disease*—Pain can be referred to anywhere in the cervical region.
- *Lymphadenopathy*—Focal pain is usually noted in the area of the enlarged lymph nodes.
- *Pancoast's Tumor*—Cervicothoracic pain is usually the rule.
- *Temporomandibular Joint Disease*—Just as with many other disorders, the pain referral pattern is nonspecific.

Thoracic Spine

- *Aortic Aneurysm*—Mid-back pain, severe with a dissecting type, is most often seen.

- *Congestive Heart Failure*—This can, but does not often, refer pain to the thoracic region.
- *Coronary Disease*—Pain referred to the mid-back is not uncommon.
- *Gallbladder Disease*—Pain is usually referred to the right paraspinal region near the tip of the scapula.
- *Herpes Zoster*—A dermatomal referral pattern associated with the level involved is the traditional pattern.
- *Hiatal Hernia*—Dull achy pain can be referred to the mid-back.
- *Kidney Disease*—Pain is usually felt in the costovertebral angle(s).
- *Lung Diseases*—Any lung disease can refer pain to the thoracic region. Such diseases can include malignancy, pneumonia, and mediastinal masses.
- *Pancreatic Disease*—These lesions usually refer straight through to the lower thoracic region. The pain can be very severe. Such diseases can include malignancy, pancreatitis, and pseudocyst.
- *Peptic Ulcer Disease*—This condition can cause sharp pain in the lower thoracic region.
- *Rib Lesions*—Lesions of the posterior ribs, such as from fractures or tumors, can result in local and radiating spine pain.
- *Spinal Cord Tumor*—Focal pain at the affected level and radiating pain above and, more commonly, below the lesion are common.

Lumbar Spine

- *Aortic Aneurysm*—Focal or diffuse pain in the region of the dilatation are not uncommon.
- *Colorectal Cancer*—Referred pain to the paraspinal regions is not unheard of.
- *Endometriosis*—The referred pain of endometriosis is dependent upon the location of the lesions.
- *Hip Disease*—These lesions can refer pain to the low back.
- *Kidney Disease*—Pain is usually noted at the costovertebral angle(s). Causes can include infection, stones, and tumors.
- *Ovarian Disease*—These conditions can refer dull, achy pain to the low back and pelvis.
- *Pelvic Inflammatory Disease*—Just as with endometriosis, the referral pattern is dependent upon the location of the disease.

- *Pregnancy*—Low back and sacroiliac pain from ligamentous laxity are relatively common sequelae of pregnancy.
- *Short Leg Syndrome*—Pain patterns are nonspecific but are usually due to altered biomechanics in the low back.
- *Spinal Cord Tumors*—Focal pain, with or without radiation, is not uncommon. The tumors can be gliomas, meningiomas, or metastatis.
- *Uterine Cancer*—Dull, achy low back and pelvic pain is not uncommon.

Mimicry Syndromes

It has been estimated that at least 33% of somatic symptoms are medically unexplained, and these symptoms are chronic or recurrent in approximately 25% of patients. Some estimates are even higher. (1) These authors suggest that the most common medically unexplained symptoms are in the gynecological signs and symptoms. They also suggest that psychiatric morbidity is not associated with these symptom complexes. These patients also tend to seek out alternative medicine approaches to what they feel are real physical ailments.

Mimicry syndromes are those constellations of symptoms that are thought to be caused by or associated with visceral diseases, but instead are caused by some other disorder, oftentimes musculoskeletal in origin.

The diagnosis of these conditions can be difficult and the patient can suffer while a well-intentioned treatment is ineffective and inappropriate. Some have suggested that these syndromes may simply be psychological manifestations of depression and anxiety, but the literature is inconclusive regarding this assertion with some authors failing to find a consistent connection. (2)

Abnormal spinal postures, such as the Straight Back Syndrome, and myofascial conditions, such as trigger points, are two conditions that can cause symptoms that are easily confused with more typical visceral diseases. These two conditions and others are discussed below.

Chronic Pelvic Pain Syndrome (CPPS)

Probably the most studied mimicry syndrome is CPPS. While chronic pain in the pelvis can certainly be caused by visceral disease in the abdomen and pelvis, there are recognized musculoskeletal abnormalities that can result in similar findings. These patients may be diagnosed with prostatitis, endometriosis, ovarian cysts, bladder dysfunction, and many other visceral diseases. These patients will not respond to medical therapy for those diseases, however. A clinical search for a musculoskeletal cause should be undertaken in these patients.

Patients with a musculoskeletal cause for CPPS have been demonstrated to have muscle spasm and pain in the levator ani, coccygeus, and psoas and groin muscles as well. (3) Men with the condition have also been found to have pain sensitization in the perineal region. (4) Some have suggested that in men with CPPS, bacterial invasion of the prostate gland could have been responsible for pain, but this has not been found clinically. (5) High white blood cell urine counts have also been shown to be as prevalent in controls as in patients with CPPS. (6)

There is preliminary evidence that manipulation and massage can be beneficial for certain cases of CPPS. (7, 8) Acupuncture has also demonstrated some effectiveness (9) as has neuromuscular reeducation, including pelvic floor muscle exercise. (10) Similar interventions have demonstrated success in the urethral syndrome and interstitial cystitis. (11)

Other poorly explained pelvic pain syndromes such as vulvodynia, orchialgia, urethral syndrome, penile pain, prostatodynia, coccygodynia, perineal pain, proctodynia, and proctalgia fugax have reportedly responded to a multidisciplinary approach, including physical medicine procedures, in anecdotal reports. (12) The authors suggest that conservative measures are appropriate, after serious pathological causes have been excluded for these syndromes. They suggest exercising caution when considering more invasive and often irreversible therapeutic procedures.

The following conditions can result in pain referral and signs and symptoms that mimic visceral disease.

Cervical Spine Dysfunction

- angina pectoris
- vertigo
- dizziness
- unsteadiness
- ocular disease
- otologic disease

Thoracic Spine Dysfunction

- angina pectoris
- dyspepsia
- gastritis
- gastroesophageal reflux disease

- peptic ulcer disease
- renal disease/colic
- pulmonary disorders (e.g., pleurisy, shortness of breath)

Lumbar Spine Dysfunction

- gynecological problems
- abdominal pain
- renal disease/colic
- gallbladder disease (cholelithiasis, cholecystitis)

SI joint dysfunction

- gynecological disorders
- prostate disorders
- sciatica

Trigger Points (with Muscle Generators)

- dizziness
- unsteadiness
- nausea
- renal colic
  –serratus posterior, quadratus lumborum, iliocostalis thoracic
- gynecologic disorders
  –external oblique, rectus abdominus, iliopsoas, iliocostalis thoracic
- headache
  –splenius capitis, trapezius, occipitalis, suboccipitals, sternocleidomastoid muscle (SCM), frontalis
- otitis
  –SCM
- toothache
  –masseter, temporalis
- temporomandibular joint disease
  –medial/lateral pterygoid
- sinusitis
  –SCM, frontalis, orbicularis oculi, frontalis, zygomaticus major
- angina pectoris
  –pectoralis major/minor, sternalis, scalenes, subclavius, external oblique

- mastitis
  –pectoralis major/minor, sternalis
- internal joint derangement (e.g., labral tear)
  –specific to body region
- sciatica
  –piriformis, biceps femoris, adductor longus, gluteus maximus/minimus
- carpal tunnel syndrome
  –opponens pollicis, adductor pollicis
- gallbladder disease (cholecystitis, cholelithiasis)
  –iliopsoas, external oblique
- pulmonary disease (e.g., pleurisy, shortness of breath)
  –pectoralis major/minor, external oblique
- abdominal pain (appendicitis, diverticulitis)
  –iliocostalis thoracis, external oblique
- orchitis
  –iliopsoas, external oblique

It is important to remember that visceral diseases can cause referral patterns similar to those noted above. An initial clinical search for primary visceral disease is critical to ascertaining whether a patient is suffering from visceral disease or a mimicry syndrome.

References

1. Nimnuan, C., Hotopf, M., & Wessely, S. Medically unexplained symptoms: an epidemiological study in seven specialities. *J Psychosom Res.* 2001 Jul;51(1):361–367.
2. Henningsen, P., Zimmermann, T., & Sattel, H. Medically unexplained physical symptoms, anxiety, and depression: a metaanalytic review. *Psychosom Med.* 2003 Jul–Aug;65(4):528–533.
3. Hetrick, D.C., Ciol, M.A., Rothman, I., Turner, J.A., Frest, M., & Berger, R.E. Musculoskeletal dysfunction in men with chronic pelvic pain syndrome type III: a case-control study. *J Urol.* 2003 Sep;170(3):828–831.
4. Yang, C.C., Lee, J.C., Kromm, B.G., Ciol, M.A., & Berger, R.E. Pain sensitization in male chronic pelvic pain syndrome: why are symptoms so difficult to treat? *J Urol.* 2003 Sep;170(3):823–826; discussion 826–827.
5. Lee, J.C., Muller, C.H., Rothman, I., Agnew, K.J., Eschenbach, D., Ciol, M.A., Turner, J.A., & Berger, R.E. Prostate biopsy culture findings of men with chronic pelvic pain syndrome do not differ from those of healthy controls. *J Urol.* 2003 Feb;169(2):584–587; discussion 587–588.

6. Nickel, J.C., Alexander, R.B., Schaeffer, A.J., Landis, J.R., Knauss, J.S., & Propert, K.J. Chronic Prostatitis Collaborative Research Network Study Group. Leukocytes and bacteria in men with chronic prostatitis/chronic pelvic pain syndrome compared to asymptomatic controls. *J Urol.* 2003 Sep;170(3):818–822.
7. Hawk, C., Long, C., & Azad, A. Chiropractic care for women with chronic pelvic pain: a prospective single-group intervention study. *J Manipulative Physiol Ther.* 1997 Feb;20(2):73–79.
8. Sinaki, M., Merritt, J.L., & Stillwell, G.K. Tension myalgia of the pelvic floor. *Mayo Clin Proc.* 1977 Nov;52(11):717–722.
9. Chen, R., & Nickel, J.C. Acupuncture ameliorates symptoms in men with chronic prostatitis/chronic pelvic pain syndrome. *Urology.* 2003 Jun;61(6):1156–1159; discussion 1159.
10. Clemens, J.Q., Nadler, R.B., Schaeffer, A.J., Belani, J., Albaugh, J., & Bushman, W. Biofeedback, pelvic floor reeducation, and bladder training for male chronic pelvic pain syndrome. *Urology.* 2000 Dec 20;56(6):951–955.
11. Weiss, J.M. Pelvic floor myofascial trigger points: manual therapy for interstitial cystitis and the urgency-frequency syndrome. *J Urol.* 2001 Dec;166(6):2226–2231.
12. Wesselmann, U., Burnett, A.L., & Heinberg, L.J. The urogenital and rectal pain syndromes. *Pain.* 1997 Dec;73(3):269–294.

Chapter 15
Clinical Conditions

Lawrence H. Wyatt, DC, DACBR, FICC

Introduction

The typical chiropractic practice focuses on the management of neuromusculoskeletal (NMS) conditions and the NMS comorbidities of other conditions. This chapter will outline some of the more common and/or ominous conditions seen in a chiropractic office. The conditions are listed alphabetically.

Abdominal Aortic Aneurysm

Incid; Etiol: >50 y/o; atherosclerosis, hypertension, trauma

Dx: >3.5 cm on plain film radiography, 90% are infrarenal, abdominal/back pain **unrelieved by position changes,** cold lower extremities, loss of distal pulses, abdominal bruit, pulsatile abdominal mass, lower extremity vascular claudication signs/symptoms

DDx: neurogenic claudication, cauda equina syndrome, bowel obstruction, pancreatitis, kidney stone

Rx: 3.5–5.0 cm and asymptomatic - careful observation; 5.0–7.0 cm and asymptomatic-elective surgery; >7.0 cm or symptomatic - nonelective surgery; high velocity manipulation is contraindicated

Achilles Tendinopathy

Incid; Etiol: active children, adults; trauma, poorly conditioned individuals, over-training, antibiotic use (especially fluoroquinolones (ciprofloxacin)) predisposes to tears

Dx: localized burning/pain, swelling, crepitation, pain with resisted and active plantarflexion and passive dorsiflexion, rupture is indicated by absence of tendon to palpation, positive Thompson Test, **"mass" in calf representing rolled-up muscles**

DDx: ankle fracture, ankle impingement syndrome (chronic pain from repeated ankle inversion injuries), ankle sprain, retrocalcaneal bursitis

Rx: rest, cryotherapy, anti-inflammatories, stretching exercises, rupture can be managed conservatively in many cases (equinus casting/boot, muscle strengthening when appropriate), surgery for rupture in athletes

Acromioclavicular (AC) Joint Separation

Incid; Etiol: active athletic types, work injury, motor vehicle accidents, falls

Dx: visible deformity/ecchymosis over AC joint, pain and tenderness, crepitation, history of trauma; Grade I–up to 50% separation, Grade II-51–99% separation, Grade III–100% separation

DDx: distal clavicle fracture, rotator cuff disease, subacromial bursitis

Rx: immobilization/bracing/taping in mild cases, surgery in severe injuries or athletes who require stabilization

Angina Pectoris

Incid; Etiol: adults >40 years old, M>F; ischemic chest pain secondary to coronary artery atherosclerosis, newer theories suggest chronic inflammatory arterial process

Dx: **substernal pain (crushing, pressure, discomfort, burning, achy, dull),** arm pain (medial), neck pain, jaw pain, epigastric pain, dizziness, syncope, brought on by exertion/stress, relieved by rest, nonexertional angina (Prinzmetal's, vasospastic), pain lasts <15 minutes, dyspnea, Levine's sign

DDx: myocardial infarction, gastroesophageal reflux disease, gastritis, esophagitis, gallbladder disease, peptic ulcer diseases, pulmonary embolism, pneumonia, Tietze's syndrome (costochondritis), mitral valve prolapse, aortic dissection, aortic stenosis, congestive heart failure

Rx: aspirin, sublingual nitroglycerin, transdermal nitroglycerin, oral nitrates, beta-blockers, calcium channel blockers, coronary artery stent placement, coronary artery bypass graft, smoking cessation, supervised exercise program, dietary changes, lifestyle modification (stress reduction)

Ankle Sprain

Incid; Etiol: sports injury, work-related injury, falls; inversion injuries are most common, causing injury to the anterior talofibular ligament (plantarflexion-inversion), calcaneofibular (neutral position-inversion) ligament and posterior talofibular ligament (dorsiflexion-inversion). The deltoid ligament is sprained with eversion injuries. Combined injuries are common.

Dx: clinical and radiographic search for instability is critical, Grade I-few fibers torn, Grade II-majority of ligament damaged, Grade III-complete rupture, if the patient has pain at the tip or posterior aspect of the lateral malleolus, pain at the tip or posterior aspect of the medial malleolus, pain/tenderness at the navicular bone, pain/tenderness at the base of the 5th metatarsal bone, or the inability to bear weight, plain film radiographs of the ankle are indicated

DDx: peroneal (lateral)/tibialis posterior (medial) strain (clinical exam), fracture (radiographs)

Rx: BRACE (see Chapter 17 on sprain/strain management for specific protocols)

Appendicitis

Incid; Etiol: young people; obstruction of ostium of vermiform appendix with resultant infection/inflammation

Dx: **diffuse/periumbilical dull achy abdominal pain that eventually migrates to right lower quadrant,** fever, rebound phenomenon (Rovsing's sign), pain at McBurney's point, severe pain followed by rapid pain reduction is a sign of rupture

DDx: endometriosis, ovarian disease (e.g., cyst), Crohn's disease, ectopic pregnancy, bowel obstruction, volvulus, intussusception

Rx: antibiotics, appendectomy

Baker's Cyst

Incid; Etiol: adults; cystic fluid-filled enlargement of the semimembranous bursa in the popliteal fossa

Dx: fluctuant swelling in the popliteal fossa at times after knee injury, ultrasound/magnetic resonance imaging (MRI) are diagnostic

DDx: abcess, soft tissue tumor, bursitis

Rx: corticosteroid injection, aspiration

Bankart Lesion

Incid; Etiol: any age, result of traumatic shoulder dislocation causing defect in inferior labrum

Dx: shoulder dislocation with continued pain especially when stressing the inferior joint capsule, positive orthopedic tests (Crank Test, O'Brien's Test), magnetic resonance imaging (MRI) is diagnostic

DDx: uncomplicated shoulder dislocation, capsular tear/capsulitis

Rx: surgery to repair lesion, subscapularis tendon shortening

Bell's Palsy

Incid; Etiol: any age, M=F; idiopathic, although occasionally associated with diabetes mellitus, hypertension, pregnancy, dental anesthesia, acute coryza

Dx: usually of sudden onset and complete within 24 hours, almost always unilateral onset, may be preceded by postauricular pain, paralysis of the upper and lower facial muscles, smooth brow, frowning and raising the eyebrows are impossible, the eye cannot be closed, when asked to close the eyes and show the teeth, the eyeball rotates upwards and outwards - Bell's phenomenon, lower lid eversion and lacrimation, drooling, loss of taste, hyperacusis

DDx: otitis media, herpes zoster, multiple sclerosis, human immunodeficiency virus (HIV), Horner's syndrome, brainstem tumor, Lyme disease

Rx: reassurance that the condition is self-limiting in >90% of patients within 4 weeks-10 months, eye drops to prevent dehydration and corneal damage, corticosteroids, facial nerve decompression

Benign Essential Tremor

Incid; Etiol: adults; often associated with beta blockers (e.g., propranolol); essential tremor is a 6–8 Hz tremor that is of varying amplitude

Dx: aggravation by posture and movement, relief by rest and alcohol (short-term improvement lasting approximately two hours), most affected are the arms, head and vocal cords, lack of rigidity, no cerebellar signs, family history

DDx: intention tremor, Parkinsonism

Rx: medications

Benign Prostatic Hyperplasia

Incid; Etiol: males, 50% of men >50 years old; benign enlargement of the prostate gland resulting in bladder outflow obstruction

Dx: urinary retention, dribbling, dysuria, nocturia, polyuria, enlarged smooth prostate on digital rectal examination

DDx: prostate carcinoma, bladder incontinence, neurogenic bladder

Rx: transurethral resection of the prostate gland, medications (Proscar)

Berry Aneurysm

Incid; Etiol: affect ~5% of population, multiple in 20–30% of patients; anterior cerebral artery most common, internal carotid artery (posterior communicating), middle cerebral artery, posterior circulation (posterior inferior cerebellar artery)

Dx: subarachnoid hemorrhage, headache, altered level of consciousness, limb weakness, visual field defects, cranial nerve III palsy (ptosis, mydriasis, sluggish pupil), facial pain, ophthalmoplegia, most remain asymptomatic throughout life

DDx: intracranial tumor, cerebrovascular accident, multiple sclerosis, migraine headache, trigeminal neuralgia

Rx: emergent surgical correction

Bicipital Tendinitis

Incid; Etiol: active young people; inflammation of biceps tendon, typically from overuse, often associated with rotator cuff disease

Dx: **marked tenderness over tendon in bicipital groove (palpate with arm rotated 30° externally),** pain with resisted flexion/supination of the elbow/forearm

DDx: rotator cuff disease, biceps tendon rupture (muscle rolled into bundle in upper arm), rupture of transverse ligament of bicipital groove (biceps tendon slips out of groove with motion)

Rx: rest, heat, transverse friction massage, corticosteroids in severe cases

Bursitis

Incid; Etiol: active patients, work-related injury, sports injury; many different locations including subacromial, deltoid, olecranon, trochanteric (hip), pes anserine (knee), (retrocalcaneal) Achilles and adventitious (not normally present, result of overuse) bursae; inflammation of bursa with swelling and pain

Dx: localized pain/tenderness, painful joint motion, history of overuse syndrome

DDx: tendinitis, sprain, strain, myofascitis

Rx: cryotherapy, contrast bath, rest, short-term immobilization, joint mobilization/manipulation, anti-inflammatory nutraceuticals

Carpal Tunnel Syndrome

Incid; Etiol: overuse syndrome, pregnancy, obesity, acute trauma; entrapment of median nerve at carpal tunnel

Dx: pain/tenderness at carpal tunnel and into thenar eminence and thumb and index finger, atrophy of thenar eminence, weakness in thumb motion, history of repetitive motion disorder, **absence of paresthesia over thenar eminence** (sensory branch of median nerve does not pass through carpal tunnel)

DDx: pronator teres syndrome, radiculopathy, radial neuropathy

Rx: joint mobilization/manipulation, orthosis/splinting, therapeutic exercise, ergonomic changes/proper wrist posture, carpal tunnel release surgery

Cerebrovascular Accident

Incid; Etiol: typically infants or elderly; atherosclerosis, hypertension, aneurysm

Dx: facial weakness/paresthesias, extremity/truncal weakness/paresthesias, aphasia (expressive (frontal lobe lesion)), receptive (temporal lobe lesion), dysarthria, dizziness/vertigo, nystagmus, cranial nerve palsies, ataxia, headache, visual disturbances

DDx: vertebrobasilar insufficiency/aneurysm, brain tumor/mass, lacunar infarcts, subarachnoid hemorrhage, acute disseminated encephalomyelitis, Bell's palsy

Rx: acute-tissue plasminogen activator, life support, resuscitation; rehabilitation-exercise, occupational therapy, speech therapy, lifestyle modifications

Cholecystitis/Cholelithiasis

Incid; Etiol: fair-skinned, obese, middle-aged females; cholelithiasis causes cholecystitis, cholecystitis causes cholelithiasis

Dx: crampy/colicky right upper quadrant pain, jaundice, low-grade fever, anorexia, nausea and vomiting, positive Murphy's sign

DDx: hepatitis, gastroesophageal reflux disease, peptic ulcer disease, cardiac disease, pulmonary embolism

Rx: low-fat diet, laparoscopic cholecystectomy

Chronic Obstructive Pulmonary Disease

Incid; Etiol: children to older adults, depending on type; emphysema, chronic bronchitis, bronchial asthma, bronchiectasis

Dx: prolonged exhalation phase of respiration, barrel chest, "blue-bloater" (edema, productive cough for at least three months, cyanosis in chronic bronchitis), "pink-puffers" (barrel-chest, acyanotic in emphysema), periodic asthma attacks (wheezing, shortness of breath), spitting up multilayered sputum (bronchiectasis), use of accessory muscles of respiration, history of smoking (emphysema, chronic bronchitis, bronchiectasis), atopy (asthma)

DDx: pneumonia, chronic restrictive lung disease

Rx: O_2 therapy, pulmonary exercises, smoking cessation, bronchodilators, possibly spinal manipulation

Cruciate Ligament Tears

Incid; Etiol: active children and adults, athletes; anterior cruciate (sharp rotation, valgus injury with external rotation or hit from behind forcing femur anteriorly), posterior cruciate (hyperextension, knee force posteriorly)

Dx: pain, almost immediate knee joint swelling, history of twisting injury where patient heard a "pop", instability (anterior/posterior drawer signs, Lachman's test, pivot shift test), MRI is confirmatory

DDx: meniscus tears, knee sprain, fracture, subchondral fracture (osteochondritis dissecans)

Rx: partial thickness tear (rest, bracing, cryotherapy, elevation, nonweight bearing), full thickness tear (arthroscopic repair)

De Quervain's Disease (Stenosing Tenosynovitis)

Incid; Etiol: adults; inflammatory tenosynovitis with reduced motion of the tendon through the sheath secondary to adhesion usually associated with repetitive motion disorder, most common in the wrist at the abductor pollicis longus and extensor pollicis brevis tendons but it may occur anywhere in the body

Dx: painful engorged tendon sheath, reduced/painful motion with passive and active motion, crepitus, positive orthopedic tests (Finkelstein's test)

DDx: tendinitis, strain, sprain, fracture

Rx: cryotherapy, nonsteroidal anti-inflammatory drugs (NSAIDs), corticosteroids (topical, injection), ultrasound, phonophoresis, joint mobilization/ manipulation, splinting

Disc Protrusion/Extrusion/Sequestration

Incid; Etiol: 30–50 year old age group most commonly; sports injury, work-related injury, falls, improper lifting techniques, axial compression loads

Dx: back/buttock/leg pain, neck/arm pain, spinal tenderness, radiculopathy, myelopathy, positive orthopedic tests suggesting nerve root tension,

MRI confirms presence of disc lesion but does not always correlate with symptomatology

DDx: facet syndrome, intracanalicular space-occupying lesions (e.g., hematoma, tumor, arteriovenous malformation), mechanical back pain

Rx: spinal mobilization/manipulation, physical medicine modalities, spinal stabilization exercises, lumbosacral orthosis, short-term rest, manipulation under anesthesia, manipulation under joint anesthesia. See chapters on back pain and neck pain for more information.

Diverticulitis

Incid; Etiol: patients >60 years old; poor bowel habits, low fiber diet, poor fluid intake

Dx: left lower quadrant pain/tenderness, hematochezia, diarrhea, anemia, weight loss, anorexia

DDx: ulcerative colitis, colorectal cancer, hemorrhoids, Crohn's disease

Rx: increase dietary fiber, adequate hydration, regular exercise, antibiotics, nutraceuticals, surgical resection in severe cases

Facet Syndrome

Incid; Etiol: adolescent, adults; typically traumatic although may be related to an old injury

Dx: low back/buttock/leg pain **(not past the knee),** neck/arm pain, **non-dermatomal pattern,** extension and rotation provoke pain, paraspinal tenderness over facet joint

DDx: herniated disc, sprain/strain

Rx: spinal mobilization/manipulation, short-term rest, physical medicine modalities, spinal stabilization exercises, manipulation under anesthesia, manipulation under joint anesthesia. See chapters on back pain and neck pain for more information.

Fever

Incid; Etiol: any age; infection, malignancy, constitutional illness, fever of unknown origin

Dx: sustained body temperature above 98.6° F/37.2° C. Most common cause of fever of unknown origin is genitourinary disease. High fevers (>102° F) are typically seen with acute bacterial infections. Low grade fevers are typically associated with acute viral, chronic bacterial, or fungal infections. Malignancy typically presents with low-grade fever with the notable exception of Ewing's sarcoma or malignancies that produce immunocompromise (leukemias).

DDx: N/A

Rx: antipyretics (acetaminophen et al.), cold forehead compress. High fevers can result in seizures, especially in children. Any patient with a fever >104° should be evaluated by a physician.

Gastroesophageal Reflux Disease

Incid; Etiol: 30–60 year olds; reflux of gastric contents through lower esophageal sphincter. Chocolate, caffeine, nicotine, peppermint, garlic, stress, and fatty foods are triggers.

Dx: dyspepsia 30–60 minutes after eating or during recumbency, hoarseness, cough, excess salivation, burning chest pain, sweating, often associated with a hiatus hernia

DDx: angina pectoris, gastritis, esophagitis, pulmonary disease, peptic ulcer disease

Rx: avoid triggers, medications (Zantac, Prilosec, et al.), nutraceuticals, eat >3 hours before reclining

Guillain-Barre Syndrome (Ascending Paralysis)

Incid; Etiol: adults 5–75 years old, but any age can be affected; idiopathic, autoimmune, viral illness causing acute radiculopolyneuritis

Dx: numbness/tingling in lower extremities, back pain, weakness in the arms/legs, diplopia, ptosis, cranial nerve deficits, absent DTRs, labored respiration, drooling, dysphagia, painful muscle contractions, **sensory loss is minimal,** elevated CSF protein levels with normal white blood cell count

DDx: poliomyelitis, transverse myelitis, botulism, polymyositis, dermatomyositis, spinal cord lesion, multiple sclerosis, amyotrophic lateral sclerosis

Rx: corticosteroids, plasmapheresis, immunoglobulin injections, rehabilitation (after resolution), most patients are temporarily paralyzed, the condition resolves in 6 months – 2 years in most cases with full recovery in 90% of patients

Headache

Table 15.1 outlines the common causes for headaches.

Headache, Cervicogenic

Incid; Etiol: adults, may be the most common headache type; headache secondary to cervical spine dysfunction

Dx: dull/achy headache precipitated by neck movement or sustained head position, pain/tenderness in suboccipital region and at C2/3 that produces/aggravates headache, restricted cervical spine range of motion, ipsilateral shoulder/upper arm pain is often concomitant, headache is usually unilateral, may radiate over top of head to orbit, no aura

DDx: cluster headache, migraine headache, muscle tension headache

Rx: spinal manipulation/mobilization, neck exercises, proper posture, physical medicine modalities

Headache, Cluster

Incid; Etiol: 20–50 year old adults, M:F-6:1; etiology unknown but possibly disordered humoral control of vasculature or centrally-mediated thalamic dysfunction

Dx: rapid onset (2–15 minutes), **unilateral excruciating/explosive/pulsatile periorbital/temporal/frontal pain,** almost always affects the same side, may be paroxysmal stabbing periorbital pain occasionally (often signals the end of the headache), +/− Horner's syndrome, lacrimation, conjunctival injection, blocked nasal passage, rhinorrhea, bradycardia, nausea, sweating, alcohol sensitivity during cluster cycle, pain generally lasts 30 minutes-2 hours (maybe longer), remissions and exacerbations with patients averaging 1–2 episodes per day for 2–6 weeks and then remission, most attacks occur at night (9 p.m.–10 a.m.)

Table 15.1 Common Causes for Headaches

Disorder	Clinical Features	Diagnostic Testing
Migraine	unilateral, nausea, familial, +/− aura	normal neuroimaging
Tension	bilateral, stress-related	normal neuroimaging
Cluster	unilateral, brief, occur in clusters, males	normal neuroimaging
Subarachnoid hemorrhage	sudden, severe, neurologic signs, altered LOC	blood in cisterns, lumbar puncture diagnostic
Intracerebral hemorrhage	sudden, severe, neurologic signs, altered LOC	computerized tomography reveals parenchymal bleed
Giant cell arteritis	>60 years old, myalgia, elevated ESR, temporal pain	temporal artery biopsy confirms
Benign Intracranial HTN	dull headache, obese, papilledema	small ventricles on MRI, high opening pressure on LP
Brain tumor/abcess	dull, achy headache, personality changes, seizures, focal neurologic findings	MRI demonstrates mass
Meningitis	meningismus, fever, altered LOC	LP confirms
Cervicogenic	unilateral, tender spine suboccipital, orbital	normal neuroimaging
Arteriovenous malformation	intermittent headache, seizures, focal neurologic findings	MRI/MRA confirms

DDx: migraine headache, cervicogenic headache, chronic paroxysmal hemicrania

Rx: prednisone, triamcinolone, ergotamine, methysergide, lithium, nifedipine, indomethacin, chlorpromazine all with varying results

Headache, Migraine (without Aura)

Incid; Etiol: adults; neurovascular etiology is surmised

Dx: prodrome may involve sweating, nausea, pale skin, irritability for hours to days before onset of headache, steady severe often throbbing unilateral headache, may last hours to days

DDx: migraine headache with aura, cluster headache, cervicogenic headache, chronic paroxysmal hemicrania

Rx: medications (ergotamine, sumatriptan, antidepressants (amitriptyline), propranolol)), ice, rest, turn off lights and sounds, biofeedback, regular exercise, spinal manipulation/mobilization

Headache, Migraine (with Aura)

Incid; Etiol: adults; neurovascular etiology suspected

Dx: aura (scintillating scotoma (flashing lights)) approximately 10–30 minutes before headache starts, unilateral steady severe often throbbing unilateral headache, usually peaks at one hour and lasts several hours, patient may also experience numbness/burning/tingling sensation, weakness, dizziness, confusion, nausea and vomiting, irritability, photophobia, phonophobia

DDx: migraine headache without aura, cluster headache, cervicogenic headache, chronic paroxysmal hemicrania

Rx: medications (ergotamine, sumatriptan, antidepressants (amitriptyline), propranolol)), ice, rest, turn off lights and sounds, biofeedback, regular exercise, spinal manipulation/mobilization

Headache, Migraine-Basilar Artery

Incid; Etiol: young women; unknown

Dx: aura (vertigo, dysarthria, ataxia, diplopia, bilateral visual impairment), remaining symptoms are similar to classic migraine

DDx: migraine headache and variants, vertebrobasilar insufficiency, vertebral artery aneurysm, brain stem tumor/infection

Rx: cold compress, over-the-counter analgesics, sumatriptan

Headache, Nervous System Etiology

Incid; Etiol: children and adults; tumors, arteriovenous malformations, aneurysm, infection, intracranial hemorrhage

Dx: **sudden onset of a "first" headache,** "worst headache I've ever had," traumatic headache, "new" headache in a patient over 50, **exercise-induced headache, awakens patient from sleep,** pain over temporal artery, headache with papilledema, headache with meningismus, headache with seizure, headache with altered consciousness, headache with cranial nerve findings, headache with focal neurologic signs, positional headache, personality changes with headache

DDx: tumor, aneurysm, arteriovenous malformation, aneurysm, subarachnoid hemorrhage, idiopathic intracranial hypertension, meningitis, encephalitis, temporal arteritis

Rx: dependent upon cause, all of the above require referral to a medical physician for management

Herpes Zoster (Shingles)

Incid; Etiol: any age, 20% of all adults suffer at some point; self-limiting inflammatory ganglion inflammation affecting the dorsal root ganglia or cranial nerve ganglia caused by herpes (varicella) zoster (chickenpox) virus, exposure to someone with chickenpox, immunosuppression, no direct contact communicability shingles to shingles, but someone who has not had chickenpox can get chickenpox from someone with shingles

Dx: dermatomal pain and paresthesia followed by erythema and then vesicular eruption that itches and burns, painful regional lymphadenopathy, patients may have severe pain after rash disappears (postherpetic neuralgia), patients may have temporary paralysis

DDx: intercostal neuralgia, trigeminal neuralgia, radiculopathy, disc herniation, other vesicular rashes

Rx: acyclovir, famciclovir, valacyclovir

Hodgkin's Lymphoma

Incid; Etiol: 15–35 and >50 years old; etiology unknown

Dx: generalized pruritis, persistent lymphadenopathy (generally localized), hilar enlargement, hepatosplenomegaly, bone pain, anemia, immunocompromise (recurrent infections), fever, night sweats, weight loss, central nervous system (CNS) dysfunction (associated with acquired immune deficiency syndrome (AIDS) related lymphoma), presence of Reed-Sternberg cells, lymph node biopsy

DDx: HIV/AIDS, Epstein-Barr virus, tuberculosis, sarcoidosis, chronic lymphocytic leukemia, non-Hodgkin's lymphoma (disseminated painless lymphadenopathy)

Rx: radiation therapy, chemotherapy, overall 5-year survival >70%

Hypertension

Incid; Etiol: adults (black males at highest risk); idiopathic (90%), renal disease, pheochromocytoma, intracranial lesion, pulmonary disease, brainstem disease

Dx: three separate elevated readings as per Table 6.5, signs and symptoms include headache, stroke, transient ischemic attack, renal failure, transient blindness

DDx: not applicable

Rx: dietary changes (low salt, low fat), supervised water-fasting, antihypertensive medications, exercise, nutraceuticals

Lateral Epicondylitis

Incid; Etiol: active adults 30–60 years old; inflammation in and around the common extensor tendon at the lateral epicondyle of the elbow, an overuse syndrome, aka tennis elbow

Dx: pain at lateral epicondyle, history of overuse (especially wrist extension (racquet sports players)), pain with resisted wrist extension with elbow extended, pain with a handshake, pain may radiate proximally or distally, positive "coffee cup sign" (gripping a coffee cup sign causes pain at lateral epicondyle), swelling/bruising

DDx: cervical radiculopathy, forearm overuse syndromes, elbow fracture, elbow instability

Rx: circumferential forearm compression strap, activity modification, physical medicine modalities, cryotherapy, elbow mobilization/manipulation, therapeutic exercises, ergonomic recommendations, anti-inflammatories

Leukemia

Incid; Etiol: < age 15 or > age 50 (60%); primary malignant neoplasm of stem cells, two types - acute (children (acute lymphoblastic leukemia)(most common malignant childhood disease), adults (acute myeloid leukemia)) and chronic (adults (chronic lymphocytic leukemia, chronic myeloid leukemia))

Dx: dependent upon type of leukemia, bone/joint pain, easy bruising, recurrent infections, recurrent epistaxis, lymphadenopathy, hepatosplenomegaly, gum hypertrophy/bleeding, headache, nonspecific chronic illness, weight loss, fever of unknown origin, hyperleukocytosis, pancytopenia

DDx: lymphoma, myelodysplasia, myeloproliferative disorders (polycythemia vera), aplastic anemia, lymphoproliferative disorders (multiple myeloma)

Rx: chemotherapy, acute leukemias have a better prognosis

Lyme Disease

Incid; Etiol: any age; tick-borne illness cause by spirochete Borrelia burgdorferi primarily in eastern and midwestern United States

Dx: tick bite, erythema chronicum migrans, fever, headache, stiff neck, arthralgia and myalgia, lymphadenopathy, fatigue, hepatomegaly, multiple secondary skin lesions, pericarditis, cardiac arrhythmia, neuritis/Bell's palsy-like syndrome, meningitis, arthritis, conjunctivitis, hepatomegaly, encephalomyelitis

DDx: inflammatory arthritis, Guillain-Barre syndrome, Bell's palsy, meningitis, infectious mononucleosis, chronic fatigue syndrome, fibromyalgia, dermatomyositis, polymyositis

Rx: antibiotics

Meniscus Tears, Knee

Incid; Etiol: active adolescents, adults; trauma

Dx: clicking sound with knee motion, knee pain, knee locking, tenderness at joint line, positive orthopedic tests, usually a twisting injury, swelling

DDx: ligament damage (anterior cruciate, posterior cruciate), osteochondral fracture

Rx: simple tears can be managed conservatively with rest, cryotherapy, manual therapy, and anti-inflammatories early on and therapeutic exercise for long-term management; complex tears often require arthroscopy

Multiple Sclerosis

Incid; Etiol: 15–45 years old, F:M-2:1; inflammatory demyelination

Dx: remissions and exacerbations of often nondescript neurologic signs and symptoms, paresthesias, weakness, ophthalmoplegia, optic neuritis, hyperactive DTRs, clonus, nystagmus, visual disturbances, fatigue, spasticity

DDx: myasthenia gravis, amyotrophic lateral sclerosis, acute disseminated encephalomyelitis, AIDs myelopathy, vitamin B-12 deficiency (subacute combined degeneration), cerebrovascular disease

Rx: physical therapy/rehabilitation, speech therapy, manipulation/mobilization, corticosteroids, interferon, Neurontin, Zanaflex

Myasthenia Gravis

Incid; Etiol: 10–70 years old, M>F in older ages, F>M in younger ages; autoimmune disorder, associated with thymoma in middle-aged patients

Dx: diplopia, ptosis, ophthalmoplegia, limb weakness (primarily upper extremities) brought on by exercise, bulbar symptoms (loss of facial expression, inability to whistle, slurred speech, dysphagia, difficulty chewing, weakness of neck muscles), shortness of breath, increased DTRs, Tensilon test is diagnostic

DDx: Lambert-Eaton myasthenic syndrome (muscles are not fatigable, decreased DTRs), motor neuron disease (ocular involvement rare), botulism

Rx: anticholinesterase medication (neostigmine, pyridostigmine), thymectomy, plasma exchange, immunosuppression, 80% of patients have remissions, those with thymoma (invasive) have 5-year survival rate of 30%

Osteochondritis Dissecans

Incid; Etiol: active adolescents-adults; subchondral fracture, often with free fragment (joint mouse) secondary to macrotrauma or repetitive microtrauma, most common in medial femoral condyle and talar dome

Dx: intermittent pain, swelling, joint effusion, joint locking, joint "giving way," premature degenerative joint disease

DDx: internal derangement of the knee (meniscus tear, ligament tear), bone contusion, sprain

Rx: activity restriction, nonweight bearing, healing may take up to two years, arthroscopy for free fragment

Osteoporosis

Incid; Etiol: adults, postmenopausal females; loss of bone density usually secondary to lowered estrogen levels, many different types exist including diffuse and regional osteoporosis (transient osteoporosis of the hip)

Dx: radiographic osteopenia, back pain, wrist pain, pelvic pain, spinal compression fractures, spinal endplate infractions, hip fracture, pelvic fracture, stress (insufficiency) fractures, bone densitometry

DDx: multiple myeloma, lytic metastasis, metabolic diseases producing osteomalacia (malabsorption syndromes), Paget's disease

Rx: calcium supplementation, exercise, smoking cessation

Pancoast's Tumor

Incid; Etiol: adults, smokers; apical lung tumor (usually squamous cell carcinoma) producing relatively typical set of signs and symptoms

Dx: neck pain, arm pain, chest pain, Horner's syndrome, cough, hemoptysis, hoarseness

DDx: thoracic outlet syndrome, cervical radiculopathy, cervical sprain/strain, carpal tunnel syndrome, complex regional pain syndrome (reflex sympathetic dystrophy), pneumonia, pulmonary embolism

Rx: surgical resection (lobectomy), radiation therapy, chemotherapy

Peptic Ulcer Disease

Incid; Etiol: 25–75-year-old adults, M:F-2:1; excess acid secretion, reduced protective mechanisms resulting in ulcers in the stomach and/or duodenum

Dx: burning epigastric pain/tenderness that may radiate to back within 1–4 hours after a meal, may be relieved by food, antacids (duodenal) and vomiting (gastric), fatigue (anemia), sudden onset of severe symptoms suggests perforation

DDx: gastroesophageal reflux disease, malignant gastric ulcer, Zollinger-Ellison syndrome (multiple gastric ulcers from a malignant gastrinoma), angina pectoris, cholecystitis/cholelithiasis, esophagitis, gastritis, hepatitis, pulmonary disease (embolism)

Rx: antacids, gastrointestinal cocktail (antacid with anesthetic and antispasmodic), H2-receptor antagonists (e.g., Tagamet), proton pump inhibitors (e.g., Prev-acid), dietary changes (reduce caffeine, NSAIDs, alcohol, nicotine), spinal manipulation (?)

Phlebitis/Thrombophlebitis

Incid; Etiol: adults; inflammation of veins, usually of lower legs, often associated with varicose veins

Dx: calf pain, swelling, palpable painful cord along course of vein, positive Homans' sign

DDx: deep vein thrombosis, calf muscle strain, radiculopathy

Rx: compression stocking, elevation of extremity, anti-inflammatories, rule out deep vein thrombosis

Piriformis Syndrome

Incid; Etiol: active/sedentary adults; compression of a portion of the sciatic nerve (peroneal branch most commonly, 20%) in/by the piriformis muscle, traumatic, developmental, post-injury muscle fibrosis, prolonged sitting, post-traumatic myositis ossificans, status-post total hip arthroplasty

Dx: nondermatomal buttock and leg pain/paresthesia, aggravated by hip rotation (passive internal, resisted external), difficulty sitting, foot on affected side may be externally rotated (protective), normal/noncontributory spine examination although many patients have lumbar spine and piriformis syndromes simultaneously, absence of superior gluteal nerve symptoms (nerve exists sciatic nerve before piriformis), spastic piriformis on palpation, positive Pace test, Beatty's maneuver, Frieberg's test

DDx: neurogenic claudication, radiculopathy, cauda equina syndrome, gluteal muscle strain, ischial bursitis, spondylolisthesis, sacroiliac joint dysfunction, sacral stress fracture, spinal canal stenosis with neurogenic claudication

Rx: muscle energy techniques, spray and stretch, hip/sacroiliac joint mobilization/manipulation, therapeutic exercise, injections, surgery in severe recalcitrant cases

Plantar Fascitis

Incid; Etiol: adults, very common foot complaint; inflammation of the plantar fascia at its insertion into the medial calcaneal tubercle, trauma, repetitive microtrauma, association with heel spurs

Dx: intense sharp medial plantar foot pain at calcaneus, pain may radiate proximally or distally, pain may be worse at the end of the day or with first step after recumbency, tenderness to palpation, pain with passive dorsiflexion of toes, pain with toe walk

DDx: tarsal tunnel syndrome, plantar fascia rupture, bone contusion, Sever's disease, calcaneal stress fracture, Reiter's syndrome, heel pad syndrome (fat atrophy with pain), foot tendinitis

Rx: stretching, cryotherapy, spray and stretch, manipulation/mobilization of the foot/ankle, deep tissue massage, therapeutic exercise (tennis ball, wall calf stretches, marble pickups with toes while heel remains on floor), splinting, rigid orthotics, taping, anti-inflammatories, injections, heel spur surgery (in recalcitrant cases)

Pronator Teres Syndrome

Incid; Etiol: adults; compression of the median nerve between the two heads of the pronator teres muscle secondary to repetitive pronation-supination of the forearm, mimics carpal tunnel syndrome

Dx: numbness in median nerve distribution, fatigue of forearm muscles (especially pronation), positive Tinel's test in the forearm, negative Phalen's test, paresthesia over thenar eminence (this does not happen with carpal tunnel syndrome), pain with resisted pronation, forearm pain with resistance to isolated flexion of the PIP joint of index and ring fingers, inability to make the "okay" sign

DDx: carpal tunnel syndrome, pronator strain

Rx: activity modification, deep tissue massage, therapeutic exercise, mobilization/manipulation, ergonomic recommendations

Raynaud's Disease

Incid; Etiol: adults, F>M; vasospastic disease

Dx: fingers, toes, nose, mouth become white then blue then red secondary to vasoconstriction, trophic changes, clubbing, gangrene

DDx: Raynaud's phenomenon, Berger's disease (thromboangiitis obliterans, middle-aged male smokers), diabetes mellitus

Rx: spontaneous resolution in ~2/3 of patients, calcium-channel blockers (nifedipine), fish oil, gamma linoleic acid, alpha-blockers (prazosin), surgical sympathectomy

Rotator Cuff Disease

Incid; Etiol: active adults >40 years old, people who work with their hands above their heads (painters), athletes; extrinsic compression of the rotator cuff by Type II/III acromion process (Type I-flat, Type II-curved, Type III-hooked) causing fraying/degeneration, with or without age-related tendon degeneration, supraspinatus muscle most commonly involved

Dx: progressive (50%) onset of superolateral shoulder pain or single traumatic event (50%), pain subsides with rest early on, night pain eventually occurs, pain is worst with arms overhead or during abduction, weakness in abduction and or external rotation, crepitus, positive impingement tests for supraspinatus (Neer, Beer Can, Codman's, Jobe), subscapularis (Gerber Liftoff, Gerber Push with Force) and infraspinatus (infraspinatus isolation, Patte); no tests exist for the teres minor, MRI is confirmatory

DDx: malignancy (night pain), subacromial bursitis, bicipital tendinitis, adhesive capsulitis, fibromyalgia, myofascial pain syndrome, thoracic outlet syndrome

Rx: analgesics, anti-inflammatories, spinal/shoulder joint mobilization/manipulation, stretching exercises, restore normal scapulohumeral rhythm, proprioceptive exercises, physical medicine modalities, joint injection, surgery for recalcitrant cases

Sacroiliac Joint Dysfunction

Incid; Etiol: any age; trauma, sprain, chronic biomechanical dysfunction of the pelvis/lower extremities

Dx: relatively specific sharp/stabbing/dull pain at PSIS, may radiate to buttock, back of thigh, worse with sitting and twisting motion, tenderness over PSIS, positive orthopedic tests (Gaenslen's, Iliac compression, Patrick-FABER), negative neurologic examination

DDx: herniated disc, lumbosacral sprain/strain, iliotibial band syndrome, piriformis syndrome, trochanteric bursitis, sacral stress fracture, sacroiliitis (inflammatory arthropathy)

Rx: manipulation/mobilization, therapeutic exercises (core stabilization), short-term rest, joint injection, manipulation under joint anesthesia

Spinal Canal Stenosis (Neurogenic Claudication)

Incid; Etiol: primarily adults >50 years old; congenitally narrow spinal canal, degenerative disc disease, facet arthrosis, large disc herniations, extradural masses (e.g., tumor, hematoma), two types - central canal stenosis and lateral recess stenosis, most common at C5-6, C6-7, L4-5, L5-S1

Dx: insidious onset of intermittent, crampy, diffuse thigh and/or leg pain/paresthesias or neck/arm/hand pain/paresthesia, inability to walk long distances (particularly downhill) without resting due to leg pain/weakness, resting, uphill walking and forward flexion relieve pain, patient can ride a bicycle without as much pain due to dynamic increase in canal diameter during flexion, physical exam is often normal unless done immediately after provocation of pain when transient neurologic findings may be present, wide-based gait, +/− Romberg's test with lumbar flexion, increased pain/weakness with lumbar extension, positive sustained Kemp's test, in severe cases signs of myelopathy may be present, MRI is confirmatory

DDx: vascular claudication, disc herniation, radiculopathy, diabetic neuropathy, mechanical low back pain, piriformis syndrome, compression fracture

Rx: many patients (~30%) will have some resolution of symptoms without intervention, spinal mobilization (flexion-distraction), William's flexion exercises, core stabilization exercises (pelvic tilts), inclined treadmill walking, decompressive surgery has a poor success rate

Thoracic Outlet Syndrome

Incid; Etiol: adults; compression of the neurovascular bundle at the thoracic outlet by the first rib, scalene muscles

Dx: shoulder/arm/hand pain/paresthesias in a nondermatomal distribution, diminished distal pulses, trophic skin changes, Raynaud's phenomenon, poor vascular return in nail beds, upper extremity weakness, specific orthopedic tests help identify causative lesion

DDx: Pancoast tumor, cervical radiculopathy/myelopathy, cervical spinal canal stenosis, myofascial pain syndromes, rotator cuff disease, adhesive capsulitis, complex regional pain syndrome (reflex sympathetic dystrophy)

Rx: shoulder joint/spinal/costovertebral mobilization/manipulation, physical medicine modalities, spray and stretch, surgical intervention in recalcitrant cases

Transient Ischemic Attack

Incid; Etiol: adults >45 years old; acute transient (usually 2–20 minutes, <24 hours maximum) of temporary and focal loss of cerebral function of vascular origin without permanent dysfunction

Dx: dysarthria, weakness/paresthesias in face, arms, legs, cranial nerve deficits, ataxia, nystagmus, dizziness/vertigo, visual disturbances

DDx: Bell's palsy, migraine headache, hypoglycemia, cerebrovascular accident, brain tumor, lacunar infarcts

Rx: antiplatelet agents (e.g., aspirin, warfarin, Persantine), supportive measures, O_2 therapy

Transitional Segment, Lumbosacral

Incid; Etiol: adults; congenital anomaly with many different types, most of which are not associated with pain, type IIB (unilateral pseudoarthrosis) is associated with increased risk of disc protrusion at L4-5

Dx: low back pain, leg pain, radiculopathy, radiography is confirmatory

DDx: lumbar facet syndrome, mechanical back pain, lumbar sprain/strain, disc protrusion/extrusion, piriformis syndrome

Rx: mobilization/manipulation, therapeutic exercise (core stabilization), heat, cryotherapy, physical medicine modalities

Trigeminal Neuralgia (Tic Douloureux)

Incid; Etiol: adults in 6th or 7th decade, M:F-1:2; aberrant vessel overlying the intracranial portion of the trigeminal nerve

Dx: paroxysmal, sharp, stabbing unilateral facial pain, usually <1 minute in duration, may be triggered by cold air, chewing, tooth brushing, skin flushing, facial sweating

DDx: acoustic neuroma invading trigeminal ganglion, antral tumors/infection, multiple sclerosis

Rx: treatment is aimed at pain relief (analgesics), surgical ablation of trigeminal ganglion in recalcitrant cases

Vascular Claudication

Incid; Etiol: elderly; narrowing of abdominal aortic lumen secondary to atherosclerosis

Dx: difficulty walking distances without rest due to leg pain, inclination of surface is immaterial, bicycling still causes pain, unaffected by position of spine, cold lower extremities, diminished pulses, trophic skin changes

DDx: neurogenic claudication, abdominal aortic aneurysm, peripheral vascular disease

Rx: thromboendarterectomy, vascular bypass, medications (Cilostazol), supervised exercise program

Vertebral Artery Dissection

Incid; Etiol: young adults <45 years old, F>M; advancing intramural vascular hematoma causing separation of arterial walls as a result of trauma, vasculitis, connective tissue diseases (Marfan's syndrome), idiopathic, fibromuscular dysplasia, hypertension, oral contraceptive use

Dx: facial dysesthesia (most common symptom), dysarthria, hoarseness, ipsilateral limb or trunk numbness, ipsilateral loss of taste, hiccoughs, vertigo, nausea and vomiting, diplopia or oscillopsia (image movement experienced with head motion), dysphagia, disequilibrium, headache ("**worst headache I've ever had**"), upper neck pain ("**worst neck pain I've ever had**"), nystagmus, Horner's syndrome, cranial nerve deficits, lateral medullary syndrome (Wallenberg's syndrome), locked-in syndrome (cerebromedullospinal disconnection)

DDx: multiple sclerosis, cerebrovascular accident, transient ischemic attack, migraine headache, subarachnoid hemorrhage, vasculitis

Rx: manipulation is contraindicated, anticoagulant therapy (e.g., warfarin, aspirin), life support

Vertigo, Benign Paroxysmal Positional (BPPV)

Incid; Etiol: adults >50 years old; presence of canaliths in the semicircular canals, most cases are idiopathic

Dx: sudden onset of positional (classically erect to supine) vertigo, nausea, vomiting, remissions and exacerbations, patient falls to side of affected ear, nystagmus, positive Dix-HallPike manuever (rotary nystagmus (top of eyes rotate to affected ear) when moving patient quickly from seated to supine position with the head turned 45°)

DDx: otosclerosis, otitis media, vestibular neuritis, CNS disease, vertebrobasilar insufficiency, acoustic neuroma, Meniere's disease, cervicogenic vertigo, labyrinthitis

Rx: Epley's maneuver (Table 15.2), watchful waiting as some cases are self-resolving, medications are not effective

Vertigo, Cervicogenic

Incid; Etiol: adults; vertigo with neck extension, thought to be the result of overstimulation of cervical facet joint mechanoreceptors

Dx: positional unsteadiness especially with neck extension, imbalance that is exacerbated by sudden neck movements, concomitant neck pain, headache, nondescript arm paresthesias, patient is placed on a revolving stool and with the neck held in the midline by the physician the body is rotated causing symptoms and/or nystagmus

DDx: BPPV, otosclerosis, otitis media, vestibular neuritis, CNS disease, vertebrobasilar insufficiency, acoustic neuroma, Meniere's disease, labyrinthitis

Rx: cervical spine mobilization/manipulation, trigger point therapy, therapeutic exercise

Vitamin B-12 Deficiency (Sub-acute Combined Degeneration)

Incid; Etiol: adults; vegan diet, alcoholism, intestinal malabsorption syndromes, atrophic gastritis, Zollinger-Ellison syndrome, Crohn's disease of the terminal ileum, medications, pregnancy

Table 15.2 Epley's Maneuver (Patient with Right-sided BPPV)

- Starting position - sitting, head turned 45° toward affected side.
- Position 1 - supine, head turned 45° toward affected side. Patient is reclined slowly to the supine position of the affected side. The rate is titrated to the point of no nystagmus and no symptoms. This normally takes about 30 seconds.
- Position 2 - supine, 15° Trendelenburg, head turned 45° toward affected side. Patient is reclined further to the Dix-Hallpike position of the affected side. This usually takes 10 seconds. Another 20 seconds are spent in the Dix-Hallpike position with the affected ear down.
- Position 3 - supine, 15° Trendelenburg, head turned 45° toward unaffected side. Next, the patient's head is turned slowly from position three toward the opposite side.
- Position 4 - lying on side with unaffected shoulder down, head turned 45° below horizon toward contralateral side. Patient's body is rolled so that the shoulders are aligned perpendicular to the floor, affected ear up. The head then is turned further so that the nose points 45° below the plane of the horizon. This typically takes another 30–45 seconds.
- Position 5 - sitting, head turned at least 90–135° toward unaffected side. Patient is raised back to the sitting position with the head turned away from the affected side.
- Procedure can be repeated if nystagmus/symptoms are not relieved.
- Patient is instructed to not aggravate condition with quick head or body movements for 48 hours.
- Ending position - finally, the head is turned back to the midline.
- Typically 1–2 sessions are required for remission.

Dx: macrocytic anemia, infections, thrombocytopenia, anorexia, weight loss, angular cheilosis, glossitis, alopecia, infertility, dementia, peripheral neuropathy (paresthesias, numbness, difficulty with ambulation, weakness), retrobulbar neuritis, optic atrophy, splenomegaly, positive Schilling's Test

DDx: multiple sclerosis, diabetic neuropathy

Rx: hydroxycobalamin supplements (oral if cause is dietary, intramuscular injection if malabsorption is present)

PART IV

Clinical Practice Protocols

Chapter 16

Ethics in Chiropractic Clinical Practice

Stephen M. Perle, DC, MS

Introduction

Ethics and morals are two terms that often are used interchangeably; both fundamentally are concerned with the boundary between good and bad behaviors in interpersonal relations. However, there are distinctions in the meaning of these words worthy of note. Ethics, from the Greek *ethos* (nature or disposition), is the term used to describe thinking about what is right and wrong. Morals, from the Latin *moris* (custom), is about the more real world vision of actions. The distinction is similar to how we might view the ancient Romans and Greeks, builder-doers and philosophers-thinkers, respectively. (1)

Caveat Emptor vs. Credat Emptor

The physician-patient relationship imposes upon the physician responsibilities not found in the typical business relationship. *Caveat emptor* (let the buyer beware) applies in business relationships because the businessperson has no special responsibility toward his or her customer. In fact, any responsibility business people have toward the customer is in reality one of benevolent self-interest. Good customer service often is offered not because the businessperson believes that he or she owes the customer the duty but because good service will hopefully ensure repeat business and word-of-mouth recommendations.

On the other hand, the physician-patient relationship is founded on the principle of *credat emptor* (let the buyer have faith). (2) Historically the professions were those occupations in which the professionals, typically physicians, lawyers, and clergy, professed to have specialized knowledge that the laity did not have. Given this specialized knowledge the patient, client, or parishioner was left with little ability to judge the validity of the advice offered by the professional. Thus, the patient must rely upon the physician's recommendations and have faith that those recommendations are made not in the physician's best interest but that the patient's best interests are foremost in the physician's mind. (2–4)

Duties

The basic duties imposed upon the physician by the physician-patient relationship are: beneficence, nonmaleficence, fidelity, justice, and veracity. (5)

Beneficence is acting in a way that results in a positive outcome for the patient. Thus, it is the basic goal of all therapeutic encounters to help the patient attain greater level of health. *Nonmaleficence* is the act of preventing harm. This is summed up in the ancient and justly venerated Hippocratic dictum *primum non nocere* (first do no harm). Left with the choice of a treatment with a greater likelihood of harming a patient or doing nothing at all, nonmaleficence dictates do nothing. Nonmaleficence and beneficence should be seen as opposite ends of a continuum, which might be rephrased as costs vs benefits. (5)

Fidelity is the duty to comply with the reasonable expectations of the patient. Obviously this entails respect for the patient as a human, which also includes respecting any agreements made between the physician and patient. Patients quite reasonably expect that their physician will be competent in both his or her skills and knowledge and that the physician will be up-to-date. (5, 6) Thus, physicians do not have the luxury of espousing beliefs that are not consistent with up-to-date knowledge (7), and given the perpetual march of entropy of knowledge physicians have an ongoing ethical duty to continually learn. (8)

Justice is simply fairness. All patients expect to be treated fairly. However, fairness is one of the most misused words in the English language. People will often say, "Please be fair," when in reality they do not want to be treated fairly, they want to be treated with some partiality. Aristotle has said that justice is treating equals equally and unequals unequally but in proportion to their relevant differences. Thus, fairness does not dictate that we treat all patients for the exact same period of time, just that patients with the same clinical need are treated similarly without regard to who they are or their ability to pay. Fairness dictates that one allows an identical period of time for every patient who has an identical clinical need but that the rate of reimbursement or the race, nationality, religion, gender, sexual orientation, etc. is not a factor that should be considered when determining the time allotted for patients. (5)

Veracity is the duty of telling the truth. At one time it was common for physicians, in a paternalistic way, to hide the truth from patients. This is no longer seen as acceptable practice. (5) When a physician gives a patient misinformation that the physician believed to be true, then there was no lie; however, one is still not in the clear, ethically. A physician's fidelity duty includes the concept that the patient expects you to provide him or her with valid information. (7)

Rights

The most fundamental right that a patient enjoys is *autonomy*. This is the right to control what happens to one's own body. The patient has the right to accept or reject a physician's recommendations without any attempts to coerce compliance with the physician's recommendations. Informed consent (see below) is a natural outgrowth of the right of autonomy. (5)

Autonomy also includes the right to control the distribution of information about oneself. Thus, one might say that the right of confidentiality in the physician-patient relationship is derived from the right of autonomy. (5) Regulations pursuant to the Health Insurance Portability and Accountability Act (HIPAA) have significant impact on confidentiality. However, ethical considerations preceded HIPAA. Codes of ethics for the chiropractic profession all demand that all information provided to the physician is confidential – "I will keep inviolate all things revealed to me as a physician." (9) Even the fact that someone is a patient might be considered to be confidential. (10)

The *right to health care* is not a universally acknowledged right. In some countries this right is public policy and universal access to health care is guaranteed. In the United States such a fundamental right has not taken its place with "the life, liberty and the pursuit of happiness." (5) However, federal law has mandated since 1985's passage of the Emergency Medical Treatment and Active Labor Act that patients do have a right to emergency care and women have the right to care if they are in labor. (11)

Regardless of a society's position on the right to health care, ethically when one has established a physician-patient relationship, the patient does have the right to expect the best health care that the physician is capable of providing. Thus, a patient should not expect that his or her ability to pay or any thing about his or her personality or who he or she is, his or her race, religion, gender, sexual orientation, etc. would have any impact on the quality of health care he or she receives from his or her physician. (5)

Self-regulation

One of the features that differentiate the professions from the laity is that professions are self-regulating. Self-regulation is granted to professionals because they are in theory the only people capable of judging the competence of other members of their profession. The monopoly that a professional license grants the professional carries with it the responsibility to the public at large to ensure that substandard professionals are not in practice. (2–4) Thus, "blowing the whistle" on an incompetent or unethical colleague is an ethical obligation common to all professionals. (5) Quality control measures, such as peer-review and the performance of independent medical examination, are duties owed to society to ensure the integrity of the profession. (5)

Informed Consent

The paternalistic relationship between physicians and patients in the past made it so that physicians often did use whatever treatments they believed were in the patient's best interest without the patient having much input into the process. This is not proper in modern health care. (12–14)

Consent has three parts: disclosure, capacity, and voluntariness. Disclosure is to provide the patient with relevant information, such as complications and benefits of a proposed treatment and of alternative treatments. Capacity refers to the patient's ability to understand the disclosure and the consequences of his or her decision. Finally, any consent must be made voluntarily without coercion or force. Consent can be explicit or implicit. Explicit consent is given orally or in writing. Implicit consent is evidenced by the patient's behavior that indicates a willingness to have a procedure. (14) In a chiropractic office implicit consent can be found in the act of lying face down on an adjusting table, after one understands the purpose of the table.

The legal requirements for informed consent vary between jurisdictions. (15) However, case law in Canada presents an interesting ethical argument. The Supreme Court of Canada found that a material risk must be disclosed. A material risk is one that, even though so slight a possibility that ordinarily would not have to be disclosed, must be disclosed if its occurrence may result in catastrophic consequences, such as paralysis or death. (16)

The risk for stroke is very rare especially when compared to over-the-counter medications, which might be an alternative treatment to cervical manipulation. (17) Such a rare event would be under Canadian law a material risk and must be disclosed to patients. However, new evidence suggests that the vertebral artery may not be stretched enough during a cervical manipulation to cause a stroke; (18) thus, a material risk may not exist. Until a definitive answer about the association between stroke and cervical manipulation is found ethically, it should be treated as a material risk.

Research Subjects

The abuse of human subjects in biomedical experiments perpetrated by physicians and scientists in the Nazi death camps led to the first universally accepted ethical rules for the protection of research subjects known as the Nuremberg Code. This Code was used to judge the behavior of the physicians and scientists involved in the experiments on the concentration camp prisoners. (19) There are 10 basic principles in the Code. Foremost among them is that consent must be voluntary, with comprehension of the risks and benefits involved. (20) In 1974 U.S. federal law created a commission to recommend rules to govern the protection of human subjects. The report of that commission, known as The Belmont Report (named for the conference center used by the commission), (19) was used by the Department of Health and Human Services (DHHS) in producing the regulations that govern the protection of human research subjects (Title 45 Part 46 of the Code of Federal Regulations) and the Food and Drug Administration's regulations (Title 25 Parts 50 and 56 of the Code of Federal Regulations).

Boundaries between Practice and Research

The Belmont Report recognized that boundary between research and practice of accepted therapy is often blurred. This is because often research is conducted on therapy methods. Also nonstandard treatments are often called "experimental" when the terms "experimental" and "research" are not carefully defined. The Report defines therapy as "interventions that are designed solely to enhance the well-being of an individual patient or client and that have a reasonable expectation of success. On the other hand the Report distinguishes "research" as "an activity designed to test a hypothesis, permit conclusions to be drawn, and thereby to develop or contribute to generalizable knowledge." (19)

"When a clinician departs in a significant way from standard or accepted practice, the innovation does not, in and of itself, constitute research. The fact that a procedure is 'experimental,' in the sense of new, untested or different, does not automatically place it in the category of research. Radically new procedures of this description should, however, be made the object of formal research at an early stage in order to determine whether they are safe and effective." (19)

Research is usually described in a formal protocol that sets forth an objective and a set of procedures designed to reach that objective. "The Report recognizes that 'experimental' procedures do not necessarily constitute research, and that research and practice may occur simultaneously. It suggests that the safety and effectiveness of such 'experimental' procedures should be investigated early, and that institutional oversight mechanisms, such as medical practice committees, can ensure that this need is met by requiring that major innovation[s] be incorporated into a formal research project." (19)

Institutional Review Boards

The Institutional Review Board (IRB) conducts oversight of research to provide for the protection of human subjects. IRBs are formed pursuant to 45 CFR 46. The members must be competent to review the science and the ethics of any study. Members of the IRB must not have any conflict of interest and thus cannot be involved in the research under review. For more information the reader is directed to The IRB Guidebook that is available free on-line at: http://ohrp.osophs.dhhs.gov/irb/irb_guidebook.htm. Other resources about protecting research subjects are available at the DHHS Office for Human Research Protections at: http://ohrp.osophs.dhhs.gov/index.html.

Abandonment

Implicit in the right to health care, which is conditional upon a physician's acceptance of a patient, is that the physician will not abandon the patient. Abandonment happens in a variety of ways. One way obviously is to withdraw from the patient's care without adequate notice. This could occur inadvertently if the physician goes on vacation or permanently closes the practice without adequate provision for continuity of care. One can also abandon a patient with poor follow-up. Thus, if a physician tells a patient to go and get a test and does not make sure the patient follows instructions, they can be accused of abandonment.

In normal business when a customer does not pay his or her bills, the businessperson is well within his or her rights to discontinue the business relationship. A painter who has a contract requiring payment in certain intervals during the course of the job who does not receive a payment can walk away from the job at will. On the other hand a physician cannot sever the physician-patient relationship on a moment's notice. When, for whatever reason, a physician chooses to sever the physician-patient relationship, notice must be given to patients with adequate time provided for them to secure the services of another physician. In addition, the physician who is withdrawing from care must provide all needed information to the new physician without regard to the patient's ability to pay for the transfer of information. While the physician has a legal and ethical right to be paid for both his or her services and for any office expenses in transferring records to a new physician, the lack of payment does not excuse the physician from helping a patient's transition to a new physician. The physician in this situation is obligated to transfer the information, and to ensure payment must probably seek legal remedy.

Boundary Issues

The physician-patient relationship is a special one. Patients confide in their physicians and provide them with access to information and to their bodies that is unprecedented outside of this relationship. All health care providers are required both ethically and legally to refrain from taking advantage of their intimate knowledge of the patient and their access to the patient's body. Physicians must maintain appropriate boundaries within this relationship. Because of both knowledge and the potential for greater intimacy with the patient that touch creates, precaution must be undertaken to ensure that patients do not see physicians stepping over the boundary of the relationship. There are many ways in which the boundary can be violated. (21, 22)

It goes without saying that a specific boundary is that any touch must be for appropriate therapeutic intent. Given the fact that chiropractors in particular are required to make contact with patients, it is conceivable that a patient may misconstrue such touch as having a motivation other than that of providing good clinical care. To ensure that no misunderstandings occur, it is important that physicians both explain carefully to patients what they intend to touch, why they intend to do so, and that they obtain permission to do so. (21, 22)

It is said that knowledge is power. In the physician-patient relationship, the physician obviously has knowledge and in particular knowledge about intimate details of the patient that gives the physician certain power. An interpersonal relationship that is developed with one party having power over the second party is not a fair and open relationship. Thus, physicians are prohibited from entering into an interpersonal relationship having started a physician-patient relationship, even if the patient consents. (21, 22)

"Gaming the System" or Fraud

Changes in the health care marketplace have resulted in physicians "gaming the system." "Gaming the system" is the phrase used to describe a situation where a healthcare provider changes diagnosis or treatment codes for the purpose of either increasing his or her own reimbursement or to help the patients obtain better reimbursement. (6) Physicians feel that there has been a shift in the balance of power over case management decisions from the patient and the physician to the managed care organization. (23) While one might rationalize "gaming" by claiming that the system is unfair and with the insurance carrier having more power to control care or control reimbursement, gaming is wrong. (6)

There is a point in time that one transitions from gaming to fraud. Altering diagnosis or treatment codes purely for the benefit of the patient might be construed as being benevolent toward the patient. Although ultimately still fraudulent when those alterations are done purely for the enrichment of the physician, gaming may be too euphemistic a term. (6)

Advertising

Consumers are interested in learning about chiropractic from advertisements. (24) However, one of the biggest problems in advertising is overstating claims of chiropractic's benefits for the patient or attempting to scare prospective patients into coming in for treatment. Advertisements must present truthful information, not just what the physician believes to be the truth. Using scare tactics, trying to make the prospective patient's symptoms seem indicative of a more serious condition than is warranted must be avoided. (22, 25–27)

Conclusion

In some way most ethical principles could be logically derived by anyone new to the profession depending upon one's upbringing. In some cases daily occurrences conspire to pollute our notions of what is right and wrong. The struggle for money puts our moral integrity at risk. Managed care threatens to wrest control of the physician-patient relationship from both the physician and patient. Boundary issues seem negated by patient consent. Physicians' beliefs often outweigh the evidence. Thus, logic might fail us and a study of ethical principles in physician-patient relationships is an important and ongoing process.

References

1. Jones, J., & Wilson, W. *An Incomplete Education.* New York: Ballantine Books; 1987. p. 608.
2. Hughes, E.C. Professions. *Daedalus.* 1963;92(Fall):655–668.

3. Pellegrino, E.D. What is a profession? *J Allied Health.* 1983;12(3):168–176.
4. Bayles, M.D. The professions. In: *Professional Ethics.* Belmont, CA: Wadsworth Pub Co; 1981. pp. 7–11.
5. Purtilo, R. *Ethical Dimensions in the Health Professions.* 3rd ed. Philadelphia: W.B. Saunders; 1999.
6. Morreim, E.H. Gaming the system. Dodging the rules, ruling the dodgers. *Arch Intern Med.* 1991;151(3):443–447.
7. Perle, S.M. Credat emptor. *Dynamic Chiropractic.* 2003;21(1):24, 33.
8. Sackett, D.L., Richardson, W.S., Rosenberg, W., & Haynes, R.B. *Evidence-based Medicine: How to Practice and Teach EBM.* New York: Churchill Livingstone; 1997.
9. Erlen, J.A., Erlen, J., & Dickstein, E. Ethical principles and professional concerns contained in chiropractic oaths. *Chirorp J Chiropr Res Clin Inves.* 1994;9(1):14–18.
10. Perle, S.M. Sign out the sign-in sheet. *Dynamic Chiropractic.* 2002;20(24):C-4.
11. Emergency Medical Treatment and Active Labor Act. In: 42 USC 1395dd; 1985.
12. Ferguson, D. Should we legislate the law of consent. *J Can Chiropr Assn.* 1990;34(2):67.
13. Burgess, M. Chiropractic informed consent. *J Can Chiropr Assn* 1990;34(1):24–26.
14. Etchells, E., Sharpe, G., Walsh, P., Williams, J., & Singer, P. Bioethics for clinicians: 1. Consent. *Can Med Assoc J.* 1996;155:177–180.
15. Gatterman, M.I., Dobson, T.P., & LeFevbre, R. Chiropractic quality assurance: standards and guidelines. *J Can Chiropr Assn.* 2001;45(1):11–17.
16. Canadian Chiropractic Association. Clinical Guidelines for Chiropractic Practice in Canada, Chapter 1 - Informed Consent. [cited 2003 Sept 28]: [8 screens]. Available from URL:*http://www.ccachiro.org/client/CCA/CCAWeb.nsf/web/1Chapter?OpenDocument.*
17. Dabbs, V., & Lauretti, W. A risk assessment of cervical manipulation vs NSAIDs for the treatment of neck pain. *J Manipulative Physiol Ther.* 1995;18(8):530–536.
18. Symons, B.P., Leonard, T., & Herzog, W. Internal forces sustained by the vertebral artery during spinal manipulative therapy. *J Manipulative Physiol Ther.* 2002;25(8):504–510.
19. National Commission for the Protection of Human Subjects of Biomedical and Behavioral Research. The Belmont Report: Ethical Principles and Guidelines for the Protection of Human Subjects of Research. Washington, DC: US Department of Health, Education, and Welfare; 1979.
20. Directives for Human Experimentation: Nuremberg Code. In: Trials of War Criminals before the Nuremberg Military Tribunals under Control Council Law No. 10, Vol. 2. Washington, DC: US Government Printing Office; 1949. p. 181–182.
21. Redleaf, A., & Baird, S.A. *Behind Closed Doors: Gender, Sexuality, and Touch in the Doctor/Patient Relationship.* Westport, CT: Auburn House; 1998.
22. Chiropractic Ethics in a Changing World. *J Am Chiropr Assoc.* 2003;40(6):11–18.
23. Manga, P. Ethical Dilemmas for Health Care Professions Under Managed Care. *Top Clin Chiropr.* 1998;5(4):53–57.

24. Johns, H.E., Kittrell, L.M., & Moser, H.R. How consumers view chiropractic advertising. *Health Market Q.* 1995;13(2):43–54.

25. Keating, J.C., Jr., & Hansen, D.T. Quackery vs accountability in the marketing of chiropractic. *J Manipulative Physiol Ther.* 1992;15(7):459–470.

26. Jenkins, A.L. Chiropractic advertising ethics. *J Am Chiropr Assoc.* 1994;31(11):64–69.

27. Grod, J.P., Sikorski, D., & Keating, J.C., Jr. Unsubstantiated claims in patient brochures from the largest state, provincial, and national chiropractic associations and research agencies. *J Manipulative Physiol Ther.* 2001;24(8):514–519.

Chapter 17

Sprain/Strain Management

Lawrence H. Wyatt, DC, DACBR, FICC

Introduction

Sprain/strain injuries are some of the most common lesions seen in the chiropractic private practice. It is essential that the treating physician be able to differentiate sprain from strain (Table 17.1), as the protocols may differ somewhat for each, especially when instability is suspected.

Sprains result from force around a joint that exceeds the tensile limits of the supportive ligaments but is less than that which would fracture the bones.

The ankle joint is an excellent example. Forces are concentrated in the ankle joint because it is the dynamic link between the leg above and the foot planted on the earth below. The large muscle masses of the lower extremity and the momentum of the body weight are concentrated on the ankle, connected to the foot, which may be firmly planted on the ground. These factors make ankle sprains the second most frequently encountered outpatient orthopedic condition. The incidence of ankle sprains has been estimated to be 1 per 10,000 people per day. (1)

Muscle strain or muscle "pull" implies damage to a muscle or its attaching tendons. Injury can occur at the origin of the muscle, the musculotendinous junction, muscle belly, or the insertion of the muscle. Strain injuries are most likely to occur when the musculotendinous junction undergoes maximum stress during an eccentric contraction.

Many factors predispose to sprain and strain injuries. These include inadequate flexibility, poor muscle strength or endurance, muscle imbalance (e.g., between the hamstrings and the knee extensors), muscle fatigue, insufficient warm-up time or stretching, and poor training/competing technique. In

Table 17.1 Differential Diagnosis of Sprain and Strain

Test	Sprain	Strain
Distraction	Pain	Pain
Active motion	Pain	Pain
Isometric (contraction)	No pain	Pain

addition, precocious return to activity before complete healing has occurred can lead to recurrence of the inury.

Sprains and strains can be graded according to their severity. Table 17.2 outlines these grading systems.

Signs and symptoms of sprains are outlined in Table 17.3 and strains in Table 17.4.

Management of Sprains and Strains

After it has been ensured that the patient suffering an acute strain injury has no fracture, dislocation, or ligamentous instability, treatment may be initiated. Radiography and advanced imaging are indicated when there is suspicion of grade III injury or when instability or fracture is suggested clinically.

Table 17.2 Sprain and Strain Grading Systems

Strain
Grade I- tear of only a few muscle and/or tendon fibers
Grade II- more severe tear without complete disruption
Grade III- complete tear

Sprain
Grade I- 1–50% tear
Grade II- 51–99% tear
Grade III- complete rupture

Table 17.3 Signs and Symptoms of Sprains

Signs and Symptoms of Sprains
Pain over the affected ligament
Painful active range of motion
Painful passive range of motion
Painless resisted range of motion
Localized swelling
Localized ecchymosis (proportional to the likelihood of fracture)
Positive orthopedic tests (see Chapter 7)

The acute phase of injury is typically ascribed to the first three days after injury. During this time, BRACE (Table 17.5) (e.g., bandage brace, rest/rehabilitation, apply ice, compression/crutches/chiropractic manipulation, elevation) is the treatment of choice. Cryotherapy early in the course of therapy has been demonstrated to be effective in earlier recovery. (2) Early mobilization has shown some positive effects when treating sprains. (3) The use of a compression bandage in the management of sprains has met with some controversy (4), but it continues to be used, primarily based on consensus opinion. Manipulation of extremity joints has demonstrated some success in the management of certain types of sprains and strains as well. (5,6)

Table 17.4 Signs and Symptoms of Strain

Signs and Symptoms of Strain
Painful active motion
Painful passive motion
Painful resisted motion
Loss of joint movement with contraction of affected muscle/tendon (Achille's rupture)
Tenderness at the injury site
Ecchymosis (the more severe the injury, the more substantial the ecchymosis)
Palpable mass (hematoma, collapsed tendon)
Palpable defect (may be felt with severe strains, but swelling may obscure this finding)

Table 17.5 Sprain/Strain Management

B—Bandage/brace
R—Rest/rehabilitation
A—Apply ice
C—Compression/crutches/chiropractic manipulation
E—Elevation

Sprain Management

The use of a brace or bandage will help with both the stability, compression, and restriction of motion in the affected extremity. The brace should not be so tight that it restricts circulation but it should be tight enough to allow compression and restriction of motion. Pulses should be taken after brace or bandage application to ensure adequate vascular status.

The proper type of brace or bandage depends on the type of injury. Rigid immobilization may be used with severe grade II and grade III injuries. Less severe sprain/strain injuries may be treated with an elastic wrap or less rigid forms of immobilization technique. Prolonged immobilization, which can result in adhesive capsulitis, should be avoided if at all possible.

Resting injured muscles, ligaments, and tendons is an integral component of therapy. Bear in mind, however, that prolonged inactivity can result in ligament fibrosis, muscle atrophy, and even disuse atrophy of bone. The injured joint should be immobilized for as little time as is clinically feasible. As pain subsides and the patient regains function, active and resisted ranges of motion with programmed rehabilitation, including proprioceptive neuromuscular facilitation and stabilization exercises, may be begun.

Cryotherapy has a number of benefits of which vascular constriction, which helps reduce capsular edema and soft tissue swelling, is only one. After the injury becomes subacute (3 days–3 weeks), a contrast bath (alternating heat and cold) is often helpful.

Compression of the involved extremity can help reduce soft tissue swelling and allows passive range of motion exercises to begin more quickly. Compression is accomplished by the application of a bandage as noted above.

The proper use of crutches, canes, and other ambulation assistance devices for lower extremity injuries helps rest the joint and provide for appropriate healing. This form of therapy is usually reserved for more severe injuries. If the patient complains that the crutches are uncomfortable, then they should be raised or lowered for better fit. Improper crutch fitting can result in brachial plexus palsies.

The use of manipulation in joint injuries is usually reserved for subacute and chronic disease. It is postulated that mobilization and manipulation help to prevent the development of fibrous adhesions within the joint and also help restore proper joint motion. Adjustment of the affected joint may be performed with caution on an acute injury. Contraindications to manipulation of a joint that has been sprained include fracture, dislocation, or an unstable joint.

Elevating the involved joint above the level of the heart, if at all possible, facilitates vascular return and helps reduce edema. Elevation should be performed whenever the patient is nonambulatory.

Strain Management

When the pain has decreased, the patient may begin painless gentle passive range of motion, as well as active-assistive range of motion. It has been suggested that even if a patient with a grade 1 injury is feeling better after a short time and wants to return to activities, particularly sports, it is usually recommended that he complete a rehabilitation program to avoid chronic injury.

The subacute phase is defined as being from 3 days to 3 weeks post-injury. The patient typically has reduced pain and swelling and should begin active range of motion exercises. Ambulation in a pool is an ideal environment for rehabilitation during this time period. Pain-free submaximal isometric exercises also are encouraged. A transcutaneous electrical nerve stimulation (TENS) unit or microcurrent therapy may be used to provide some pain relief and enhanced healing at this time. The patient should continue applying ice to decrease pain and inflammation. The patient also should resume nonweight bearing or limited-weight bearing cardiovascular training. This may include stationary bicycling, swimming, and nonaffected extremity exercises.

The remodeling phase, which occurs from 1–6 weeks, is when the patient is able to perform isometric exercises at 100% effort without pain. Isotonic exercises can now generally be safely added to the TENS unit and ice. Begin using low weight and high numbers of repetitions.

Once the patient can perform these exercises without pain, isokinetic exercises can be instituted. If isokinetic exercises are tolerated well, then eccentric strengthening exercises performed with a weight that is 10% greater than the 10-repetition concentric contraction maximum can be initiated. In other words, if the maximum weight that the patient can tolerate without pain for 10 repetitions is 10 pounds, then add 10% to that amount, making 11 pounds the proper weight to eccentric strengthening.

Proprioceptive neuromuscular facilitation can also be utilized for joint stabilization and muscle reeducation. For example, in a patient with ankle injury, standing in a doorway (for support if needed), on the affected foot alone, will fire the muscles of the lower extremity and help support the ankle joint. The chapter on physical medicine and rehabilitation outlines other procedures used in this process.

Another approach for ankle injuries is the use of a wobble board. A ¾–inch thick piece of wood, which is as long and as wide as the foot, and has one half of a 3- or 4-inch diameter plastic or wooden ball fixed to the center of one surface of the board, can be made inexpensively. It can be used at home for six weeks of self-directed exercises.

The wobble board affords two levels of range of motion. The patient steps on it with the half of a ball down on the floor to perform 10 sets of ankle motion in plantarflexion and then dorsiflexion. Then the foot is placed on the board crosswise, and side-to-side motions are performed 10 times. These sets of exercises are performed twice a day.

These exercises are typically performed easily after approximately 2–3 weeks. When range of motion is increased, the board can then be used in the opposite fashion. The plantarflexion and dorsiflexion motions can be performed with the foot sideways on the proprioceptive board. The side-to-side movements can be performed with the foot on the board so it fits the foot.

Care must be taken with these exercises to avoid causing another ankle sprain, which is what the proprioceptive exercises are designed to prevent. These patients must be compliant and motivated and the exercises should be demonstrated in the office. The patient should not begin the exercises at home until the physician is comfortable with the patient's performance. This proprioceptive board also helps with the stretching and strengthening exercises.

Prognosis

Most patients with sprain/strain type injuries can return to normal activities within 3 weeks to 6 months, depending upon the severity of the injury and the proposed activities. In most patients with grade I injuries, return occurs within approximately 4–6 weeks. Clinical judgment regarding return to activities is patient-specific, however.

Indications for surgical intervention in these types of injuries are generally limited to severe grade II and grade III injuries. Patients with clinically demonstrable instability are often best served by surgical intervention, although some studies have demonstrated similar outcomes in surgical and nonsurgical interventions. (7)

References

1. Trevino, S.G., Davis, P., & Hecht, P.J. Management of acute and chronic lateral ligament injuries of the ankle. *Orthop Clin North Am.* 1994 Jan;25(1):1–16.
2. Hocutt, J.E., Jr., Jaffe, R., Rylander, C.R., & Beebe, J.K. Cryotherapy in ankle sprains. *Am J Sports Med.* 1982 Sep–Oct;10(5):316–319.
3. Eiif, M.P., Smith, A.T., & Smith, G.E. Early mobilization versus immobilization in the treatment of lateral ankle sprains. *Am J Sports Med.* 1994 Jan–Feb;22(1):83–88.
4. Linde, F., Hvass, I., Jurgensen, U., & Madsen, F. Compression bandage in the treatment of ankle sprains. A comparative prospective study. *Scand J Rehabil Med.* 1984;16(4):177–179.
5. Pellow, J.E., & Brantingham, J.W. The efficacy of adjusting the ankle in the treatment of subacute and chronic grade I and grade II ankle inversion sprains. *J Manipulative Physiol Ther.* 2001 Jan;24(1):17–24.
6. Struijs, P.A., Damen, P.J., Bakker, E.W., Blankevoort, L., Assendelft, W.J., & Van Dijk, C.N. Manipulation of the wrist for management of lateral epicondylitis: a randomized pilot study. *Phys Ther.* 2003 Jul;83(7):608–616.
7. Evans, G.A., Hardcastle, P., & Frenyo, A.D. Acute rupture of the lateral ligaments of the ankle: to suture or not to suture. *J Bone Joint Surg.* 1984; 66-B: 209.

Suggested Readings

Best, T.M. Soft-tissue injuries and muscle tears. *Clin Sports Med.* 1997 Jul;16(3):419–434.

Garrett, W.E., Jr. Muscle strain injuries. *Am J Sports Med.* 1996;24(6 Suppl):S2–8.

Chapter 18

Cervical Spine Trauma Management

Lawrence H. Wyatt, DC, DACBR, FICC

Introduction

Over 10 million motor vehicle accidents occur in the United States annually, and many of these result in acceleration-deceleration (whiplash) injuries. In addition, falls, sports injuries, and other forms of trauma can result in cervical spine injury. The diagnosis in a patient who presents with acute cervical spine trauma can be enigmatic, if not handled properly. Sequelae, from chronic pain to quadriplegia and even death, can occur if the patient is improperly dealt with during examination and treatment.

A patient who has sustained trauma to the neck, usually from a motor vehicle accident, is often in a great deal of pain. It is ironic that at times the amount of pain has little to do with the severity of the problem. Patients have sustained life-threatening injuries in simple "fender bender" accidents where little-to-no pain was experienced.

The precise pathophysiologic mechanism resulting in pain associated with whiplash-type injuries is poorly understood. Recent studies, which used human cadavers, suggest that the suboccipital pain associated with these injuries is due to the stretch of dorsal root ganglia at C1 and C2. In addition, it is suggested that the lower cervical pain is due to compression of the cervical facet joints. (1) As a result of these findings, it is thought that the upper cervical spine injury occurs during flexion and the lower cervical spine injury during extension.

Studies using primate models of acceleration-deceleration injury to the cervical spine have identified several abnormalities on pathologic examination. These include muscle tears, ligament tears, disk herniations, lacerations of the pharynx and larynx, and esophageal hematomas. (2) It is difficult to extrapolate from these models what actually happens during a real situation in a human being.

The role of seat belts in precipitating or preventing whiplash injuries is unclear. Some evidence suggests an increase in whiplash injuries since the introduction of mandatory seat belt legislation. (2) It has been suggested that seat belts limit the movement of the torso thereby increasing the forces applied to the neck after a rear-end collision. In other studies, investigators have found no difference in the incidence of whiplash in passengers with or without seat belts. (3) While head restraints may prevent whiplash, studies have shown that they often are used incorrectly and may even contribute to injuries.

Examination

Since approximately 10–20% of patients with cervical spine trauma present with overt neurologic signs, the primary goal of examination of the patient with cervical spine trauma is to rule out unstable injuries. An unstable injury is one where, unless appropriate treatment is employed, serious neurologic damage is likely to result.

Figure 18–1 outlines the evaluation of acute cervical spine trauma.

The first procedure to be performed on a patient with macrotrauma to the neck is to place the patient in a cervical collar when appropriate. The collar should not be removed until it is verified that the patient does not have any serious injury that may be unstable and result in neurologic damage.

The initial examination should include a history of the trauma and a search for any contributory past medical history, such as previous accidents, fractures, or conditions that might predispose the patient to more severe injury from a trauma to the neck.

A brief and concise neurologic history and an examination are also of paramount importance. The patient should be questioned as to neurologic deficit such as sensory and/or motor losses, dizziness, vertigo, visual disturbances, loss of consciousness, and mental status (orientation). There are a number of signs and symptoms that should lead the physician to believe that serious consequences may follow. (Table 18.1)

Three features of accident mechanisms are most often associated with more severe injuries. These include an unprepared occupant, rear-end collision, and head rotation or inclination at the time of impact. (4)

Neck pain occurs in most patients who sustain cervical spine trauma, and it is the hallmark symptom. The pain can radiate into the occiput, shoulder, or mid-

Figure 18.1 Evaluation of the Acute Cervical Spine Trauma Patient

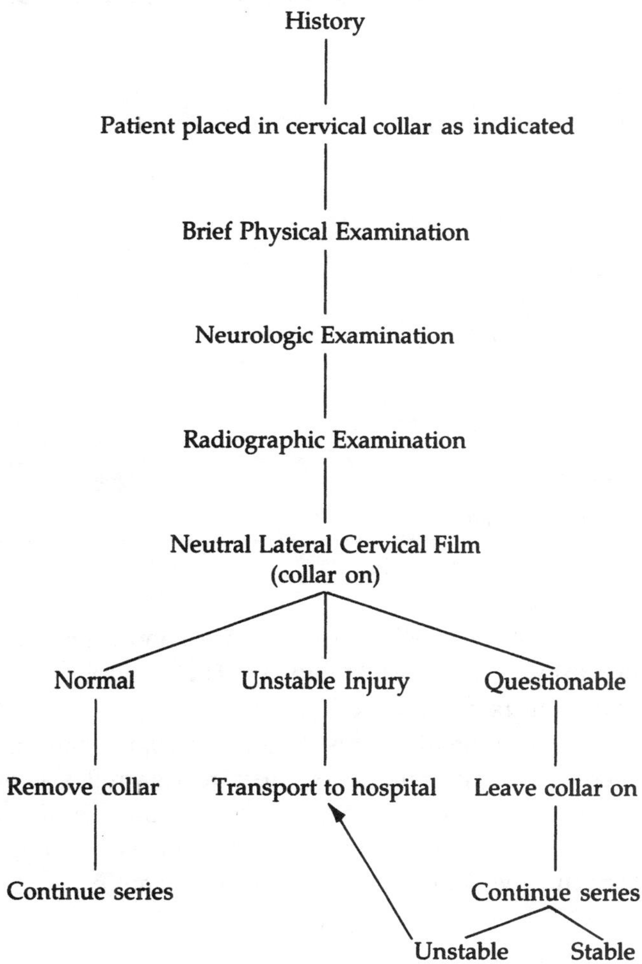

scapular area in addition to causing pain in the anterior neck as well. Headaches are typically located in the suboccipital region. Other common complaints include thoracolumbar back pain and paresthesias of the upper extremities in almost 50% of patients. A variety of theories have been proposed to explain these paresthesias, including facet syndrome, thoracic outlet syndrome, myofascial injuries, stretch injuries of the brachial plexus, and central cord injuries. Dysphagia,

Table 18.1 Signs/Symptoms of Neurologic Sequelae in Cervical Spine Trauma Patients

Midline spine pain
Altered mental status
Loss of consciousness
Neurologic deficit
Severe headache
Visual field loss
Seizure
Blood behind tympanum
Serous otorrhea/rhinorrhea
Battle's sign
Raccoon eyes
Hemiplegia/paraplegia/quadriplegia
Loss of bowel and/or bladder control

dizziness, vertigo, visual and auditory disturbances, and cognitive impairment also have been reported to occur after whiplash. The pathophysiologic explanation for these symptoms remains unexplained.

A brief neurologic examination consisting of pupillary examination and response to light, cranial nerve examination, deep tendon reflexes, otoscopic examination (rhinorrhea), and motor and sensory screening examinations should also be performed. If patient complaints of visceral damage are suggested by the neurologic history, the involved areas should also be examined.

Radiography

Radiography of the cervical spine in patients with neck trauma has long been the mainstay of the initial investigation. Recent evidence, although controversial, suggests that plain film radiography is only indicated to rule out serious injury when the patient has specific physical findings, including altered mental status, midline spine pain, or neurologic deficit. (5, 6) In patients who have these findings, computerized tomography or magnetic resonance imaging (MRI) appear to be the procedures of choice for the investigation of serious injuries. Unfortunately, a consistent correlation between MRI changes and symptoms of whiplash never has been well defined. (7)

The primary study for the investigation of cervical spine trauma has been the Davis series. (Table 18.2) Some institutions will also include articular pillar views as an ancillary portion of the examination. This view is excellent for demonstration of the articular facets.

In patients where plain film radiography is indicated, the radiographs should be performed within a very specific serial arrangement, beginning with the neutral lateral cervical projection. If the patient is in a collar, she/he should remain in the cervical collar until at least this view is completed. This film is then developed and screened for any gross pathology, as it is the best projection for depicting unstable injuries. If it is deemed that no instability exists, the collar can be removed, if warranted. If not, the remainder of the radiographic examination should be performed in the collar.

The anteroposterior (AP) open mouth view should be performed and developed next. A search is made for odontoid fractures and burst fracture of C1 in addition to any signs of ligamentous instability. The AP lower cervical, flexion and extension laterals, and obliques complete the study. Articular pillar views are added if a subtle injury of the articular facets is suspected.

After it is confirmed that there are no contraindications to manipulation and the patient can benefit from conservative care, a treatment regimen can begin.

Table 18.2 **Davis Series Radiographs**

Davis Series Radiographs
Neutral lateral
AP open mouth
AP lower cervical
Flexion
Extension
Right oblique
Left oblique

Ancillary Diagnostic Testing

Several investigators have used other diagnostic tests, such as electroencephalography, brainstem auditory evoked responses, electromyography, somatosensory evoked responses, positron emission tomography, and single-photon emission computed tomography. (7, 8, 9) Because none of these diagnostic tests have provided consistent findings, none can currently be recommended to confirm the diagnosis of whiplash injury.

Treatment

Traditional management of cervical spine injury has been conservative, provided that there is no neurologically unstable injury. Management consists of rest, analgesia, early mobilization, and therapeutic exercise. Immobilization of the neck with use of a soft cervical collar for 2 to 4 weeks also has been recommended but recently has been called into question by investigators. (10) Mealy and associates (11), in a prospective randomized trial comparing use of a soft cervical collar and analgesic medications with a regimen of active therapy, found that the group treated actively had significant improvement in both neck pain and mobility compared with the group treated with a soft collar. Another prospective randomized study demonstrated significant improvement in neck pain in early-mobilization groups compared with the group that rested. (12)

It is important to recognize the benefits of early mobilization in the treatment of these injuries. In a trial by Borchgrevink and coworkers (3), patients were divided into two groups. Group 1 was encouraged to continue to engage in normal preinjury activities, and group 2 was given time off from work and immobilized with a soft collar for 14 days. The groups were then evaluated for six months for the presence of subjective symptoms. Patients who were encouraged to continue with their normal activities of daily living had a better outcome than patients treated with immobilization and time off from work.

A number of other treatment strategies have been used, including subcutaneous trigger-point injections, cervical-facet injections, and low-energy, high-frequency pulsed electromagnetic therapy. The results of these strategies have been variable, depending on the study, and therefore strong recommendations regarding their use cannot be justified.

There is evidence that manipulation and mobilization of the cervical spine in patients without contraindications has demonstrated benefit in the management of neck pain. (13, 14, 15, 16)

It is also critically important to counsel the patient regarding fear-avoidance beliefs. Patients should be reassured that their injury is not serious and will heal adequately provided that they participate actively in their care. Encouraging early mobilization and return to activities of daily living is paramount. (17)

Prognosis

Cervical spine trauma can vary in severity from simple injuries with no substantial osseous or ligamentous injury with normal range of motion to full-thickness ligament tears, severely restricted range of motion, fractures, herniated discs, and neurologic sequelae. Treatment duration can vary from one to two weeks for simple uncomplicated injuries to months for more severe injuries with confounding comorbidities. Most patients respond to treatment within approximately three months.

A number of comorbidities can have a substantial impact on the clinical outcome of patients with neck trauma. These factors may lengthen the amount of time necessary for the therapeutic regimen to be effective. These include advancing age, herniated nucleus pulposus, paresthesias, objective neurologic signs, spondylosis, facet arthrosis, inflammatory arthritis, thoracolumbar pain, prior spinal surgery, spinal canal/foraminal/lateral recess stenosis, and previous spinal injury. (18, 19)

Malingering for monetary gain is a concern in whiplash patients. Currently, instruments are being designed to ferret out these patients. (20)

Ancillary Therapies

Therapies that are used in the management of neck pain are summarized in Table 18.3. The use of analgesics such as aspirin, ibuprofen, and acetaminophen can be helpful in cases of moderate pain.

Therapeutic exercise has also demonstrated effectiveness for patients suffering from chronic neck pain, particularly when combined with manipulation. (21)

Electromagnetic therapy has demonstrated some beneficial effects as well. (22)

After careful scrutiny that no life-threatening sequelae are apparent, the patient should be assured that common side effects following this type of injury (Table 18.4) are troublesome but will dissipate in time, in most cases. This type of reassurance along with assistance with avoiding fear-avoidance beliefs can help prevent these patients from progressing to chronic whiplash syndrome.

Table 18.3 Therapy in the Management of Traumatic Neck Pain

Analgesia
Manipulation
Early mobilization
Patient education
Counseling on side effect subsidence
Therapeutic exercise
Electromagnetic therapy
Cognitive behavioral therapy (chronic whiplash syndrome)

Chronic whiplash syndrome has been demonstrated to involve varied biopsychosocial issues that must be addressed in these patients. (23) If the patient progresses to chronic whiplash syndrome, cognitive behavioral therapy may be beneficial. A study that evaluated the response of patients with chronic whiplash syndrome to cognitive behavioral therapy documented improvement of symptoms in nearly all patient-reported outcome measures (e.g., visual analogue pain scale, self-reported Quebec Back Pain Disability Scale). At 6-month

Table 18.4 Side Effects of Cervical Spine Trauma

Dizziness
Vertigo
Headaches
Temporomandibular pain
Nausea & vomiting
Visual defects
Ataxia
Sleep disturbance

follow-up, 65% of patients had returned to full-time work, and 81% of patients had not sought any medical care for symptom relief, such as conventional physical or chiropractic therapy. (24) Randomized clinical trials are needed before definitive conclusions can be made about the role of cognitive behavioral therapy in the treatment of chronic whiplash syndrome.

Conclusion

Serious physical injury in whiplash patients is rare, and reassuring patients concerning the relatively good prognosis in these injuries is important. Long-term intensive in-office care is often detrimental to long-term recovery and should be avoided, when appropriate. Those therapies that demonstrate the most effectiveness include early return to normal activities of daily living, therapeutic exercise, and manual therapy. Instructions to patients regarding fear-avoidance beliefs are helpful in regaining normal pre-accident activity levels. Importantly, excess rest, cervical collar usage, and negative attitudes can significantly delay recovery and contribute to chronicity. (25)

References

1. Cusick, J.F., Yoganadan, N., & Pintar, F.A. Whiplash syndrome: kinematic factors influencing pain patterns. Presented at the 27th annual meeting of the Cervical Spine Research Society. Dec 1999; Seattle.
2. Cabbell, K., & Papadopoulos, S.M. Whiplash syndrome. In: Menezes AH, & Sonntag VK, eds. *Principles of Spinal Surgery.* Vol 2. New York: McGraw-Hill, 1996:801–806.
3. Borchgrevink, G.E., Kaasa, A., McDonagh, D., et al. Acute treatment of whiplash neck sprain injuries. A randomized trial of treatment during the first 14 days after a car accident. *Spine.* 1998;23(1):25–31.
4. Sturzenegger, M., DiStefano, G., Radanov, B.P., et al. Presenting symptoms and signs after whiplash injury: The influence of accident mechanisms. *Neurology.* 1994;44(4): 688–693.
5. Griffen, M.M., Frykberg, E.R., Kerwin, A.J., Schinco, M.A., Tepas, J.J., Rowe, K., & Abboud, J. Radiographic clearance of blunt cervical spine injury: plain radiograph or computed tomography scan? *J Trauma.* 2003 Aug;55(2):222–226; discussion 226–227.
6. Bandiera, G., Stiell, I.G., Wells, G.A., Clement, C., De Maio, V., Vandemheen, K.L., Greenberg, G.H., Lesiuk, H., Brison, R., Cass, D., Dreyer, J., Eisenhauer, M.A., Macphail, I., McKnight, R.D., Morrison, L., Reardon, M., Schull, M., & Worthington, J. Canadian C-Spine and CT Head Study Group. The Canadian C-spine rule performs better than unstructured physician judgment. *Ann Emerg Med.* 2003 Sep;42(3): 395–402.

7. Pearce, J.M. A critical appraisal of the chronic whiplash syndrome. *J Neurol Neurosurg Psychiatry.* 1999;66(3):273–276.
8. Otte, A, Ettlin, T.M., Nitzsche, E.U., et al. PET and SPECT in whiplash syndrome: a new approach to a forgotten brain? *J Neurol Neurosurg Psychiatry.* 1997;63(3):368–372.
9. Bicik, I., Radanov, B.P., Schafer, N., et al. PET with 18 fluorodeoxyglucose and hexamethylpropylene amine oxime SPECT in late whiplash syndrome. *Neurology.* 1998;51(2):345–350.
10. Rosenfeld, M., Gunnarsson, R., & Borenstein, P. Early intervention in whiplash-associated disorders: A comparison of two treatment protocols. *Spine.* 2000 Jul 15;25(14): 1782–1787.
11. Mealy, K., Brennan, H., & Fenelon, G.C. Early mobilization of acute whiplash injuries. *Br Med J.* (Clin Res Ed). 1986;292(6521):656–657.
12. McKinney, L.A. Early mobilization and outcome in acute sprains of the neck. *BMJ.* 1989;299(6706):1006–1018.
13. Hurwitz, E.L., Morgenstern, H., Harber, P., Kominski, G.F., Yu, F., & Adams, A.H. A randomized trial of chiropractic manipulation and mobilization for patients with neck pain: Clinical outcomes from the UCLA neck-pain study. *Am J Public Health.* 2002 Oct;92(10):1634–1641.
14. Wood, T.G., Colloca, C.J., & Matthews, R. A pilot randomized clinical trial on the relative effect of instrumental (MFMA) versus manual (HVLA) manipulation in the treatment of cervical spine dysfunction. *J Manipulative Physiol Ther.* 2001 May;24(4):260–271.
15. McMorland, G., & Suter, E. Chiropractic management of mechanical neck and low-back pain: a retrospective, outcome-based analysis. *J Manipulative Physiol Ther.* 2000 Jun;23(5):307–311.
16. Kjellman, G.V., Skargren, E.I., & Oberg, B.E. A critical analysis of randomized clinical trials on neck pain and treatment efficacy. A review of the literature. *Scand J Rehabil Med.* 1999 Sep;31(3):139–152.
17. Verhagen, A.P., Peeters, G.G., de Bie, R.A., & Oostendorp, R.A. Conservative treatment for whiplash. *Cochrane Database Syst Rev.* 2001;(4):CD003338.
18. Croft, A.C. Treatment paradigm for cervical acceleration/deceleration injuries (whiplash). *Am Chiro Assoc J.* 1993;30(1):41–45.
19. Norris, S.H., & Watt, I. The prognosis of neck injuries resulting from rear-end vehicle collisions. *J Bone Joint Surg Br.* 1983;65(5):608–611.
20. Sartori, G., Forti, S., Birbaumer, N., & Flor, H. A brief and unobtrusive instrument to detect simulation and exaggeration in patients with whiplash syndrome. *Neurosci Lett.* 2003 May 15;342(1–2):53–56.
21. Evans, R., Bronfort, G., Nelson, B., & Goldsmith, C.H. Two-year follow-up of a randomized clinical trial of spinal manipulation and two types of exercise for patients with chronic neck pain. *Spine.* 2002 Nov 1;27(21):2383–2389.
22. Gross, A.R., Aker, P.D., Goldsmith, C.H., & Peloso, P. Physical medicine modalities for mechanical neck disorders. *Cochrane Database Syst Rev.* 2000;(2):CD000961.

23. Ferrari, R. Prevention of chronic pain after whiplash. *Emerg Med J.* 2002 Nov; 19(6):526–530.
24. Vendrig, A.A., Van Akkerveeken, P.F., & McWhorter, K.R. Results of a multimodal treatment program for patients with chronic symptoms after a whiplash injury of the neck. *Spine.* 2000;25(2):238–244.
25. McClune, T., Burton, A.K., & Waddell, G. Whiplash associated disorders: A review of the literature to guide patient information and advice. *Emerg Med J.* 2002 Nov; 19(6):499–506.

Chapter 19

Low Back Pain Management

Lawrence H. Wyatt, DC, DACBR, FICC

Introduction

Low back pain (LBP) is a common morbid condition resulting in a large number of visits to health care providers, second only to upper respiratory infection as a reason for office visits to primary care physicians. Newton et al. (1) have shown that, in a population with back pain, over 70% of those patients had acute symptoms lasting less than three months, and that only 15% of cases of back pain were work-related. In addition they also demonstrated that patients fell into one of the following categories:

- acute low back strain (32%)
- "radicular" syndromes (28%)
- chronic low back strain (14%)
- sacroiliac syndromes (10%)
- facet syndrome (6%)
- multiple syndromes (10%)

It has been previously suggested that most patients with acute LBP will have spontaneous resolution of their symptoms. More recent evidence suggests that while many patients' pain will resolve, recurrences are quite common. (2) These authors demonstrated that only 9% of patients who had LBP for more than 30 days in the first year of the study were pain free at the end of the study five years later. They conclude that most cases of LBP are not, in fact, self-resolving, but rather represent periodic remissions and exacerbations. A recent systematic review reached similar conclusions. (3) Most patients with uncomplicated mechanical back pain will resolve with conservative management (4) and will not require more invasive interventions such as surgery. In fact, surgery for low back and leg pain is wrought with poor outcomes (5, 6) with complication rates as high as 40% for 360° fusion (7) including a high rate of re-operation for certain surgical procedures. (8) Interestingly, these authors suggest that patients with well-contained disc herniations were three times more likely to require re-operation than those with extruded or sequestered disc fragments. More recent interventions, including epidural steroid injections (9), percutaneous intradiscal radiofrequency thermocoagulation (10), and percutaneous diskectomy (11) have also demonstrated poor results.

The diagnostic and therapeutic approach to LBP is, to say the least, fragmented at times. This chapter presents an approach based on a compilation of many different disciplines.

Diagnostic Evaluation

Investigation of the complaints of a patient with LBP can be well accomplished if a simple rule is remembered. In the case of acute pain, it is important to rule out lesions such as fracture and instability first and then concentrate on arriving at the final diagnosis. In other words, are there any contraindications to manipulation of the patient's lumbar spine?

One of the essential considerations in the management of LBP is the exclusion of serious pathologic causes for the patient's complaints. The following signs and symptoms should raise concern that the patient is not suffering from uncomplicated mechanical LBP.

- fever
- pain unrelieved by changes in patient position
- night pain
- high-grade leg weakness
- loss of bowel and/or bladder control
- progressive neurologic deficit(s)

Figure 19.1 Investigation of Low Back Pain

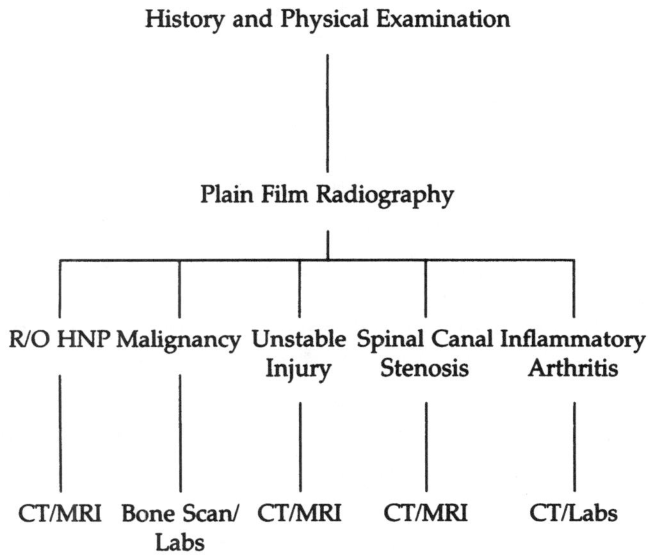

Figure 19–1 will help guide the investigation of the patient presenting with LBP.

Treatment

There are multiple therapeutic goals for the conservative management of LBP including pain relief, return to activities of daily living, and reduction of disability. Patients undergoing conservative management for back pain, including spinal manipulation, by chiropractors are typically very satisfied with their treatment. (12)

While it is beyond the scope of this text to list all the specific techniques, both manipulative and otherwise, for managing LBP, typically techniques that utilize high velocity low amplitude manipulation provide the best results. (13) The clinical judgment of the physician will serve as the best indicator of which therapies will most effectively serve each patient's particular therapeutic needs.

Acute Low Back Pain

While the therapeutic approach to chronic LBP can take many paths, treatment of acute LBP is initially directed at reducing pain, decreasing muscle spasm, and reducing soft tissue and capsular swelling so that the patient can return to the normal activities of daily living. The therapy listed below is one suggested approach to the initial treatment of acute low back pain. (Table 19.1)

Centralization of pain is a critical component of the management of LBP. Use of this phenomenon involves placing the patient into positions that relieve extremity pain, which appears to be effective in applying manipulative therapy. (14) A common use of the centralization phenomenon is the prone antigravity position, with the patient prone and the buttocks elevated above the head and feet. Positions that centralize pain will vary from patient to patient, so individual selection is critical.

Cryotherapy, 20 minutes every two hours, will help reduce swelling. It is often combined with interferential current and can relieve some, if not all, of the pain. (15,16) A rigid lumbar support can be helpful, provided the pa-

Table 19.1 Acute Low Back Pain Treatment

Acute Low Back Pain Treatment
Centralization of pain (antigravity position)
Cryotherapy (20 minutes every two hours)
Interferential current
Lumbosacral support
Bed rest (short-term, if at all)
Stool softener
Analgesics
Transcutaneous electrical nerve stimulation unit
Microcurrent therapy
Manipulation/mobilization

tient is compliant. (17) Short periods of bed rest with bathroom privileges as needed can be useful in patients with physically demanding jobs, but generally speaking, a rapid return to activity is as effective, if not more, than bed rest in most patients. (18) A stool softener may be useful in the management of patients with a positive Valsalva maneuver, and natural analgesics such as willow-bark extract (19, 20) and phytoanti-inflammatory supplements (21) can be helpful therapeutic adjuncts. Microcurrent therapy has also demonstrated some promise in the management of LBP. (22)

Only 22% of family practitioners would refer patients for manipulation. In addition, they do not tend to follow the recommended guidelines for the management of acute LBP. (23) Other therapies such as radiofrequency facet joint denervation have proven ineffective. (24) Manipulation of the patient with acute LBP has demonstrated to be quite effective. (13, 25, 26) In selected instances, manipulation can be performed on the first visit, but this decision must be made on a case-by-case basis.

Therapeutic exercise has been demonstrated to be more effective than normal activities in patients with back pain. (27) Spinal stabilization exercises should be instituted and have demonstrated to be effective in the long-term management of back pain. (28, 29)

There is some recent evidence that continuous low-level heat wrap therapy can be effective for patients with LBP as well. (30, 31, 32) This therapy involves the placement of a low-intensity long-duration heat wrap with hook and loop closures. It heats to 104° within 30 minutes, remains useful for eight hours, and should be worn until the heat dissipates.

This treatment for acute LBP can be performed once daily until there is a significant reduction in pain and return to functional capacity. Most patients with uncomplicated mechanical LBP can be expected to have a substantial reduction in pain within four weeks. (33) It is of paramount importance to recognize, however, that confounding co-morbidities (34,35) such as diabetes mellitus, smoking, obesity, cardiovascular and pulmonary status, length of disability, concurrent injury in some other body region, systemic musculoskeletal disease, and psychosocial stresses can alter this course and may require an increase in duration of care and/or co-management of the patient with another health care provider. (36, 37, 38) This list is not all inclusive and should be tailored to fit each individual patient.

Treatment may be performed in an intensive care area in the office until it is deemed that the patient may be released with appropriate home care instructions. Thereupon, the treatment schedule should be modified to patient needs.

Chronic Low Back Pain

The treatment of chronic LBP is usually directed at restoring functional capacity, relieving pain, and eliminating any disability that the patient may be suffering.

Manipulation (39, 40, 41), therapeutic exercise (41, 42) including spinal stabilization, and ergonomic recommendations (43) have all demonstrated effectiveness in the management and prevention of chronic LBP. Other conservative modalities that have demonstrated effectiveness include acupuncture (40, 44) and microcurrent therapy. (22) Pain relief can be accomplished by utilizing standard manipulative techniques and soft tissue therapy, such as massage and passive stretching.

Patients who have pain with sitting and then have trouble standing may benefit from the use of a weighted (10–20 pounds) backpack while walking, as wearing the backpack actually reduces spine loading by acting as a counterweight and prevents loading with a partially flexed posture secondary to pain.

Patients with lumbar spinal canal stenosis, who are not candidates for surgical intervention, have also been demonstrated to respond well to a manual therapy therapeutic regimen. (45,46) This program includes mobilization/manipulation, therapeutic exercise, restoring neural mobility, and restoring muscle function.

Neural mobilization technique involves mobilization of neural structures by tension development at the interfaces where they are restricted due to inflammation, scarring, chronic muscle spasm, and surgery. It has shown promise in the management of mechanical neuromusculoskeletal disorders. It is discussed further in the chapter on physical medicine and rehabilitation.

Patients with spinal canal stenosis, provided that there are no serious or progressive neurologic deficits, can be placed on a course of conservative management for an appropriate period of time. Should the patient fail to respond appropriately to conservative management, neurosurgical consultation can be helpful.

Physical therapy modalities, such as interferential current, galvanic current, ultrasound, traction, and heat, can be helpful alone or in combination with each other. It is best to use what is most comfortable for the patient and what yields the best therapeutic results. These therapies are discussed in-depth in the chapter on physical medicine and rehabilitation.

Prognosis for Manipulative Therapy Success

In a recent study, Flynn et al. suggested that patients with a specific set of five findings were determined to have the best chance of response from manipulative therapy. The findings included symptom duration less than 16 days, lumbar hypomobility, at least one hip internal rotation range of motion >35°, no symptoms beyond the knee, and lack of fear-avoidance beliefs such as fear of pain and avoidance of activity. They concluded that patients who had four of the five variables had a 95% chance of success with spinal manipulative therapy (SMT) of the lumbar spine and pelvis, and if the patient had three of four, a 68% rate. Completely random selection resulted in a 45% success rate. (47)

In addition, while long thought to be an important part of SMT, it has recently been suggested that the audible pop associated with cavitation is not particularly important in terms of positive patient outcomes. (48) This creates an interesting situation for the clinician in that there is often an expectation from patients for the audible pop. Clinicians can now inform their patients that SMT can be effective even without achieving cavitation of the joints involved.

The findings of these studies and others like them can aid the clinician in accurately predicting the likelihood of success for patients with LBP.

References

1. Newton, W., Curtis, P., Witt, P., & Hobler, K. Prevalence of subtypes of low back pain in a defined population. *J Fam Pract.* 1997 Oct;45(4):331–335.
2. Hestbaek L., Leboeuf-Yde, C., Engberg, M., Lauritzen, T., Bruun, N.H., & Manniche, C. The course of low back pain in a general population. Results from a 5-year prospective study. *J Manipulative Physiol Ther.* 2003 May;26(4):213–219.
3. Pengel, L.H.M., Herbert, R.D., Maher, C.G., & Refshauge, K.M. Acute low back pain: Systematic review of its prognosis. *BMJ.* 2003;327:323.
4. Cox, J.M., Fromelt, K.A., & Shreiner, S. Chiropractic statistical survey of 100 consecutive low back pain patients. *J Manipulative Physiol Ther.* 1983 Sep;6(3): 117–128.

5. Long, D.M. Failed back surgery syndrome. *Neurosurg Clin N Am.* 1991 Oct;2(4): 899–919.
6. Schoeggl, A., Maier, H., Saringer, W., Reddy, M., & Matula, C. Outcome after chronic sciatica as the only reason for lumbar microdiscectomy. *J Spinal Disord Tech.* 2002 Oct;15(5):415–419.
7. Fritzell, P., Hagg, O., & Nordwall, A. Complications in lumbar fusion surgery for chronic low back pain: Comparison of three surgical techniques used in a prospective randomized study. A report from the Swedish Lumbar Spine Study Group. *Eur Spine J.* 2003 Apr;12(2):178–189.
8. Morgan-Hough, C.V., Jones, P.W., & Eisenstein, S.M. Primary and revision lumbar discectomy. A 16-year review from one centre. *J Bone Joint Surg Br.* 2003 Aug;85(6):871–874.
9. Valat, J.P., Giraudeau, B., Rozenberg, S., Goupille, P., Bourgeois, P., Micheau-Beaugendre, V., Soubrier, M., Richard, S., & Thomas, E. Epidural corticosteroid injections for sciatica: A randomized, double-blind, controlled clinical trial. *Ann Rheum Dis.* 2003 Jul;62(7):639–643.
10. Barendse, G.A., van Den Berg, S.G., Kessels, A.H., Weber, W.E., & van Kleef, M. Randomized controlled trial of percutaneous intradiscal radiofrequency thermocoagulation for chronic discogenic back pain: Lack of effect from a 90-second 70 C lesion. *Spine.* 2001 Feb 1;26(3):287–292.
11. Shapiro, S. Long-term follow-up of 57 patients undergoing automated percutaneous discectomy. *J Neurosurg.* 1995 Jul;83(1):31–33.
12. Hertzman-Miller, R.P., Morgenstern, H., Hurwitz, E.L., Yu, F., Adams, A.H., Harber, P., & Kominski, G.F. Comparing the satisfaction of low back pain patients randomized to receive medical or chiropractic care: Results from the UCLA low back pain study. *Am J Public Health.* 2002 Oct;92(10):1628–1633.
13. Gatterman, M.I., Cooperstein, R., Lantz, C., Perle, S.M., & Schneider, M.J. Rating specific chiropractic technique procedures for common low back conditions. *J Manipulative Physiol Ther.* 2001 Sep;24(7):449–456.
14. Lisi, A.J. The centralization phenomenon in chiropractic spinal manipulation of discogenic low back pain and sciatica. *J Manipulative Physiol Ther.* 2001 Nov–Dec; 24(9):596–602.
15. Shao, Z.H. Cryotherapy for low back pain. Zhonghua Wai Ke Za Zhi. 1992 Nov; 29(12):721–723, 796.
16. Borenstein, D.G. A clinician's approach to acute low back pain. *Am J Med.* 1997 Jan 27;102(1A):16S–22S.
17. Jellema, P., van Tulder, M.W., van Poppel, M.N., Nachemson, A.L., & Bouter, L.M. Lumbar supports for prevention and treatment of low back pain: A systematic review within the framework of the Cochrane Back Review Group. *Spine.* 2001 Feb 15;26(4):377–386.

18. Rozenberg, S., Delval, C., Rezvani, Y., Olivieri-Apicella, N., Kuntz, J.L., Legrand, E., Valat, J.P., et al. Bed rest or normal activity for patients with acute low back pain: A randomized controlled trial. *Spine.* 2002 Jul 15;27(14):1487–1493.
19. Marz, R.W., & Kemper, F. Willow bark extract—effects and effectiveness. Status of current knowledge regarding pharmacology, toxicology and clinical aspects. *Wien Med Wochenschr.* 2002;152(15–16):354–359.
20. Chrubasik, Sigrun, et al. Treatment of low back pain exacerbations with willow bark extract: A randomized double-blind study. *Am J Med.* 2000;109(1):9–14.
21. Ernst, E., & Chrubasik, S. Phytoanti-inflammatories. A systematic review of randomized, placebo-controlled, double-blind trials. *Rheum Dis Clin North Am.* 2000 Feb;26(1):13–27, vii.
22. Lambert, M.I., Marcus, P., Burgess, T., & Noakes, T.D. Electromembrane microcurrent therapy reduces signs and symptoms of muscle damage. *Med Sci Sports Exerc.* 2002 Apr;34(4):602–607.
23. Di Iorio, D., Henley, E., & Doughty, A. A survey of primary care physician practice patterns and adherence to acute low back problem guidelines. *Arch Fam Med.* 2000;9:1015–1021.
24. Leclaire, R., Fortin, L., Lambert, R., Bergeron, Y.M., & Rossignol, M. Radiofrequency facet joint denervation in the treatment of low back pain. A placebo-controlled clinical trial to assess efficacy. *Spine.* 2001;26:1411–1416.
25. Swenson, R., & Haldeman, S. Spinal manipulative therapy for low back pain. *J Am Acad Orthop Surg.* 2003 Jul–Aug;11(4):228–237.
26. Koes, B. et al. Spinal manipulation for low back pain. An updated systematic review of randomized clinical trials. *Spine.* 1996; 21(24):2860–2871.
27. McLain, K., Powers, C., Thayer, P., & Seymour, R.J. Effectiveness of exercise versus normal activity on acute low back pain: An integrative synthesis and meta-analysis. Online. *J Knowl Synth Nurs.* 1999 Sep 13;6:7.
28. Janeck, K., Reuven, B., & Romano, C.T. Spinal stabilization exercises for the injured worker. *Occup Med.* 1998 Jan–Mar;13(1):199–207.
29. Hides, J.A., Jull, G.A., & Richardson, C.A. Long-term effects of specific stabilizing exercises for first-episode low back pain. *Spine.* 2001 Jun 1;26(11):E243–48.
30. Nadler, S.F., Steiner, D.J., Petty, S.R., Erasala, G.N., Hengehold, D.A., & Weingand, K.W. Overnight use of continuous low-level heat wrap therapy for relief of low back pain. *Arch Phys Med Rehabil.* 2003 Mar;84(3):335–342.
31. Nadler, S.F., Steiner, D.J., Erasala, G.N., Hengehold, D.A., Abeln, S.B., & Weingand, K.W. Continuous low-level heat wrap therapy for treating acute nonspecific low back pain. *Arch Phys Med Rehabil.* 2003 Mar;84(3):329–334.
32. Nadler, S.F., Steiner, D.J., Erasala, G.N., Hengehold, D.A., Hinkle, R.T., Beth Goodale, M., Abeln, S.B., & Weingand, K.W. Continuous low-level heat wrap therapy provides more efficacy than ibuprofen and acetaminophen for acute low back pain. *Spine.* 2002 May 15;27(10):1012–1017.

33. Seferlis, T., Nemeth, G., Carlsson, A.M., & Gillstrom, P. Conservative treatment in patients sick-listed for acute low back pain: A prospective randomized study with 12 months' follow-up. *Eur Spine J.* 1998;7(6):461–470.
34. Hestbaek, L., Leboeuf-Yde, C., & Manniche, C. Is low back pain part of a general health pattern or is it a separate and distinctive entity? A critical literature review of comorbidity with low back pain. *J Manipulative Physiol Ther.* 2003 May;26(4): 243–252.
35. Wright, D., Barrow, S., Fisher, A.D., Horsley, S.D., & Jayson, M.I. Influence of physical, psychological and behavioral factors on consultations for back pain. *Br J Rheumatol.* 1995 Feb;34(2):156–161.
36. Nordin, M., Hiebert, R., Pietrek, M., Alexander, M., Crane, M., & Lewis, S. Association of comorbidity and outcome in episodes of nonspecific low back pain in occupational populations. *J Occup Environ Med.* 2002 Jul;44(7):677–684.
37. van der Weide, W.E., Verbeek, J.H., Salle, H.J., & van Dijk, F.J. Prognostic factors for chronic disability from acute low back pain in occupational health care. *Scand J Work Environ Health.* 1999 Feb;25(1):50–56.
38. Infante-Rivard, C., & Lortie, M. Prognostic factors for return to work after a first compensated episode of back pain. *Occup Environ Med.* 1996 Jul;53(7):488–494.
39. Nyiendo, J., Haas, M., Goldberg, B., & Sexton, G. Pain, disability, and satisfaction outcomes and predictors of outcomes: A practice-based study of chronic low back pain patients attending primary care and chiropractic physicians. *J Manipulative Physiol Ther.* 2001 Sep;24(7):433–439.
40. Giles, L.G., & Muller, R. Chronic spinal pain: A randomized clinical trial comparing medication, acupuncture, and spinal manipulation. *Spine.* 2003 Jul 15;28(14): 1490–1502.
41. Aure, O.F., Nilsen, J.H., & Vasseljen, O. Manual therapy and exercise therapy in patients with chronic low back pain: A randomized, controlled trial with 1-year follow-up. *Spine.* 2003 Mar 15;28(6):525–531; discussion 531–532.
42. Harris, G.R., & Susman, J.L. Managing musculoskeletal complaints with rehabilitation therapy: Summary of the Philadelphia Panel evidence-based clinical practice guidelines on musculoskeletal rehabilitation interventions. *J Fam Pract.* 2002 Dec;51(12):1042–1046.
43. Staal, J.B., Hlobil, H., van Tulder, M.W., Koke, A.J., Smid, T., & van Mechelen, W. Return-to-work interventions for low back pain: a descriptive review of contents and concepts of working mechanisms. *Sports Med.* 2002;32(4):251–267.
44. Meng, C.F., Wang, D., Ngeow, J., Lao, L., Peterson, M., & Paget, S. Acupuncture for chronic low back pain in older patients: A randomized, controlled trial. *Rheumatology* (Oxford). 2003 Jul 30 [Epub ahead of print].
45. Whitman, J.M., Flynn, T.W., & Fritz, J.M. Nonsurgical management of patients with lumbar spinal stenosis: A literature review and a case series of three patients managed with physical therapy. *Phys Med Rehabil Clin N Am.* 2003 Feb;14(1):77–101, vi–vii.

46. Snow, G.J. Chiropractic management of a patient with lumbar spinal stenosis. *J Manipulative Physiol Ther.* 2001 May;24(4):300–304.
47. Flynn, T., Fritz, J., Whitman, J., Wainner, R., Magel, J., Rendeiro, D., Butler, B., Garber, M., & Allison, S. A clinical prediction rule for classifying patients with low back pain who demonstrate short-term improvement with spinal manipulation. *Spine.* 2002 Dec 15;27(24):2835–2843.
48. Flynn, T.W., Fritz, J.M., Wainner, R.S., & Whitman, J.M. The audible pop is not necessary for successful spinal high-velocity thrust manipulation in individuals with low back pain. *Arch Phys Med Rehabil.* 2003 Jul;84(7):1057–1060.

Chapter 20

Joint Manipulation and Mobilization

Lawrence H. Wyatt, DC, DACBR, FICC

"In the field of scientific discovery chance only favors the prepared mind."

Louis Pasteur

Introduction

Spinal manipulation has been practiced for some 4000 years. The earliest records indicate that it was initially performed in Asia. While spinal manipulation was not first practiced by chiropractors, it has been the mainstay of therapy in chiropractors' offices since the development of the profession in the late 19th and early 20th centuries. This form of therapy, while beneficial for many neuromusculoskeletal conditions, is not without controversy.

Most chiropractors utilize high velocity low amplitude (HVLA) manipulation in the management of spinal disorders. (1) Much research into the almost 200 various and sundry therapeutic techniques utilized by chiropractors is often proprietary and not published in peer-reviewed scientific journals. There does remain a large body of evidence into the use of HVLA manipulation for common neuromusculoskeletal conditions. In addition, manual force mechanically assisted (e.g., drop table, flexion-distraction) as well as mechanical force manually assisted procedures (MeFMA) (instrument adjusting) have been studied. Gatterman et al. report research-based consensus ratings on the various chiropractic manipulative techniques used for low back pain. (2) Their findings are outlined in Table 20.1.

This chapter provides documentation of the rationale, indications, contraindications, benefits, and adverse reactions for these types of joint manipulation.

Table 20.1 Evidence for Manual Techniques for Low Back Pain

Relatively strong
HVLA without drop table assist (lateral decubitus/side-posture)
Flexion-distraction
Segmental mobilization
HVLA prone with drop table assist
Moderate evidence
Pelvic blocking
MeFMA (instrument) manipulation
Relatively poor evidence
Upper cervical technique
Non-thrust/reflex low force technique
HVLA prone without drop table assist

Rationale for Spinal Manipulation

Most patients who visit chiropractors have spinal manipulative therapy (SMT) as a part of their therapeutic regimen. The most common conditions seen are low back pain and neck pain. (3) Most of these patients respond favorably to SMT, but no definitive reproducible mechanical lesion has been identified. Most often, this manipulation is provided to correct a putative spinal "subluxation." Often, these patients have multiple comorbidities such as degenerative disc disease, facet syndrome, and disc protrusion/extrusion, so it is difficult to isolate the patient's pain to a singular mechanical lesion.

More recently, researchers have suggested that mechanical spinal dysfunction is based on solid biomechanical principles. Triano (4) utilizes the term "functional spinal lesion," suggesting that patients with spine pain have mechanical buckling within functional spinal units (FSU). An FSU is akin to a vertebral motion segment. Buckling of an FSU refers to the production of symptoms that result from an uncontrolled localized mechanical response to loads being placed upon the spine. In other words, the FSU cannot sustain the loads placed upon it as would be expected, but instead, the tissues deform beyond the boundaries of expected normal displacement. Much research still needs to be performed until a definitive mechanical spinal lesion can be defined, if one in fact even exists.

Indications for Joint Manipulation

There are a number of clinical indications for spinal manipulation, and most of them are neuromusculoskeletal in origin. As was mentioned previously, the functional spinal lesion is often found along with other comorbidities which together produce the patient's symptoms.

Generally, uncomplicated low back pain is most easily managed. Other conditions that have been found to be amenable to SMT include sacroiliac joint dysfunction (2), low back pain with/without buttock or leg pain (2, 5, 6), nonorganic headaches (7, 8), thoracic spine pain (9), and disc herniations. (10, 11, 12) Provided that there are no contraindications, Table 20.2 outlines the more common conditions that respond to SMT. The presence of pain only in the buttock or leg without back pain, radiculopathy, peripheral neuropathy, and other conditions such as these are less amenable to SMT.

Generally speaking, acute low back pain is more readily managed by manipulation (2) than chronic low back pain, but recent evidence suggests a beneficial effect on chronic low back pain as well. (13)

Table 20.2 Common Indications for Joint Manipulation

Arthralgia (uncomplicated)
Decreased regional joint range of motion
Degenerative joint disease
Disc bulge/herniation
Functional spinal lesion
Headaches (nonorganic)
Internal joint derangement (nonsurgical)
Muscle spasm
Myofasciitis
Neuralgias
Sacroiliac joint dysfunction
Scoliosis (pain management)
Sprain/strain

Appropriate utilization of reasonable indications for SMT by chiropractors in patients with low back pain was studied by Shekelle et al. (14) This study was based on a retrospective review of manipulation on over 1,300 patients against preset criteria for appropriateness that were developed from a systematic review of the literature and by a nine-member panel of chiropractic and medical specialists. The appropriateness criteria reflected a reasonable balance between risk and benefit. They determined that in only 22% of cases, manipulation was inappropriate for the patient's clinical status. Larequi-Lauber and associates demonstrated that the inappropriateness of surgery for low back pain was 38%. (15)

Contraindications to Joint Manipulation

Joint manipulation has been purported to have many beneficial effects. Some of the more well-researched ones are listed in Table 20.3. (16, 17, 18, 19, 20) It cannot, however, be performed on all patients. (21) The contraindications listed in this chapter should be considered before applying a manipulative thrust to any patient.

There are two categories of contraindications to SMT: absolute contraindications and relative contraindications.

An absolute contraindication is one where, under no circumstances, should high force forms of manipulation be performed on the area of disease until the reason for the contraindication is corrected. This does not imply that low

Table 20.3 Benefits of Manipulation

Pain relief
Restoration of range of motion
Relief of disability
Return to activities of daily living
Muscle strengthening
Improved gait
Improved posture
Visceral effects (?)

force techniques and/or manipulation in other areas of the spine cannot be performed.

A relative contraindication, on the other hand, is one where certain types of manipulation or the force by which the manipulation is given must be altered to compensate for the problem.

The lists that follow are not all inclusive, and it must be remembered that clinical judgment in each individual case is the best indication or contraindication for manipulative treatment. In other words, because a condition is listed in this chapter does not by itself mean a patient with that condition should not be manipulated.

Absolute Contraindications

Patients with the following problems should not have dynamic high force manipulation in the area(s) of disease.

Entire Spine

- Benign bone tumors (aggressive types)
- Aneurysmal bone cyst
- Giant cell tumor
- Osteoblastoma
- Osteoid osteoma
- Cord tumor
- Dislocation
- Fracture (acute)
- Inflammatory arthritis (acute)
- Infection (osteomyelitis/septic discitis)
- Instability
- Hematoma (cord or intracanalicular)
- Malignancy
- Meningeal tumor
- Myelopathy
- Osteogenesis imperfecta
- Radiculopathy (with atrophy, severe muscle weakness)

In addition to the above contraindications, which apply to the entire spine, there are a number of conditions that should not be manipulated in each spinal region.

Cervical Spine

- Anomalies (e.g., unstable os odontoideum, dens hypoplasia)
- Arnold-Chiari malformation (Type II-III) (upper cervical spine)
- Atlantoaxial instability (upper cervical spine)
- Basilar invagination (upper cervical spine)
- Cerebral ischemic syndromes (e.g., vertebrobasilar artery insufficiency)

Thoracic Spine

- Aortic aneurysm
- Diastematomyelia

Lumbar Spine

- Abdominal aortic aneurysm
- Cauda equina syndrome
- Conus medullaris syndrome

Relative Contraindications

This section lists those diseases that mandate that the type and/or force used for manipulation must be altered to prevent serious injury to the patient. In most cases, patients with the following conditions can be safely manipulated, but caution must be used.

- Anticoagulant therapy
- Benign bone tumors (nonaggressive types)
- Ehlers-Danlos syndrome
- Fibrous dysplasia
- Hemangioma
- Cerebrovascular accident (history of)
- Clotting/bleeding disorders
- Spinal canal stenosis
- Intervertebral foraminal stenosis
- Fracture (healed injury without instability)
- Lateral recess stenosis
- Marfan's syndrome
- Osteoporosis

- Pregnancy
- Seizures
- Spondylolisthesis (progressive unstable types)
- Syringomyelia

Adverse Reactions to Manipulation

Until recently, there have been no well-done systematic reports of the complications or risks of spinal manipulation, and all that was known came from case reports and clinical trials. Recently, however, data from a prospective Norwegian study of side effects of spinal manipulation performed by chiropractors have become available. (22) During the course of six manipulations, 55% of the patients reported at least one negative reaction. The most commonly reported reactions were: local discomfort (53%), headache (12%), tiredness (11%), and radiating discomfort (10%). Only 15% of these reactions were considered "severe" and no seriously morbid or mortal complications were reported. Most reactions appeared within four hours of treatment and had disappeared within 24 hours.

Negative reactions are more likely to be reported by women, following the first treatment, when multiple spinal regions are treated and when only the thoracic spine is treated. (23) A causal relationship between manipulation and adverse reactions has not been definitively established. In fact, it is possible that some of the reactions attributed to manipulation were, in fact, coincidental. Another possible explanation is that some of these reactions are, in fact, part of the normal process of healing when manipulation is used as part of the therapeutic regimen. In other words, there are expected normal reactions to manipulation.

No systematic reports of the rate of serious complications of spinal manipulation have been conducted in the United States. Only anecdotal reports and "surveys" are available for critical analysis. Case reports may overestimate or underestimate the true number of adverse events, including serious ones. Some case reports and surveys are so poorly documented that a true cause-and-effect relationship is not established. (24, 25)

The total number of people who have received spinal manipulation is unknown. Because of this fact, estimates using data from case reports on the number of complications and epidemiologic estimates of the number of spinal manipulations are used. For example, Shekelle (21) roughly estimated the rate of occurrence of the cauda equina syndrome as about 1 case per 100 million manipulations.

It is important to note that no serious complications have ever been reported from any of the clinical trials investigating manipulation conducted to date.

Serious complications of cervical spine manipulation are also rare. Some suggest that complications from SMT in this spinal region appear to be more common and severe than complications of lumbar manipulation.

The most serious complication of cervical spine manipulation is related to vertebrobasilar artery damage, which can lead to cerebrovascular accident involving the brainstem or even death. As with lumbar manipulation, the limited data pool prohibits an exact estimate of the frequency of this complication. In addition, no definitive risk factors have been identified and it appears most often to be an idiosyncratic event. (26, 27) A recent study, however, suggests a link between hyperhomocystinemia and manipulation-related stroke. (28) This case series was small with only four patients, so no definitive conclusions can be drawn. In a retrospective case review of patients seen in a chiropractic college clinic, no evidence of manipulation-related stroke was seen. (29)

It cannot be said that no link exists. A population-based case-control study perfomed by Rothwell et al. suggests that a link exists. (30) To date, however, no well-designed prospective studies have been performed that document a relationship between cervical spine manipulation and stroke.

It has been postulated that perhaps some of these incidents are in fact coincidental; in other words, the patient seeks chiropractic care for a headache or neck pain that is the result of an arterial dissection in progress. It is for this reason that the signs and symptoms associated with vertebrobasilar insufficiency are outlined in Table 20.4. It is hoped that careful history and physical examination of these patients will expedite appropriate care for these patients.

Previously, George's battery of vascular tests were used to screen patients for cervico-cranial vascular disease. These tests demonstrate poor reliability and a poor predictive value as well. False positive tests often inappropriately limit care and patient activities, and false negative tests give the physician a false sense of security. It is recommended that these tests be abandoned for these reasons.

Differential diagnosis of the signs and symptoms commonly associated with vertebrobasilar artery ischemia/dissection are included in Table 20.5.

Some anecdotal evidence suggests that the risk for stroke from combined rotation and extension manipulation is higher than for other types of manipulation. In addition, patients who have suffered manipulation-related vertebrobasilar artery compromise have different clinical characteristics than patients who suffer vertebrobasilar stroke due to atherosclerotic disease. Patients who suffer manipulation-related stroke are generally younger and otherwise in good health. There have been suggestions that smoking, use of oral contraceptive agents, hypertension, diabetes mellitus, and cervical spondylosis might be implicated in manipulation-related stroke, but this has yet to be confirmed. (27)

Table 20.4 **Clinical Findings Associated with Vertebrobasilar Ischemia/Dissection**

Severe headache ("worst headache I've ever had")
Severe upper cervical spine pain ("worst neck pain I've ever had")
Relatively rapid insidious onset of pain
Vertigo/dizziness/lightheadedness
Ataxia
Nausea/vomiting
Diplopia and other visual disturbances
Unilateral facial dysesthesia or hemidysesthesia
Dysarthria
Dysphagia
Drooling

Estimates of the incidence of vertebrobasilar artery compromise related to cervical spine manipulation are that it occurs approximately once in 1 million manipulations, but estimates do vary widely. (31, 32)

Low back pain, neck pain (33), and many other musculoskeletal conditions are managed successfully by chiropractors utilizing many conservative

Table 20.5 **Differential Diagnosis for Vertebrobasilar Ischemia/Dissection**

Basilar migraine
Transient ischemic attack
Drop attack
Traumatic neck pain
Tension headache
Cervicogenic headache
Benign paroxysmal positional vertigo

measures including manipulation. It must be remembered that, while spinal manipulation has its risks and benefits, so do other treatments for back and neck pain. For example, medications commonly used for back pain can cause significant complications (34, 35, 36) as can lumbar surgery. (37, 38)

The risks of conservative treatments in the treatment of spine pain are low, particularly given that most randomized clinical trials directly comparing spinal manipulation with other types of conservative nonoperative treatment have reported no major complications. At present, the risks and benefits of spinal manipulation have not been compared to those for surgery for spinal lesions. It is known that there is a high failure rate for patients operated on for disc disease including a relatively high rate of surgical reintervention (39), in some series reaching over 15% (40), and continued low back pain. (41) Even the use of antiadhesion barrier gels to prevent postoperative fibrosis, a leading cause of continued postoperative pain, are not effective. (42) Recent evidence even suggests that cases of complications associated with lumbar discectomies are underreported. (43)

Optimal care of musculoskeletal pain patients will require balancing the risks and benefits of all available treatments.

Manipulation under Anesthesia/Conscious Sedation

In patients who fail to respond to more conservative in-house and home care, manipulation under anesthesia or conscious sedation offers an effective viable alternative (44, 45, 46) for chronic neck and back pain.

This procedure involves the use of therapeutic passive stretching and range of motion exercise along with manipulation while the patient is under anesthesia. General anesthesia is not utilized and patients are not intubated during the procedure. More recently, conscious sedation, similar to that used for some endoscopic procedures, has been utilized.

While patients are under conscious sedation, muscle relaxation and lack of anxiety make the application of these procedures more easily accomplished.

This procedure is not without risk, as is any procedure involving the use of anesthesia or conscious sedation.

Joint Mobilization

The treatment of musculoskeletal injuries often involves the application of passive physiological movement. The concept of mobilizations with movement

(MWMs) is the application of both physician-applied accessory and patient-generated active physiological movements. First used in the cervical spine, MWMs quickly found their way into the treatment of peripheral joint dysfunctions and have undergone clinical refinement and expansion to all areas of the spine and most extremity joints.

Principles of Mobilization

In the application of manual therapy techniques, it must be acknowledged that contraindications to manipulation and mobilization exist and should be heeded at all times. *Primum Non Nocere.* Although always guided by the basic rule of never causing pain, the basic rules for the application of manual therapy techniques should be followed.

Mobilization Grades

Grade I- minimal movements near the beginning of range of motion

Grade II- moderate movements to the mid-range of pain-free motion

Grade III- large movements to the end of range of motion

Grade IV- sustained large movements to the end of range of motion

Grade V- manipulation

Types of Mobilization

Mobilization can be performed at specific spinal levels or within specific portions of a joint or it can be generalized.

There are three types of general passive mobilization: graded oscillatory mobilization (GOM), continuous stretch mobilization (CSM), and progressive stretch mobilization (PSM). GOM utilizes alternating pressure and release within the passive range of motion to restore pain-free range of motion. CSM involves the use of continuous incrementally increasing joint stretching, and PSM utilizes progressive low-amplitude pressure-release motions.

GOM is utilized when mechanoreceptor stimulation, with resultant pain reduction, is the goal, while CSM is used to stretch soft tissues and PSM is utilized for resolution of soft-tissue biomechanical restriction.

Manually-assisted motion mobilization techniques include MWMs, natural apophyseal glides (NAGs), and sustained natural apophyseal glides (SNAGs).

Mobilization with Movements (MWMs)

Specific to the application of MWMs in clinical practice, the following basic principles have been developed:

1. Indications for mobilization include, but are not limited to, a loss of joint movement, pain associated with movement, or pain associated with specific functional activities (i.e., lateral elbow pain with resisted wrist extension).
2. A passive accessory joint mobilization is applied following either parallel or perpendicular to the joint plane and this accessory glide should be pain-free. Simple passive joint mobilization can occur in any normal range of motion.
3. Utilizing a knowledge of joint anatomy and motion, a well-developed sense of tissue tension, and clinical reasoning, the physician should investigate various combinations of parallel or perpendicular glides to find the correct treatment plane and grade of accessory movement that the patient tolerates without pain.
4. While sustaining the accessory glide, the patient is requested to perform active joint motion. This active motion should become significantly improved (e.g., increased range of pain-free active motion and muscle contraction).
5. Failure to improve pain-free motion should indicate that the correct treatment plane, grade of mobilization, spinal segment, or other factor is not correct or that the mobilization is not indicated.
6. The previously restricted and/or painful range of motion or activity is repeated by the patient while the appropriate accessory glide movements are performed by the physician. Further gains are expected with repetition during a treatment session, particularly when pain-free overpressure is applied. Patients can be instructed in home-treatment methods by using MWM principles with sports type adhesive tape and/or elastic banding. Pain must always be the patient's barometer of therapy. Successful MWM techniques should render the joint motion painless while significantly improving function during the application of the technique. Sustained improvements are necessary to justify ongoing intervention. (47)

Natural Apophyseal Glides (NAGs)

In the cervical spine, Mulligan describes an oscillatory mid-to-end range manual therapy technique performed in seated weight-bearing position. The gliding force is always performed parallel to the surface of the relevant apophyseal joints under treatment, so this form of therapy has been termed Natural Apophyseal Glides or "NAGs."

The patient is placed in the seated position, and force is directed along the facet joint planes near the end of range of motion.

Their application is well described by Mulligan, and physicians utilizing these techniques have demonstrated excellent clinical results in both the mid and lower cervical spine dysfunction, as well as dysfunction in the upper thoracic spine. (48)

NAGs provide the opportunity to both assess and treat a patient in the closed kinetic chain weight-bearing position. This is the position where most patients experience their symptoms.

NAGs are often indicated in the elderly and are highly useful in the management of the acute post-injury patient (e.g., whiplash) when other manual therapy techniques (high velocity manipulation) would be poorly tolerated or contraindicated.

Sustained Natural Apophyseal Glides (SNAGs)
Another spinal manual therapy treatment technique involves the concurrent application of both physican-applied accessory apophyseal joint gliding and end-of-passive range of motion and active physiological movement on the part of the patient. In this technique, because the movements are sustained at the end of available pain-free range of motion and still follow the plane of the apophyseal joints under treatment, they have gained the name "Sustained Natural Apophyseal Glides".

SNAGs are performed exclusively in weight bearing and are applicable to all spinal joints. The technique is similar to NAGs but the physician-applied gliding motion is sustained at the end of pain-free range of motion. Studies have demonstrated immediate and sustained gains in pain-free function. (49)

Peripheral MWMs
MWM in the peripheral joints also involves the simultaneous combination of physician-applied accessory gliding techniques parallel of perpendicular to the joint plane and patient and/or physician-generated physiological movements. They are applicable to most extremity joints. Research suggests that their use results in immediate and sustained improvement in mobility and function of extremity joints. (50)

Clinical Examples of Mobilization

The patient is seated in a supportive chair with the physician positioned behind him. The current range of cervical extension is checked for range, rhythm, deviation, and limiting factors such as increasing pain during motion, pain at end of the available range, or painless stiffness at the end of a reduced range of motion.

The physician uses the medial border of one thumb reinforced by the pad of the other thumb to apply an anterior-superior accessory glide through the involved motion segment. The direction of this mobilization must follow the plane described by the surfaces of the apophyseal joints under treatment. The cervical apophyseal joint planes are directed anteriorly-superiorly with the inclination increasing at lower levels. A general rule of thumb is that the planes of the cervical apophyseal joints converge near the eyes of the patient.

While sustaining this pain-free accessory glide, the patient is instructed to actively perform cervical extension. The expectation is that the range displayed will significantly increase and any pain previously experienced will be virtually abolished.

As the patient progresses through the increasing physiological range, the physician should "track" with the spinous process to maintain his/her glide parallel to the changing treatment plane. As such, the physician's forearms circumscribe an arc whose apex faces anteriorly-superiorly. The end-range physiological movement is sustained for several seconds. Overpressure may be given at the end of range by the patient to enhance the effect, and the procedure is repeated in sets of five to ten.

The patient's post-treatment range should now be reevaluated to observe the overall gain without the application of the mobilization component. Between one to four sets of this maneuver are performed, depending on patient tolerance.

Other examples of MWMs for peripheral joint dysfunction include posterior glide of the head of the humerus within the glenoid cavity for a painful arc of active shoulder elevation, a lateral glide of the forearm in relation to the distal humerus for patients with pain experienced at the lateral elbow with resisted wrist extension, and/or hand grip and long-axis distraction of the hip with internal hip rotation for hip joint pain and dysfunction. Myriad other techniques are available.

Lateral Decubitus Traction/Extension mobilization is a procedure that should cause no discomfort to the patient. The patient is asked to report any increase in pain or peripheralization of symptoms (radiation into the extremities), in which case the procedure should be discontinued.

The patient is asked to lie with the knees together, painful side down with the hips flexed to approximately 45 degrees. The head is supported on the headpiece to keep the spine in as straight a line in the coronal plane as is possible. The pelvis and thorax are in neutral position.

The physician is positioned behind the patient, facing toward the patient's feet. The heel of the hand is placed on the lumbar spine centrally at the level of the intervertebral disc between L4-5. The supraspinous ligament is nestled between the physician's pisiform and trapezium. His elbow is braced against the anterior-superior iliac spine. For a left side-lying patient, force is directed with the right hand/right hip. For a right side-lying patient, force is directed with the left hand/left hip.

The height of the table should be such that the force of traction is coming from the hips, horizontally via the forearm, using his or her body weight. A series of five to ten firm but not forceful sustained tractions of approximately five seconds duration are performed. There is normally not a great deal of movement with this mobilization. Ideally there should be a sensation of taking up the slack in the tissues, then releasing after four seconds. During this entire procedure, the patient should not feel any increased discomfort or peripheralization of symptoms.

After traction, the patient's pelvis is stabilized with the other hand, and extension mobilizations performed. The physician now faces the patient's head and changes contact hands. These mobilizations are in a posteroanterior plane, the force coming from the physician's free hand, which is clenched into a fist and a V formed between the thumb and the flexed index finger. The lumbar spinous process fits into the V and the force is transmitted to the articular pillars via the physician's horizontal forearm. The elbow can be braced against the hip as described above, to increase stability and force. The extension mobilizations are performed at the level of L4-5 with the patient still in lateral decubitus position. Typically, five to six mobilizations will suffice. While it is always wise to start with a gentle grade I mobilization, there will often be a surprising degree of pain-free mobility of the segment and, many times, a stronger mobilization causes no discomfort.

After the extension mobilization, a repeat set of eight tractions is given. The patient can then be reassessed for range of motion and pain before being sent home with instructions regarding posture and maintaining the lumbar lordosis.

Oscillatory cervical lateral glide mobilization is a technique whereby the patient is in the supine position with the head supported by the physician's hands, while he stands at the head of the table. The head and neck are then moved right to left in a smooth gliding motion with generally increasing levels of lateral flexion induced with each glide.

Progressive or continuous thoracic extension stretching mobilization involves the placement of the physician's hand in the middle of the thoracic spine while placing the other hand under the patient's elbows, which are in front of his face while he is seated. The clinician then raises the patient's elbows while exerting either continuous progressively increasing force or pressure-release motions.

Progressive or continuous lumbar rotation stretching mobilization has the patient prone on the table with a rolled up towel under the patient's waistline to elevate the buttocks. The more cephalic of the physician's hands is placed on the thoracolumbar junction while the other hand reaches under the patient's pelvis and grasps the anterior-superior iliac spine. Pressure-release or continuously increasing pressure is applied exerting a rotational force on the lumbar spine by lifting the pelvis off the table and exerting cephalic traction on the thoracolumbar region.

The aforementioned techniques can also be used at specific vertebral levels for specific joint motions or in the extremities as well. Simple changes in hand placement make these techniques quite adaptable.

Attempts are made with these mobilization techniques to increase the patient's diminished range(s) of motion and decrease the patient's pain, discomfort, and stiffness. Mobilization may also be used as a premanipulative stretching technique that may make manipulation more easily accomplished and comfortable for the patient.

References

1. Christensen, M.G., & Delle Morgan, D.R., editors. Job analysis of chiropractic. Greeley (CO): National Board of Chiropractic Examiners; 1993.
2. Gatterman, M.I., Cooperstein, R., Lantz, C., Perle, S.M., & Schneider, M.J. Rating specific chiropractic technique procedures for common low back conditions. *J Manipulative Physiol Ther.* 2001 Sep;24(7):449–456.
3. Hurwitz, E.L., Coulter, I.D., Adams, A.H., Genovese, B.J., & Shekelle, P.G. Use of chiropractic services from 1985 through 1991 in the United States and Canada. *Am J Pub Health.* 1998;88:771–776.
4. Triano, J.J. The Functional Spinal Lesion. An evidence-based model of subluxation. *Topics in Clin Chiro.* 2001;8(1):16–28.
5. Hadler, N.M., Curtis, P., Gillings, D.B., & Stinnett, S. A benefit of spinal manipulation as adjunctive therapy for acute low back pain: A stratified controlled trial. *Spine.* 1987;12:702–706.
6. Meade, T.W., Dyer, S., Browne, W., et al. Randomized comparison of chiropractic and hospital outpatient management for low back pain: Results from extended follow-up. *BMJ.* 1995;311:349–351.
7. Boline, P.D., Kassak, K., Nelson, C., Bronfort, G., & Anderson, A. Spinal manipulation vs amitriptyline for the treatment of chronic tension-type headaches: A randomized clinical trial. *J Manipulative Physiol Ther.* 1995;18:148–154.
8. Nilsson, N., Christensen, H.W., & Hartvigsen, J. The effect of spinal manipulation in the treatment of cervicogenic headache. *J Manipulative Physiol Ther.* 1997 Jun;20(5):326–330.
9. Schiller, L. Effectiveness of spinal manipulative therapy in the treatment of mechanical thoracic spine pain: A pilot randomized clinical trial. *J Manipulative Physiol Ther.* 2001 Jul–Aug;24(6):394–401.
10. BenEliyahu, D.J. Magnetic resonance imaging and clinical follow-up: Study of 27 patients receiving chiropractic care for cervical and lumbar disc herniations. *J Manipulative Physiol Ther.* 1996 Nov–Dec;19(9):597–606.
11. Quon, J.A., Cassidy, J.D., O'Connor, S.M., & Kirkaldy-Willis, W.H. Lumbar intervertebral disc herniation: Treatment by rotational manipulation. *J Manipulative Physiol Ther.* 1989 Jun;12(3):220–227.

12. Floman, Y., Liram, N., & Gilai, A.N. Spinal manipulation results in immediate H-reflex changes in patients with unilateral disc herniation. *Eur Spine J.* 1997;6(6):398–401.
13. Giles, L.G., & Muller, R. Chronic spinal pain: A randomized clinical trial comparing medication, acupuncture, and spinal manipulation. *Spine.* 2003 Jul 15;28(14): 1490–1502.
14. Shekelle, P.G., Coulter, I., Hurwitz, E.L., Genovese, B., Adams, A.H., Mior, S.A., & Brook, R.H. Congruence between decisions to initiate chiropractic spinal manipulation for low back pain and appropriateness criteria in North America. *Ann Int Med.* 1998;129:9–17.
15. Larequi-Lauber, T., Vader, J.P., Burnand, B., Brook, R.H., Kosecoff, J., Sloutskis, D., Fankhauser, H., Berney, J., Tribolet, N., & Paccaud, F. Appropriateness of indications for surgery of lumbar disc hernia and spinal stenosis. *Spine.* 1997;22(2):203–209.
16. Suter, E., McMorland, G., Herzog, W., & Bray, R. Conservative lower back treatment reduces inhibition in knee-extensor muscles: A randomized controlled trial. *J Manipulative Physiol Ther.* 2000 Feb;23(2):76–80.
17. Herzog, W., Conway, P.J., Zhang, Y.T., Gal, J., & Guimaraes, A.C. Reflex responses associated with manipulative treatments on the thoracic spine: A pilot study. *J Manipulative Physiol Ther.* 1995 May;18(4):233–236.
18. Vernon, H.T., Dhami, M.S., Howley, T.P., & Annett, R. Spinal manipulation and beta-endorphin: A controlled study of the effect of a spinal manipulation on plasma beta-endorphin levels in normal males. *J Manipulative Physiol Ther.* 1986 Jun;9(2):115–123.
19. Kjellman, G.V., Skargren, E.I., & Oberg, B.E. A critical analysis of randomized clinical trials on neck pain and treatment efficacy. A review of the literature. *Scand J Rehabil Med.* 1999 Sep;31(3):139–152.
20. Haas, M., Jacobs, G.E., Raphael, R., & Petzing, K. Low back pain outcome measurement assessment in chiropractic teaching clinics: Responsiveness and applicability of two functional disability questionnaires. *J Manipulative Physiol Ther.* 1995 Feb;18(2): 79–87.
21. Shekelle, P.G., Adams, A.H., Chassin, M.R., Hurwitz, E.L., & Brook, R.H. Spinal manipulation for low back pain. *Ann Intern Med.* 1992 Oct 1;117(7):590–598.
22. Senstad, O., Leboeuf-Yde, C., & Borchgrevink, D. Frequency and characteristics of side effects of spinal manipulative therapy. *Spine.* 1997;22:435–441.
23. Senstad, O., Leboeuf-Yde, C., & Borchgrevink, C. Frequency and characteristics of side effects of spinal manipulative therapy. *Spine.* 1997 Feb 15;22(4):435–441.
24. Dupeyron, A., Vautravers, P., Lecocq, J., & Isner-Horobeti, M.E. Complications following vertebral manipulation—a survey of a French region physician. *Ann Readapt Med Phys.* 2003 Feb;46(1):33–40.
25. Lee, K.P., Carlini, W.G., McCormick, G.F., & Albers, G.W. Neurologic complications following chiropractic manipulation. A survey of California neurologists. *Neurology.* 1995;45:1213–1215.
26. Haldeman, S., Kohlbeck, F.J., & McGregor, M. Stroke, cerebral artery dissection, and cervical spine manipulation therapy. *J Neurol.* 2002 Aug;249(8):1098–1104.

27. Haldeman, S., Kohlbeck, F.J., & McGregor, M. Unpredictability of cerebrovascular ischemia associated with cervical spine manipulation therapy: A review of 64 cases after cervical spine manipulation. *Spine.* 2002 Jan 1;27(1):49–55.
28. Pezzini, A., Del Zotto, E., & Padovani, A. Hyperhomocystinemia: A potential risk factor for cervical artery dissection following chiropractic manipulation of the cervical spine. *J Neurol.* 2002 Oct;249(10):1401–1403.
29. Wyatt, L.H., & Basaraba, B. Morbidity and mortality associated with spinal manipulation performed at a chiropractic college health center. Proceedings of the 124th Annual Meeting of the American Public Health Association. November 1996.
30. Rothwell, D.M., Bondy, S.J., & Williams, J.I. Chiropractic manipulation and stroke: A population-based case-control study. *Stroke.* 2001 May;32(5):1054–1060.
31. Hurwitz, E.L., Aker, P., Adams, A.H., Meeker, W., & Shekelle, P.G. Mobilization and manipulation of the cervical spine: A systematic review of the literature. *Spine.* 1996;21:1746–1760.
32. McGregor, M., Haldeman, S., & Kohlbeck, F.J. Vertebrobasilar compromise associated with cervical manipulation. *Top Clin Chiropr.* 1995;2:(3):63–73.
33. Hoving, J.L., Koes, B.W., de Vet, H.C., van der Windt, D.A., Assendelft, W.J., van Mameren, H., Deville, W.L., Pool, J.J., Scholten, R.J., & Bouter, L.M. Manual therapy, physical therapy, or continued care by a general practitioner for patients with neck pain. A randomized, controlled trial. *Ann Intern Med.* 2002 May 21;136(10):713–722.
34. Anker, A.L., & Smilkstein, M.J. Acetaminophen concepts and controversies. *Emerg Med Clin North Am.* 1994;12:335–349.
35. Bjarnason, I., Hayllar, J., MacPherson, A.J., & Russell, A.S. Side effects of nonsteroidal anti-inflammatory drugs on the large and small intestines in humans. *Gastroenterology.* 1993;104:1832–1847.
36. van Tulder, M.W., Touray, T., Furlan, A.D., Solway, S., & Bouter, L.M. Muscle relaxants for nonspecific low back pain: A systematic review within the framework of the Cochrane Collaboration. *Spine.* 2003;28:1978–1992.
37. Kraemer, R., Wild, A., Haak, H., Herdmann, J., Krauspe, R., & Kraemer, J. Classification and management of early complications in open lumbar microdiscectomy. *Eur Spine J.* 2003 Jun;12(3):239–246.
38. Katonis, P., Christoforakis, J., Aligizakis, A.C., Papadopoulos, C., Sapkas, G., & Hadjipavlou, A. Complications and problems related to pedicle screw fixation of the spine. *Clin Orthop.* 2003 Jun;(411):86–94.
39. Fritsch, E.W., Heisel, J., & Rupp, S. The failed back surgery syndrome: Reasons, intraoperative findings, and long-term results: A report of 182 operative treatments. *Spine.* 1996 Mar 1;21(5):626–633.
40. Osterman, H., Sund, R., Seitsalo, S., & Keskimaki, I. Risk of multiple reoperations after lumbar discectomy: A population-based study. *Spine.* 2003 Mar 15;28(6):621–627.
41. de Kleuver, M., Oner, F.C., & Jacobs, W.C. Total disc replacement for chronic low back pain: Background and a systematic review of the literature. *Eur Spine J.* 2003 Apr;12(2):108–116.

42. Ganzer, D., Giese, K., Volker, L., Pietzner, U., Follak, N., & Merk, H. Two-year results after lumbar microdiscectomy with and without prophylaxis of a peridural fibrosis using Adcon-L. *Arch Orthop Trauma Surg.* 2003 Feb;123(1):17–21.
43. Romano, P.S., Chan, B.K., Schembri, M.E., & Rainwater, J.A. Can administrative data be used to compare postoperative complication rates across hospitals? *Med Care.* 2002 Oct;40(10):856–867.
44. West, D.T., Mathews, R.S., Miller, M.R., & Kent, G.M. Effective management of spinal pain in 177 patients evaluated for manipulation under anesthesia. *J Manipulative Physiol Ther.* 1999 Jun;22(5):299–308.
45. Palmieri, N.F., & Smoyak, S. Chronic low back pain: A study of the effects of manipulation under anesthesia. *J Manipulative Physiol Ther.* 2002 Oct;25(8):E8–E17.
46. Herzog, J. Use of cervical spine manipulation under anesthesia for management of cervical disk herniation, cervical radiculopathy, and associated cervicogenic headache syndrome. *J Manipulative Physiol Ther.* 1999 Mar–Apr;22(3):166–170.
47. Exelby, L. Mobilizations with movement, a personal view. *Physiotherapy.* 1995 Dec 81;12.
48. Mulligan, R.B. NAGS - Modified Mobilization Techniques for the Cervical and Upper Thoracic Spines. *New Zealand Journal of Physiotherapy.* 1982:Aug.
49. Mulligan, B.R. Manual Therapy, "NAGS", "SNAGS", "MWMS". 1995, Plane View Press, Wellington.
50. Mulligan, B.R. Mobilizations with movement (MWMS). *J Man and Manip Ther.* 1993 1;4.

Chapter 21

Physical Medicine and Rehabilitation

Lawrence H. Wyatt, DC, DACBR, FICC

Introduction

The use of physical medicine and rehabilitation in chiropractic practice is commonplace. Such modalities can have a beneficial effect on the clinical outcome of patients in many cases. They must be used judiciously, however, as they are not without side effects and contraindications.

Effects of Physical Medicine Modalities

The basic effects of physical medicine modalities can be divided into three categories: thermal, chemical, and kinetic. The type of effect desired is the basis for deciding what therapy to use. Many of the modalities have more than one effect. For example, if the desired effects are a decrease in soft tissue swelling and analgesia, cryotherapy would be helpful in obtaining both. Table 21.1 lists the more commonly used modalities and their suggested primary and secondary effects.

Specific Physical Medicine Modalities

This section will outline the use of the various modalities with regard to their indications, contraindications, and physical application.

Table 21.1 Physical Modalities and Their Suggested Effects

Modality	Effect
Cryotherapy	Hypothermia Decongestion Vasoconstriction Analgesia
Heat	Hyperthermia Vasodilatation Analgesia Muscle relaxation
Ultrasound	Heating (continuous mode) Micromassage (pulsed mode)
Galvanic current	Electrochemical Decongestion
Sinusoidal current	Muscle contraction Decongestion

Cryotherapy

The use of ice has been a primary treatment for acute musculoskeletal injuries for many years. Its purported effects include vasoconstriction, tissue decongestion, and an anti-inflammatory/analgesic effect. Ice is used most commonly in the treatment of acute diseases to reduce swelling, provide analgesia, and reduce the secondary damage from an injury by lowering the local metabolic rate over which the coolant is placed. (1, 2) (Table 21.2). There is also evidence that the effective depth of cold temperatures is affected by the type of therapy used. (3) From this study it was determined that ice bags, where the ice actually undergoes physical change to water during the therapy, was more effective than chemical-based flexible cold packs that do not undergo this change.

Ice should not be used in patients with a number of different diseases, and these contraindications are outlined in Table 21.3. Ice should be applied over an area with protection by a towel or wrap of some sort. This helps prevent the onset of frostbite. Treatment times vary from 10 to 20 minutes. Home cryotherapy can also be useful if clinically indicated.

Table 21.2 Indications for Cryotherapy (Acute Diseases)

Sprains
Strains
Bursitis
Arthritis
Tendinitis
Myositis

A special form of cryotherapy, called ice massage, is used in acute sprain/strain injuries. It is helpful in creating anesthesia after massaging ice over an area for a period of about 5–10 minutes. The patient will experience four separate sensations from an ice massage: cold, burning, aching, and finally anesthesia. Care should be taken with this therapy as frostbite is more easily accomplished secondary to the convection utilized in this therapy.

Spray and Stretch Technique

The use of coolant sprays such as fluorimethane have become popular in recent years and are used in combination with passive stretching. This represents the "spray and stretch" technique. Ice may be used in place of vapocoolants.

The coolant stream should be directed at the skin from about 18 inches away. You will notice that the mixture vaporizes almost immediately. Use three to six

Table 21.3 Contraindications for Cryotherapy

Advanced cardiovascular disease
Diabetes mellitus
Raynaud's phenomenon
Sensory loss involving cold perception
Vasospastic diseases

sweeping strokes of one to two seconds each, in one direction. Frosting the skin should be avoided.

Stretch the muscles with your free hand by moving the joints over which they or their tendons pass. For back muscles, rock the back, while sitting, or bend over a chair. It is not enough to cover the area where the patient feels pain, as often times this is referred pain from a trigger point. Sweep from the trigger points or muscle origins to the insertions and over the region where the patient tells you he or she feels pain. For example, if pain is in the biceps muscle, spray from origin at the anterior shoulder to the lower end of the humerus anteriorly, while at the same time gently extending the elbow. Stretch the muscle just short of producing pain or to its resting length.

The rationale behind spray and stretch is that the cold stream apparently produces impulses that move faster from skin receptor organs along large afferent nerves than do painful impulses. Both sets of impulses are relayed by the lateral spinothalamic tracts to the brain, perhaps at the level of the thalamus. Arriving first, the cooling impulses set up a refractory state that blocks reception of the slower pain impulses. This permits the muscle to relax and to be stretched to resting length. The muscle is then in its normal physiological position.

There are contraindications to spray and stretch technique, and they are generally the same as for other cryotherapeutic techniques. In addition, this technique should be reserved for patients with pain of myofascial origin, not true neuropathy.

Heat Therapy

Heat has a number of useful effects including vasodilation, increased phagocytosis, relief of muscle spasm, and analgesia. The use of heat is usually confined to subacute and chronic diseases and is most often provided by Hydrocollator packs. (Table 21.4) Some recent evidence suggests that a continuous 8-hour low-level heat wrap during the overnight hours is helpful for low back pain. (4, 5, 6)

Heat should not be applied in patients whose sensation is diminished, as well as in the conditions listed in Table 21.5.

Heat is applied with a towel or wrap between the heat source and the patient to prevent burns. The patient should be questioned periodically as to comfort. Treatment times vary from 10 to 20 minutes. Dry heat is usually less beneficial than moist heat.

Specialized forms of therapeutic heat include diathermy, whirlpool bath (where there is convection and also a massaging effect), and infrared therapy. Diathermy provides the deepest tissue heating of the various modalities whereas infrared heat is most superficial.

Table 21.4 Indications for Heat Therapy

Indications for Heat Therapy
Subacute/Chronic
Sprains
Strains
Arthritis
Tendinitis
Bursitis
Myositis
Premanipulation relaxation
Premassage relaxation
Muscle spasm/myofasciitis

Contrast Bath

The use of alternating heat and cold has the effect of causing vasodilatation and vasoconstriction with all of its concomitant benefits. This modality is best used in the subacute stage of an injury when decongestion of tissues and the influx of blood to the injured area are the main goals of therapy. Common indications for contrast bath are outlined in Table 21.6.

Table 21.5 Contraindications to Heat Therapy

Contraindications to Heat Therapy
Acute inflammation
Hemorrhage
Neoplasia
Gravid uterus
Encapsulated swelling (abscess)
Diabetes mellitus
Acute infection
Sensory deficit to heat

Table 21.6 Common Indications for Contrast Bath

Subacute/chronic/remission phase
Sprain/strain
Inflammatory arthritides
Myofasciitis
Stasis edema
Peripheral vascular disease (use on unaffected extremity from consensual vasodilation)
Degenerative joint disease

Contrast baths should always begin and end with heat and alternate in a cycle for a sustained period of time. For example, treatment with 4 minutes of heat followed by 1 minute of cold for four cycles is then completed with 4 minutes of heat. The treatment may also be started with a 10-minute warm bath with cycling afterwards.

The cold bath should be between 50 and 60 degrees and the hot bath between 105 and 110 degrees.

Ultrasound

Applying high frequency sound waves to the body tissues can produce both a micromassage (pulsed) and deep heating (continuous), depending upon which type of ultrasound is used. The list of lesions treatable by ultrasound is long but, generally speaking, when lesions are chronic, ultrasound can be used for both massage and heating effects. (Table 21.7) The use of this therapy in acute injuries is confined to micromassage to reduce swelling, although there is cursory evidence of its effectiveness.

Because continuous ultrasound generates heat by bouncing off internal structures, it should not be used in the diseases listed in Table 21.8.

Ultrasound should be performed with a conducting gel placed on the skin over the area to be treated or used underwater. These techniques are necessary because the crystal inside the ultrasound head will be destroyed if transmission of the sound waves is attempted without a liquid medium. The sound head should also be constantly moving and it should not be used over bony prominences in order to prevent tissue burning. The intensity of the dosage may be safely varied between 0.5 and 2.5 watts/centimeter^2. Acute conditions are usu-

Table 21.7 **Indications for Ultrasound**

Acute (pulsed only)
Sprain/strain
Bursitis
Traumatic arthritis
Chronic (continuous)
Sprain/strain
Bursitis
Arthritis
Myalgia/myositis
Tendinitis

Table 21.8 **Contraindications for Ultrasound**

Hemorrhage
Malignancy
Over the stellate ganglion
Gonads
Over a gravid uterus
Eye
Over a developing epiphyses
Over bony prominences
Infections
Advanced cardiovascular disease
Diabetes mellitus
Sensory deficit to heat

ally treated with low intensity (0.5–1.5) and chronic conditions with relatively high intensity (1.5–2.5). The intensity should be increased by 0.5 if the technique is used underwater. The time of treatment varies from 5 to 15 minutes.

A special form of ultrasound, called phonophoresis, can be used to drive chemicals, usually analgesics, into the affected area.

Galvanic Current

Direct electrical current has chemical and mechanical properties, depending upon the type of current used. Because the modality is polar, ion transfer occurs, which results in acid and alkaline changes in the body tissues. When interrupted current is used, muscle contraction results, thereby providing the mechanical effects.

Galvanic current has a number of different uses, many of which are outlined in Table 21.9. Generally speaking, the positive pad is used when analgesia is necessary and the negative pad is used for the other effects of this treatment.

Contraindications include malignancy, loss of sensation, passage of the current through the brain, eye, carotid sinus or heart, and use in patients with cardiac pacemakers.

The application of galvanic current includes the use of a wet dispersal pad and a smaller active pad. The current is much greater at the active pad; this is the pad that should be used for iontophoresis, the driving of ions into the affected area. Remember that the same polarity as the ion must be used on the small pad to repel the ions into the body. The machine should be turned off any time changes in settings, including polarity, are made. This will prevent injury to the patient. Treatment times vary from 10 to 20 minutes, and the intensity is to patient tolerance.

Sinusoidal Current

Alternating electrical current is primarily used to stimulate muscle contraction. It is best used on muscles weakened by some disease state although there are

Table 21.9 Indications for Galvanic Current

Chronic myalgia/myositis
Adhesions
Muscle spasm

Table 21.10 Indications for Sinusoidal Current

Muscle weakness/atrophy
Muscle spasm
Chronic myalgia/myositis

other indications, as noted in Table 21.10. Contraindications are listed in Table 21.11.

The use of AC current is facilitated by the use of wet pads and applications over the motor points of muscles. It is best not to prolong therapy to the point of dangerous muscle fatigue.

Interferential Current (IFC)

This form of electrical stimulation is characterized by the crossing of two electrical mediums using independent frequencies that work together to effectively stimulate large impulse nerve fibers. These frequencies interfere with the transmission of pain messages at the spinal cord level. The interferential wave meets low impedance when crossing the skin to enter the underlying tissue so it allows for deeper tissue penetration. It can be adjusted to stimulate parasympathetic nerve fibers, for example, to increase blood flow. Interferential current stimulation differs from transcutaneous electrical nerve stimulation (TENS) because it provides for deeper penetration of the tissues with more comfort and increased

Table 21.11 Contraindications for Sinusoidal Current

Hemorrhage/hematoma
Use through the heart
Abscess
Malignancy
Fracture

circulation in the region being treated. This may explain why IFC may be most suitable for treating patients with deep pain, for promoting osteogenesis in delayed and nonunion fractures, and for stimulating deep skeletal muscle to augment the muscle pump mechanism in venous insufficiency.

Pain control is the primary use for IFC. Anecdotal evidence suggests that it may be useful for patients who have not had relief from TENS therapy. Other common indications include joint injuries, muscle spasm, cumulative/repetitive trauma disorders, and increasing circulation to a body region.

Table 21.12 outlines the typical treatment protocols for IFC, and Table 21.13 outlines contraindications for this therapy.

Microcurrent Therapy (MCT)

The use of small amounts of electrical current, measured in microamperes (typically 20–500), can be used as a long-term therapy for conditions such as fibromylagia and delayed onset muscle soreness (DOMS). Patients have no perceivable sensations from MCT.

It is theorized that this therapy can stimulate healing on a more cellular level as microcurrents can increase cellular energy and protein production in addition to improve the function of cell membranes, so that nutrients can be exchanged more readily across cell walls.

In addition to fibromyalgia and DOMS, certain cases of myofascial pain syndromes, carpal tunnel syndrome, headaches, trigger points, and neck and back pain seem to respond to MCT. (7) In addition, it has been suggested MCT appears to hasten skin ulcer healing and retard bacterial growth as well. Typical treatment time consists of 5- to 120-minute applications one to four times per day. Some patients are placed on MCT for years at a time. Strength of the current

Table 21.12 Interferential Current Treatment Protocols

	Acute Conditions	Chronic Conditions
Treatment frequency	high, 75–100 Hz narrow spectrum	low, 20–50 Hz wide spectrum
Treatment time	short, 3–10 min.	long, 5–30 min.
Current intensity	low	high
Number of sessions	1–2 per day	2–3 per week

Table 21.13 Contraindications for Interferential Current Therapy

Bleeding
Tumors
Blood clots
Over the gravid/menstruating uterus
Electronic/metal implants (e.g., pacemaker)
Along with short-wave or microwave diathermy

is typically between 25–100 microamperes and frequency is 0.5 Hz to 40 Hz, depending upon the desired effects. Lower frequencies are used for a healing response, where higher frequencies are used for control of pain and swelling.

Contraindications are similar to those for any electrical current. Some patients do report sensitivity to the electrode pads.

Traction

Two types of traction are used in the physical rehabilitation of a patient: sustained and intermittent. Sustained traction is best used to splint an area or cause tissue stretching that will result in relaxation. Intermittent traction is used to "pump" an affected area, such as the intervertebral discs in patients with some form of disc disease. (8, 9)

Contraindications to traction are listed in Table 21.14.

The application of traction is best accomplished in the cervical spine with 5 percent of the patient's body weight and in lumbar traction with 25 percent of the patient's weight. All attachments should be snug but not too tight, and the patient should be positioned so that the maximal effect will be gained.

Massage

The main therapeutic effect of massage is mechanical, although there may be some reflex visceral changes as well. The purported physiologic effects of massage include relaxation, adhesion breakdown, edema reduction, and analgesia. There are many different forms of massage, including pétrissage (muscle kneading), effleurage (stroking massage), tapotement (percussion massage), transverse friction massage, and vibration.

Table 21.14 Contraindications for Mechanical Traction
Acute inflammatory arthritis
Severe muscle spasms
Acute inflammation
HNP (intermittent traction)
Osteomyelitis
Fracture
Malignancy
Osteoporosis
Spinal cord disease
Pregnancy (lumbar spine traction)

Massage has received mixed results in the literature regarding its effectiveness, but certain conditions have responded well including muscle-tension headaches (10), cancer pain (11), and labor pain. (12) There has also been a demonstrable increase in the level of serum beta-endorphin levels in patients in pain who receive massage. (13) Interestingly, normal patients who received massage did not show a similar increase. (14)

Transverse friction massage (TFM) involves the use of the physician's fingers to massage across the longitudinal axis of the muscle/tendon/ligament being treated to separate the fibers and/or microadhesions of the structure being massaged. The depth of massage should not create pain beyond patient tolerance. Treatments typically last from 5–15 minutes. Treatments should be separated by at least 24–48 hours.

The indications for massage are listed in Table 21.15 and the contraindications in Table 21.16.

Muscle Energy Techniques

Muscle energy techniques are essentially forms of proprioceptive neuromuscular facilitation (PNF) and include techniques such as post-isometric relaxation (PIR), reciprocal inhibition, contract-relax (CR), post-facilitation stretch, and the oculocephalogyric reflex (OCGR).

Table 21.15 Common Indications for Massage

Sprain
Strain
Tendinitis
Myositis/Myalgia
Arthritis
Bursitis
Labor pain
Cancer pain management
Psychological stress

Indications include improving local circulation and respiratory function, lengthening and/or normalizing restricted muscles and fascia and helping to mobilize restricted joints. Conditions commonly treated include muscle strains, capsulitis, thoracic cage restriction, and mechanical joint dysfunction.

With PIR, the physician slowly moves and gently stretches the patient's affected body part to the end of its painless unrestricted range of motion (ROM). At this point the patient exerts a mild muscle contraction against the physician's pull, creating an isometric contraction, for approximately 5 seconds. The patient

Table 21.16 Contraindications for Massage

Malignancy
Osteomyelitis
Hemorrhage
Vascular disease (phlebitis)
Skin infection/ulceration
Varicose veins

relaxes the body part and the physician continues into the ROM. This technique is performed for 3–5 cycles or until full pain-free ROM is attained, whichever is less.

Reciprocal inhibition involves having the patient contract the antagonist muscle to the one being treated, utilizing the reciprocal inhibition mechanism to relax the affected muscle without actually touching it. This technique is typically used in patients with acute strains, who cannot tolerate contracting the affected muscle to use PIR.

For CR therapy, have the patient perform a contraction of the affected muscle, at approximately 75% of full-strength, for 5 seconds. The physician then slowly and gently stretches the muscle to the end of its painless unrestricted ROM as the patient performs a very light contraction of the affected muscle.

Post-facilitation stretching is a more aggressive therapy for patients who need muscle stretching. The patient is instructed to perform a full-strength contraction of the muscle to be stretched for approximately 10 seconds. The muscle is then allowed to fully relax, whereupon a rapid stretch of the affected muscle is performed and held in position by the physician for 15 seconds. This cycle can then be repeated 3–5 times after the patient relaxes the muscle and then begins a full-strength contraction again.

The OCGR is used to cause inhibition of either the anterior or posterior cervical musculature by moving the eyes either up or down. Moving the eyes into an upward vertical gaze position relaxes the anterior cervical muscles, and moving the eyes to the downward vertical gaze position relaxes the posterior cervical musculature.

Contraindications for the active forms of muscle energy techniques (MET) include fracture, severe sprains and strains where instability may be a concern, and an uncooperative or unresponsive patient.

Trigger Point (TrP)/Tender Point Therapy

Trigger points can occur in muscles, fascia, skin, and ligaments. They are assumed to be small foci of chemical irritants that irritate local nociceptive fibers and are often associated with ropy hardened bands in the soft tissues of the structures noted above. These lesions can be quite painful. By definition, a TrP refers pain; a tender point does not.

TrPs are thought by some to be the genesis of the so-called "mimicry syndromes." Mimicry syndromes are conditions that mimic more typical medical conditions (angina pectoris, renal colic) without the actual presence of the medical condition. They can be quite frustrating when a patient presents with signs and symptoms of chest pain, for example. Patients can have extensive cardiovascular diagnostic work-ups, where the findings point to no cardiovascular cause. It is in these instances that a search for TrPs should be undertaken.

Therapy for TrPs includes direct ("ischemic") compression, PNF/MET techniques, local electrical muscle stimulation, and "dry-needling," a form of acupuncture.

Direct compression of a TrP includes the following steps: the affected muscle is slowly stretched and direct pressure is placed on the TrP to the patient's pain tolerance until the pain begins to subside, whereupon more pressure, to patient tolerance, is applied. Direct compression should be held for no longer than 60 seconds. Hot packs can be applied to the area either before or after direct compression. Ice massage or cooling sprays can be used over an exquisitely tender TrP before the use of direct compression, to facilitate the patient's tolerance to pain in the area.

Spinal Stabilization Exercises

A spinal stabilization exercise program is a protocol involving the use of back exercises designed to teach patients strengthening and flexibility within a pain-free ROM. While its primary thrust is to help the patient with efficient movement, it also improves the patient's physical condition and symptoms. It provides the patient with a keen awareness of movement of his or her spine, knowledge of safe spinal postures, and functional muscular strengthening and coordination that promotes healthy management of back pain.

These exercise protocols have been demonstrated to be effective in the management of back pain in a number of studies. (15,16)

The initial phase of the spinal stabilization protocol begins with isolated muscle contractions. Stabilization training begins with the patient being instructed in the neutral spine position. This position is where the spine is in ideal alignment and is found by envisioning the face of a clock on the abdomen, with 12:00 at the umbilicus and 6:00 at the symphysis. Pelvic tilts are then accomplished by having the patient alternately tilt the pelvis so that the umbilicus rocks toward the floor and then the symphysis pubis rocks toward the floor. These pelvic tilts are performed 10 times, slowly and gently, in each direction. The neutral spine position is the point within that range of pelvic tilts where the patient is the most comfortable. It is then emphasized that this position should be maintained for all movements performed during stabilization activities as well as during the patient's normal activities of daily living.

Once the patient can consistently assume the neutral spine position, isolated contraction of the transversus abdominus muscle is begun. This muscle is trained by having the patient pull his navel into his spine, and/or having him exhale completely. The patient must maintain the neutral spine position during the entire exercise.

Once the patient can perform the transversus abdominus exercise, the exercises outlined in Table 21.17 can be attempted until the patient is confident. This is simply a sample of a spinal stabilization program for the low back.

After this basic spinal stabilization exercise protocol is mastered, further nonweight-bearing and/or weight-bearing exercises can be instituted. As always the patient should try to maintain a comfortable neutral spine position. When training a patient in the performance of these protocols, it is critical to remember that it is the quality of the exercise that is performed that is most effective and not the quantity of exercises performed. Coordination and stability are the core goals of this therapy.

It is important for the physician to have the patient isolate the key spinal stabilizer muscles such as the abdominal, gluteal, and quadricep muscle groups. When a patient has soreness after the exercises without an increase in back or extremity pain, the program is considered successful. Other components of this

Table 21.17 Early Spinal Stabilization Exercise Protocols

Step 1- Achieve and maintain neutral spine position while supine

Step 2- Supine pelvic tilts

Step 3- Supine transversus abdominus contractions

Step 4- Supine, arms flat on floor, left knee bent
- -Tighten abdominals and buttocks, keeping back in neutral position
- -Raise right leg 12 inches, knee straight
- -Hold three counts
- -Lower leg. Repeat 10 times
- -Repeat with left leg
- -Progress to making circles and squares with raised leg

Step 5- Kneeling position
- -Maintain neutral spine position
- -Tighten abdominal and buttock muscles
- -Place hands on hips
- -Raise right foot and place on floor, kneeling on left knee
- -Lunge forward, moving at hips (maintain neutral spine position)
- -Hold for three seconds
- -Return to kneeling position
- -Repeat 10 times
- -Repeat on opposite side

protocol include the use of an exercise ball, range of motion exercises, proprioceptive neuromuscular facilitation, and strength training exercises.

Orthoses and Mechanical Supports

The use of orthotics such as braces, heel lifts, lumbosacral supports, and cervical collars is commonplace in the practice of chiropractic medicine. It is well beyond the scope of this text to describe all the types of supports, as there are so many that are used many different ways.

Table 21.18 lists some of the more commonly used supports and their indications. If supports are used, they should, in general, be used for the least amount of time necessary. Prolonged use of a support may lead to muscle atrophy, weakness, and even adhesive capsulitis.

Joint Mobilization

Joint mobilization can be utilized to increase range of motion, relieve pain, and help restore a patient to his or her normal activities of daily living. Below are the outlines of closed-packed joint positions (position in which the joint is most stable and least moveable), open-packed joint positions (position where joint is freely moveable), capsular patterns (patterns of painful motion that suggest disease [sprain, synovitis] of the joint capsule), and mobilizations for spine and upper and lower extremity joints.

Table 21.18 Orthoses and Their Indications

Appliance	Indication
Cervical collar	Whiplash injury
Heel lift	Lower extremity pain Spine pain Leg length inequality
Lumbosacral orthosis	HNP Sprain/strain
Braces (extremity)	Acute injury Prophylaxis

Motion during joint mobilization should essentially be pain-free. Increases in joint ROM should be identified as the mobilization progresses. If there are not increases in ROM and a decrease in pain, then a reevaluation of the clinical joint mechanics should be perfomed to assure that the appropriate type/direction of mobilization is being performed.

The general types of mobilization include:

- Mobilization with Movement (MWM): stretch mobilizations in accessory motion planes (parallel to joint plane, perpendicular to joint plane, long axis distraction) with active movement by the patient in ROMs as directed by the clinician. These mobilizations are regional in the spine and joint motion specific in the appendicular skeleton.
- Graded Oscillatory Mobilization (GOM): pressure-release movement with accessory glide within the passive ROM (e.g., lateral bending with accessory lateral glide in the cervical spine). These mobilizations are regional in the spine and joint motion specific in the appendicular skeleton.
- Continuous Stretch Mobilization (CSM): continuously increasing joint stretching within the passive ROM (e.g., lumbar rotation in lateral decubitus [side posture] position). These types of mobilizations are regional in the spine and joint motion specific in the appendicular skeleton.
- Progressive Stretch Mobilization (PSM): progressive pressure-release low-amplitude motions within the passive ROM. These types of mobilizations are regional in the spine and joint motion specific in the appendicular skeleton.

Spinal Joints

- Open-packed positon: midway between flexion and extension
- Close-packed position: full extension
- Capsular patterns:

  -atlantooccipital joint: loss of flexion, then extension

  -C1-C2: loss of rotation

  -C3-T2: loss of lateral flexion and rotation, then extension

  -T3-T12: loss of lateral bending and rotation, then extension, then flexion

  -L1-L5: loss of lateral bending and rotation, then extension, then flexion

  -SI joint: painful when stress is placed on the joint

- Mobilizations:

  -Natural Apophyseal Glides: pressure-release along plane of facet joints, typically done with the thumbs; regional or segmental

  -Sustained Natural Apophyseal Glides: sustained pressure along plane of facet joints; regional or segmental

  -Mobilization with Movement (MWM): stretch mobilizations in accessory motion planes (parallel to joint plane, perpendicular to joint plane, long axis distraction) with movement by the patient; regional

  -GOM: e.g., lateral bending with accessory lateral glide

  -CSM: e.g., lumbar rotation in lateral decubitus (side posture) position

  -PSM: e.g., cervical rotation/flexion/extension/lateral bending in supine position

Hip Joint

- Loose-packed position: 30° flexion, 30° abduction, slight external rotation
- Close-packed position: full extension, abduction, and internal rotation
- Capsular pattern: loss of flexion then internal rotation, abduction
- Mobilizations:

  -posterior glide MWM flexion and internal rotation

  -anterior glide MWM with extension and external rotation

  -long axis distraction with internal/external rotation

  -internal/external rotation GOM with lateral/medial glide

  -internal/external rotation and flexion/extension CSM/PSM

Knee Joint (Femoral-Tibial)

- Loose-packed position: 25° flexion
- Close-packed position: full extension and external rotation
- Capsular pattern: loss of flexion, then extension
- Mobilizations:

  -posterior glide MWM with flexion

  -anterior glide MWM with extension

  -lateral glide GOM with rotation of lower leg

  -flexion/extension CSM/PSM

Knee Joint (Tibiofibular)

- Loose-packed position: N/A
- Open-packed position: N/A
- Capsular pattern: painful when stressing the joint
- Mobilizations:
  -anterior glide MWM with ankle inversion
  -posterior glide MWM with ankle eversion

Ankle Mortise

- Loose-packed position: 10° plantarflexion
- Close-packed position: full dorsiflexion
- Capsular pattern: loss of plantarflexion, then dorsiflexion
- Mobilizations:
  -anterior glide MWM with flexion
  -posterior glide MWM with extension
  -long axis distraction MWM with flexion/extension
  -flexion/extension CSM/PSM

Subtalar Joint

- Loose-packed position: 10° plantarflexion
- Close-packed position: full inversion
- Capsular pattern: loss of inversion, then eversion
- Mobilizations:
  -medial glide MWM with inversion
  -lateral glide MWM with eversion
  -inversion/eversion CSM/PSM

Transverse Tarsal Joint (Calcaneocuboid, Talonavicular)

- Open-packed position: 10° plantarflexion
- Close-packed position: full inversion
- Capsular pattern: loss of inversion, then eversion
- Mobilizations:
  -plantar glide MWM with inversion
  -dorsal glide MWM with eversion
  -inversion/eversion CSM/PSM

Tarsometatarsal Joints

- Open-packed position: midway between inversion and eversion
- Close-packed position: full inversion
- Capsular pattern: loss of inversion then eversion
- Mobilizations:

  -plantar glide MWM with inversion

  -dorsal glide MWM with eversion

  -inversion/eversion CSM/PSM

Metatarsophalangeal Joints (MPJ)

- Open-packed position: neutral (10° extension)
- Close-packed position: full extension
- Capsular patterns: MPJ 1 is loss of extension, then flexion; MPJs 2–5 are flexion
- Mobilizations:

  -plantar glide MWM with plantarflexion

  -dorsal glide MWM with dorsiflexion

  -long axis distraction MWM with plantarflexion/dorsiflexion

  -plantarflexion/dorsiflexion/rotation CSM/PSM

Interphalangeal Joints

- Open-packed positon: slight flexion
- Close-packed position: full extension
- Capsular pattern: loss of extension
- Mobilizations:

  -plantar glide MWM with plantar flexion

  -dorsal glide MWM with dorsiflexion

  -long axis distraction with plantarflexion/dorsiflexion

  -plantarflexion/dorsiflexion/rotation CSM/PSM

Glenohumeral Joint

- Loose-packed position: 55° abduction, 30° horizontal adduction
- Close-packed position: full abduction and external rotation
- Capsular pattern: loss of external rotation, then abduction, then internal rotation

- Mobilizations:
  -inferior glide MWM with abduction
  -anterior glide MWM with extension and external rotation
  -posterior glide MWM with flexion and internal rotation
  -internal/external rotation CSM/PSM
  -flexion/extension CSM/PSM

Acromioclavicular Joint

- Loose-packed position: arm resting at side
- Close-packed position: 90° of shoulder abduction
- Capsular pattern: loss of full elevation
- Mobilizations:
  -anterior glide MWM with shoulder elevation

Sternoclavicular Joint

- Loose-packed position: arm resting at side
- Close-packed position: shoulder maximally elevated
- Capsular pattern: loss of maximal elevation
- Mobilizations:
  -superior glide MWM with shoulder elevation

Scapulothoracic Joint

- Not a true joint, but allows scapular retraction, protraction, elevation, depression, tipping, and winging
- Mobilizations:
  -lateral decubitus position; scapular CSM/PSM in all ranges

Elbow (Humeroulnar Joint)

- Loose-packed position: 70° elbow flexion, 10° supination
- Close-packed position: full elbow extension and supination
- Capsular pattern: loss of elbow flexion, then extension
- Mobilizations:
  -long axis traction with elbow flexion
  -elbow flexion/extension CSM/PSM

Elbow (Humeroradial Joint)

- Loose-packed position: full elbow extension and supination
- Close-packed position: 90° flexion, 5° supination
- Capsular pattern: loss of flexion, then extension
- Mobilizations:
  -dorsal glide MWM with extension
  -ventral glide MWM with flexion
  -elbow flexion/extension/supination/pronation CSM/PSM

Elbow (Proximal Radioulnar Joint)

- Loose-packed position: 70° flexion, 35° supination
- Close-packed position: full extension, 5° supination
- Capsular pattern: elbow supination and pronation equally limited
- Mobilizations:
  -dorsal glide MWM with pronation
  -ventral glide MWM with supination
  -supination/pronation CSM/PSM

Wrist (Distal Radioulnar Joint)

- Loose-packed position: 10° supination
- Close-packed position: 5° supination
- Capsular pattern: supination and pronation equally limited
- Mobilizations:
  -dorsal glide MWM with supination
  -ventral glide MWM with pronation
  -supination/pronation CSM/PSM

Wrist (Radiocarpal Joint)

- Loose-packed position: slight ulnar deviation
- Close-packed position: full wrist extension and radial deviation
- Capsular pattern: flexion and extension equally limited
- Mobilizations:
  -ventral glide MWM with wrist extension
  -dorsal glide MWM with wrist flexion

-radial glide MWM with ulnar deviation

-ulnar deviation/radial deviation/flexion/extension CSM/PSM

-glide radius on fixed scaphoid ventrally to increase flexion

-glide scaphoid on a fixed radius ventrally to increase extension

-glide radius on a fixed lunate ventrally to increase flexion

Carpometacarpal (CMC), Metacarpophalangeal (MCP), and Interphalangeal Joints (IPJ) of Fingers 2–5

- Loose-packed position: CMC=midway between all ranges; MCP=slight flexion with ulnar deviation; IPJ proximal=10° flexion; IPJ distal=30° flexion
- Close-packed position: CMC=full opposition; MCP=full flexion; PIP and DIP=full extension
- Capsular pattern: CMC=equally in all directions; IPJ=loss of flexion then extension
- Mobilizations:

  -ventral glide MWM with flexion

  -dorsal glide MWM with extension

  -flexion/extension CSM/PSM

Carpometacarpal Joint of the Thumb

- Loose-packed position: midway in all positions
- Close-packed position: full opposition
- Capsular pattern: loss of abduction greater than extension
- Mobilizations:

  -ulnar glide MWM with flexion

  -radial glide MWM with extension

  -long axis distraction MWM with flexion/extension/abduction/adduction

  -ventral glide/dorsal glide/abduction/adduction CSM/PSM

Neural Mobilization

Neural mobilization is the use of specific body movements to functionally lengthen the dynamic motion of nerves that have become adherent within the spinal or peripheral structures secondary to inflammation. Recent evidence has suggested that spinal nerves have the ability to chemically "dissolve" tissues that are impinging them. It would follow then that if the nerves have the ability to move as originally intended that this process would occur more effectively. This is the premise behind neural mobilization.

The process is one of tensioning the nerves from one end of the body while releasing them from the other and then switching the movement pattern so that the roots are released during this back and forth motion.

The following procedure is indicated in patients with chronic sciatica. The patient sits on a table with the lower legs dangling off the table. While flexing the neck, the patient then also flexes the knee of the affected leg. Then, while extending the neck, the patient also extends the knee of the affected leg. These two motions create the back and forth motion necessary for mobilization of the nerves.

Care must be taken when using this technique as these patients are suffering with some form of compressive or adhesive nerve compression that is causing their sciatica. The procedure should be done with only slight movements at first. If at any point, any of these motions exacerbate the patient's symptoms, the procedure should be stopped immediately. If, on the other hand, the patient improves, the amount of mobilization can be increased, always keeping in mind the patient's response to this therapy.

References

1. Thompson, C., Kelsberg, G., & St Anna, L. Heat or ice for acute ankle sprain? *J Fam Pract.* 2003 Aug;52(8):642–643.
2. Rubley, M.D., Denegar, C.R., Buckley, W.E., & Newell, K.M. Cryotherapy, sensation, and isometric-force variability. *J Athl Train.* 2003 Jun;38(2):113–119.
3. Merrick, M.A., Jutte, L.S., & Smith, M.E. Cold modalities with different thermodynamic properties produce different surface and intramuscular temperatures. *J Athl Train.* 2003 Mar;38(1):28–33.
4. Nadler, S.F., Steiner, D.J., Petty, S.R., Erasala, G.N., Hengehold, D.A., & Weingand, K.W. Overnight use of continuous low-level heatwrap therapy for relief of low back pain. *Arch Phys Med Rehabil.* 2003 Mar;84(3):335–342.
5. Nadler, S.F., Steiner, D.J., Erasala, G.N., Hengehold, D.A., Abeln, S.B., & Weingand, K.W. Continuous low-level heatwrap therapy for treating acute nonspecific low back pain. *Arch Phys Med Rehabil.* 2003 Mar;84(3):329–334.
6. Nadler, S.F., Steiner, D.J., Erasala, G.N., Hengehold, D.A., Hinkle, R.T., Beth Goodale, M., Abeln, S.B., & Weingand, K.W. Continuous low-level heatwrap therapy provides more efficacy than ibuprofen and acetaminophen for acute low back pain. *Spine.* 2002 May 15;27(10):1012–1017.
7. Lambert, M.I., Marcus, P., Burgess, T., & Noakes, T.D. Electromembrane microcurrent therapy reduces signs and symptoms of muscle damage. *Med Sci Sports Exerc.* 2002 Apr;34(4):602–607.

8. Ramos, G., & Martin, W. Effects of vertebral axial decompression on intradiscal pressure. *J Neurcsurg.* 1994 Sep;81(3):350–353.
9. Krause, M., Refshauge, K.M., Dessen, M., & Boland, R. Lumbar spine traction: evaluation of effects and recommended application for treatment. *Man Ther.* 2000 May;5(2):72–81.
10. Hammill, J.M., Cook, T.M., & Rosecrance, J.C. Effectiveness of a physical therapy regimen in the treatment of tension-type headache. *Headache.* 1996 Mar;36(3):149–153.
11. Weinrich, S.P., & Weinrich, M.C. The effect of massage on pain in cancer patients. *Appl Nurs Res.* 1990 Nov;3(4):140–145.
12. Chang, M.Y., Wang, S.Y., & Chen, C.H. Effects of massage on pain and anxiety during labor: A randomized controlled trial in Taiwan. *J Adv Nurs.* 2002 Apr;38(1):68–73.
13. Kaada, B., & Torsteinbo, O. Increase of plasma beta-endorphins in connective tissue massage. *Gen Pharmacol.* 1989;20(4):487–489.
14. Day, J.A., Mason, R.R., & Chesrown, S.E. Effect of massage on serum level of beta-endorphin and beta-lipotropin in healthy adults. *Phys Ther.* 1987 Jun;67(6):926–930.
15. Timm, K.E. A randomized-control study of active and passive treatments for chronic low back pain following L5 laminectomy. *JOSPT.* 1994;20:276–286.
16. Saal, J.A., & Saal, J.S. Nonoperative treatment of herniated lumbar intervertebral disc with radiculopathy. *Spine.* 1989;14:431–437.

Appendix A

Abbreviations

The following is a list of abbreviations and acronyms and their meanings. These will help make medical recordkeeping much less time consuming and hence, more efficient. This list is certainly not all encompassing but should serve as a helpful guide. Entertain the possibility of modifying and adding to this list so that it fits your practice specifically.

$\bar{a}$—ante, "before"
A—abnormal
aa—artery, arteries
AAA—abdominal aortic aneurysm
AAF—African-American Female
AAM—African-American Male
A&O×4—alert and oriented to person, place, time, and situation
Ab—antibody
ABD—abdomen
a.c.—*ante cibum* (before eating)
ACJ—acromioclavicular joint
acid phos—acid phosphatase
ACTH—adrenocorticotrophic hormone
ADH—anti-diuretic hormone
ADL—activities of daily living
ad lib—*ad libitum* (as much as wanted)
AFB—acid-fast bacilli
AFP—alphafeto protein

ag—antigen
A/G—albumin/globulin ratio
AIDS—acquired immune deficiency syndrome
alk phos—alkaline phosphatase
ALS—amyotrophic lateral sclerosis
ALT—alanine aminotransferase (formerly SGPT)
a.m.—morning
AMA—against medical advice
amb—ambulate
AMPLE—allergies, medications, PMH, LMP, events of illness
ANA—antinuclear antibody
ant—anterior
AP—anteroposterior
APGAR—appearance, pulse, grimace, activity, respirations
ARC—AIDS-related complex
AROM—active range of motion
AS—ankylosing spondylitis
ASA—acetylsalicylic acid (aspirin)
ASAP—as soon as possible
ASD—atrial septal defect
ASO—antistreptolysin O
AST—aspartate aminotransferase (formerly SGOT)
ASVD—atherosclerotic vascular disease
AXR—abdomen X-ray

B—bilateral
BBB—bundle branch block
BCP—birth control pill
BE—barium enema
b.i.d.—*bis in die* (twice a day)
bili—bilirubin
BM—bowel movement
BMR—basal metabolic rate
BP—blood pressure
BPH—benign prostatic hypertrophy
bpm—beats per minute
BRBPR—bright red blood per rectum (hematochezia)
BRP—bathroom privileges
BS—bowel sounds, breath sounds
BUN—blood urea nitrogen

Bx—biopsy
B9—benign

$\overline{c}$—*cum* (with)
C—celcius, centigrade
CA—cancer
Ca—calcium
CABG—coronary artery bypass graft
CAD—coronary artery disease
CADS—cervical acceleration/deceleration syndrome
cap—capsule
CAT—computerized axial tomography
CBC—complete blood count
CC—chief complaint
cc—cubic centimeter
CDA—crystal deposition arthropathy
CF—cystic fibrosis
CHF—congestive heart failure
CI—contraindication
Cl—chloride
cm—centimeter
CMC—carpometacarpal joint
CMT—chiropractic manipulative therapy
CNI-CNXII—cranial nerves one through twelve
CNS—central nervous system
c/o—complaining of
C_o—occiput
coc—coccyx
COPD—chronic obstructive pulmonary disease
CP—cerebral palsy
CPK—creatine phosphokinase
CPBB—brain band
CPMB—myocardial band
CPMM—muscle band
CPPD—calcium pyrophosphate arthropathy
CPR—cardiopulmonary resuscitation
CRP—C-reactive protein
CSF—cerebrospinal fluid
CT—computerized tomography
CTA—connective tissue arthropathies

CV—cardiovascular
CVA—cerebrovascular accident
CVAT—costovertebral angle tenderness
c/w—consistent with
CXR—chest X-ray
C1-C7—first through seventh cervical vertebrae

DAMA—discharged against medical advice
D&C—dilation and curettage
d/c—discontinue
DDx—differential diagnosis
diff—differential count (in the CBC)
DIP—distal interphalangeal joint
DISH—diffuse idiopathic skeletal hyperostosis
DJD—degenerative joint disease
DKA—diabetic ketoacidosis
DM—diabetes mellitus
DP—dorsalis pedis (artery)
DPT—diphtheria, pertussis, tetanus
d/t—due to
DTR—deep tendon reflex
DVT—deep vein thrombosis
Dx—diagnosis
Dz—disease

EBV—Epstein-Barr virus
ECG—electrocardiogram
ED—emergency department
EDC—estimated date of confinement
EEG—electroencephalogram
(E) ENT—(eyes), ears, nose, throat
EMG—electromyogram
EMS—electrical muscle stimulation
EMT—emergency medical technician
EOA—erosive osteoarthritis
EOMI—external ocular muscles intact
EORP—end of range pressure
ESR—erythrocyte sedimentation rate
Etiol—etiology

ETOH—ethanol (intoxication)
exac—exacerbation
ext—extension

F—farenheit
FBS—fasting blood sugar
FCNS—fever, chills, night sweats
FD—flexion distraction, fibrous dysplasia
FEV1—forced expiratory volume in one second
FHx—family history
flex—flexion
FN—finger to nose test
FTA-ABS—fluorescent treponemal antibody absorption
F/U—follow-up
FUO—fever of unknown origin
Fx—fracture

g—gram
GC—gonorrhea
GGT—gamma-glutamyl transpeptidase
GHJ—glenohumeral joint
GI—gastrointestinal
G/P/A—gravida/para/aborta
GPF—gross physical findings
gr—grain
GSW—gunshot wound
gt., gtt.—*gutta, guttae* (drop, drops)
GTT—glucose tolerance test
GU—genitourinary
gyn—gynecologist

h—hour(s)
HA—headache
HADD—hydroxyapatite deposition disease
H&P—history and physical examination
HBP—high blood pressure
HCG—human chorionic gonadotropin
HCO3—bicarbonate
Hct—hematocrit
HDL—high-density lipoprotein

HEENT—head, eyes, ears, nose, throat
Hg—mercury
Hgb—hemoglobin
H/H—hemoglobin/hematocrit
HIV—human immunodeficiency virus (or human T-lymphocyte virus)
HLA—histocompatibility locus antigen
HNP—herniated nucleus pulposus
H/O—history of
HPI—history of present illness
HR—heart rate
HS—heel to shin test
h.s.—*hora somni* (hour of sleep—at bedtime)
HSM—hepatosplenomegaly
ht.—height
HTLV-III—human lymphotropic virus-type III
HTN—hypertension
HVG—high volt galvanism
H/W—height/weight
Hx—history

I&O—intake and output
IC—intermittent claudication
ICS—intercostal space
ICU—intensive care unit
IDDM—insulin-dependent diabetes mellitus
IFC—interferential current
Ig—immunoglobulin
IgA—albumin
IgD—beta
IgE—gamma
IgG—alpha-1
IgM—alpha-2
IM—intramuscular (injection)
Incid—incidence
inf—inferior
INH—isoniazid (antituberculous drug)
IPJ—interphalangeal joint
IU—international unit
IV—intravenous
IVC—inferior vena cava

IVP—intravenous pyelogram
IVU—intravenous urogram

JCA—juvenile chronic arthritis
JODM—juvenile onset diabetes mellitus
JVD—jugular venous distension

K+—potassium
Kg—kilogram
KUB—kidneys, ureter, bladder (abdomen X-ray)
kVp—kilovoltage potential

L—left
Lab—laboratory
LAE—left atrial enlargement
LAM—laminectomy
LAO—left anterior oblique
LAT—lateral
lat flex—lateral flexion
lb.—pound
LBP—low back pain
LDH—lactate dehydrogenase
LDL—low-density lipoprotein
LE—lower extremity
LE prep—lupus erythematosus cell preparation
ll—ligament
LLF—left lateral flexion
LLL—left lower lobe (lung)
LLQ—left lower quadrant (abdomen)
LMNL—lower motor neuron lesion
LMP—last menstrual period
LOC—level of consciousness
LP—lumbar puncture
LPO—left posterior oblique
LR—left rotation
LR—left to right
L/S—lumbosacral
LUL—left upper lobe
LUQ—left upper quadrant
LVG—low volt galvanism

LVH—left ventricular hypertrophy
L1-L5—first through fifth lumbar vertebrae

M—murmur
mA—milliampere
mAs—milliampere seconds
MCH—mean corpuscular hemoglobin
MCHC—mean corpuscular hemoglobin concentration
MCL—mid-clavicular line
MCP—metacarpophalangeal joint
MCV—mean corpuscular volume
meds—medications
mets—metastasis
MFTP—myofascial trigger point
mg—milligrams
MI—myocardial infarction
ml—milliliter
mm—millimeter
MM—multiple myeloma
MMI—maximum medical improvement
MMR—measles, mumps, rubella
mo—month
MRI—magnetic resonance imaging
MS—multiple sclerosis
MTP—metatarsophalangeal joint
MVA—motor vehicle accident

N—normal
Na+—sodium
NAD—no apparent distress
NARE—no apparent residual effects
NCV—nerve conduction velocity
neg—negative
neuro—neurological examination
NIDDM—non-insulin-dependent diabetes mellitus
NKA—no known allergies
NKCIM—no known contraindications to manipulation
NKDA—no known drug allergies
NMS—neuromusculoskeletal
NPH—neutral protamine Hagedorn (insulin)

n.p.o.—*nil per os* (nothing by mouth)
NSAID—nonsteroidal anti-inflammatory drugs
NSR—normal sinus rhythm
N/T—numbness and tingling
N&V—nausea and vomiting

O_2—oxygen
OA—osteoarthritis
OB/GYN—obstetrician/gynecologist
obl.—oblique
OCA—oral contraceptive agent
OCG—oral cholecystogram
o.d.—*oculus dexter* (right eye)
OOB—out of bed
OP—osteopenia, osteoporosis
OPLL—ossification of posterior longitudinal ligament
OR—operating room
orthos—orthopedic tests
o.s.—*oculus sinister* (left eye)
OTC—over the counter (medications)
O.U.—*oculus uterque* (both eyes)
oz.—ounce

p—post, after
PA—posterior-anterior
PAT—paroxysmal atrial tachycardia
Path—pathogenesis
p.c.—*post cibum* (after meals)
PDR—*Physicians' Desk Reference*
PE—physical examination, pulmonary embolism
PERLA—pupils equal and react to light and accommodation
PFT—pulmonary function tests
pH—hydrogen ion concentration
PID—pelvic inflammatory disease
PIP—proximal interphalangeal joint
p.m.—evening
PMH—past medical history
PMI—point of maximum impulse
PMN—polymorphonuclear leukocyte (neutrophil)
pn—pain

PND—paroxysmal nocturnal dyspnea
PO_4—phosphorous
p.o.—*per os* (by mouth)
polys—neutrophils
PON—physical, orthopedic, neurologic examination
post—posterior
PPD—purified protein derivative (TB test)
p.r.n.—*pro re nata* (as needed)
PROM—passive range of motion
PSS—progressive systemic sclerosis
PT—physical therapy
Pt—patient
PTA—prior to admission
PTH—parathyroid hormone
PTPW—patient tolerated procedures well
PUD—peptic ulcer disease
PVC—premature ventricular contraction
PVD—peripheral vascular disease
Px—prognosis

$\overline{q}$—quaque (every)
qAM—every morning
q.d.—quaque die (every day)
q.h.—quaque hora (every hour)
q.i.d.—quater in die (four times a day)
q.o.d.—every other day
qPM—every evening

R—right
RA—rheumatoid arthritis
Rad—radiology
RAO—right anterior oblique
RBC—red blood cell count
RDA—recommended daily allowance
RF—rheumatoid factor
RHD—rheumatic heart disease
RIA—radioimmunoassay
RICE—rest, ice, compression, elevation
RL—right to left
RLF—right lateral flexion
RLL—right lower lobe (lung)

RLQ—right lower quadrant (abdomen)
RML—right middle lobe (lung)
R/O—rule out
ROM—range of motion
ROS—review of systems
rot—rotation
RPO—right posterior oblique
RR—right rotation
RRR—regular rate and rhythm
RTC—return to clinic
RUL—right upper lobe (lung)
RUQ—right upper quadrant (abdomen)
Rx—treatment

$\overline{s}$—*sine* (without)
S&A—sugar and acetone
SC—subcutaneous
sec—seconds
SGOT—serum glutamic-oxaloacetic transaminase
SGPT—serum glutamic-pyruvic transaminase
Sgy—surgery
SI—sacroiliac joint
SIDS—sudden infant death syndrome
Sig.—*signa* (write on label)
SL—spondylolisthesis
SLE—systemic lupus erythematosus
SMAC—sequential multiple analysis chemistry (serum chemistry)
SNSA—seronegative spondyloarthropathies
SOAP—subjective, objective, assessment, plans
SOB—shortness of breath
SP—spinous process
S/P—*status post* (the state after)
SPE—(serum) protein electrophoresis
spondylo—spondylolisthesis
sp/st—sprain/strain
S/S—signs and symptoms
STAT—*statim* (immediately)
STD—sexually transmitted disease
STM—soft tissue manipulation
STS—soft tissue swelling
subQ—subcutaneous

sup.—superior
SVC—superior vena cava
Sx—symptom
S1-S5—first through fifth sacral segments

T3/T4/T7—abbreviations for thyroid hormone assays
T3—triiodothyronine
T4—thyroxine
T.AB.—therapeutic abortion
tab—tablet
TAH—total abdominal hysterectomy
TAHBSO—TAH with bilateral salpingo-oophorectomy
T&A—tonsillectomy and adenoidectomy
T&T—taut and tender
TB—tuberculosis
TBR—total bed rest
tbsp.—tablespoon
temp.—temperature
TENS—transcutaneous electrical nerve stimulation
TFT—transverse friction therapy
TGs—triglycerides
THEREX—therapeutic exercise
TIA—transient ischemic attack
TIBC—total iron binding capacity
t.i.d.—*ter in die* (three times a day)
TMJ—temporomandibular joint
TMT—tarsometatarsal joint
TNTC—too numerous to count
TO—telephone orders
TP—trigger point, transverse process
TPRBP—temperature, pulse, respiration, blood pressure
TPT—trigger point therapy
TSH—thyroid-stimulating hormone
TURP—transurethral resection of the prostate
tw—twice a week
Tx—treatment

U—unilateral
UA—uric acid
U/A—urine analysis
ud—*ut dictum* (as directed)

UE—upper extremity
UGI—upper gastrointestinal series
UMNL—upper motor neuron lesion
URI—upper respiratory infection
US—ultrasound
UTI—urinary tract infection

VD—venereal disease
VDRL—Venereal Disease Research Laboratory (syphilis test)
VFI—visual fields intact
VLDL—very low-density lipoproteins
VO—voice orders
VS—vital signs
vv—vein(s)

$\overline{w}$—which
WBC—white blood cell count
w/cm2—watts per square centimeter
WDWN—well-developed, well-nourished
WF—white female
wk.—week
WM—white male
WNL—within normal limits
wt.—weight
W/U—work-up

$\overline{x}$—except
⊗—functional spinal lesion; joint dysfunction
XR—X-ray

y/o—years old
yr.—year

⊖—negative, patient denies
⊕—positive
Δ—changes
$>$—greater than
$<$—less than
/—per
+/− —plus or minus
i, ii, iii—one, two, three, etc.

Index

NOTE: page numbers followed by *f* indicates figures, *t* indicates tables.

A

Abandonment, 334–335
Abasia, 183
Abbreviations, 417–429
Abdomen. *See also* Chest
  normal vasculature, 82*f*
  pain in, 86
  physical examination of, 79–81, 83–84, 83*t*
  radiograph interpretation, 237, 238*t*
  radiographic evaluation of, 210
    adrenal calcification, 216
    dysphagia, 218–219
    hematemesis, 222
    hematochezia, 222
    hepatomegaly, 222
    mass (adult), 222
    melena, 222
    pancreatic calcification, 222
    pneumoperitoneum, 223
    renal calcification, 223
    splenic calcification, 223
    splenomegaly, 223
    vas deferens calcification, 223
Abdominal aortic aneurysms (AAA), 83–84, 301. *See also* Aneurysms
Abdominal mass (adult), 222
Abulia, 180
Acanthocytes, 188
Acataphasia, 180
Achilles' tendon, 134*f*, 302
Acid phosphatase, 193, 275
Acid phosphatase, normal values for, 194*t*
Acoria, 180
Acromioclavicular (AC) joint, 302, 412
Acronyms (abbreviations chart), 417–429
Activity, as element in orders, 17
Acupuncture, for low back pain, 364
Adam's position, 102*f*
Adenocarcinoma, 284
Adenoma, 284
ADHD (attention deficit hyperactivity disorder), 44
Adie's tonic pupil, 180
Adolescents, pre-athletic participation examination for, 34–36
Adrenal calcification, radiographic interpretation of, 216
Adson's test, 112*f*
Advertising, ethics and, 336
Ageusia, 180
Aging. *See also* Geriatrics/geriatric patients
  characteristic neuromusculoskeletal changes with, 24–25*t*
  theories on, 21, 23
Agnosia, 180
Agraphesthesia, 180
Agraphia, 180
AIDS (acquired immunodeficiency syndrome), 75. *See also* HIV
Akathisia, 180
Akinesia, 180
Akoria, 180
Alalia, 180
Alanine aminotransaminase (ALT), 194*t*
Albumin, 193, 194*t*, 195
Albumin/globulin ratio, 194*t*, 195
Alcoholic neuropathy, 179
Alexia, 180
Alkaline phosphatase, 194*t*, 195–196, 275
Alkaptonuria, 73
Allen's test, 113*f*
Allergies, 43, 57, 74
Allesthesia, 180
Alpha fetoprotein (AFP), 194*t*, 196, 274
Amblyopia, 176, 180
Amelodia, 180, 181
Amenorrhea, female athlete triad and, 36
Amentia, 181
Amnesia, 181
AMPLE (mnemonic), 59*t*
Amusia, 181

Amylase, 194*t*, 196
Amyotrophic lateral sclerosis (ALS), 177, 178
Anacusia, 181
Analgesia, 181, 353
Anaplasia, 284
Anarithmetria, 183
Anemias, 188
Anesthesia
  ice massage and, 393
  joint manipulation under, 380
Aneurysmal bone cysts
  contraindications to joint manipulation with, 283
Aneurysms
  abdominal aortic, 83–84, 301
  aortic, referred spine pain and, 293, 294
  berry, 305
  diagnosis of, 83
  visual evoked potentials and, 176
Angina pectoris, 302–303
Anhedonia, 181
Anisocoria, 72, 172, 181
Anisocytosis, 188
Ankle
  anterior drawer sign of, 133*f*
  fractures of, differential diagnosis of, 216*t*
  joint mobilization, 410
  posterior drawer sign of, 134*f*
  sprain, 303
  tests of foot and, 133–135*f*
Ankylosing spondylitis, 262, 288–289
Anomia, 181
Anopsia, 181
Anorexia, 181
Anosmia, 181
Anosognosia, 181
Anterior cord syndrome, 160*t*
Anterior cruciate ligament, 129*f*, 131*f*, 132*f*. *See also* Cruciate ligament tears
Anterior spine, 157
Antibiotics, ototoxic, 74
Anti-coagulation therapy
  contraindications to joint manipulation, 376
  electromyography and, 178
Anti-dsDNA (anti-double stranded DNA antibody), 196
Antigravity position, for low back pain, 362
Anti-nuclear antibodies (ANA), 196, 260
Antistreptolysin-o titre (ASO), 194*t*, 196
Anuria, 89
Aortic aneurysms, referred spine pain and, 293, 294
Apastia, 181
Aphasia, 181
  receptive or expressive, 167
Aphemia, 181
Aphonia, 181, 183
Apices, lung, auscultation of, 76
Apley's compression test, 130*f*
Apley's distraction test, 130*f*
Apley's scratch test A, 114*f*
Apley's scratch test B, 114*f*
Apophyseal injuries, in children *versus* adults, 39
Appendicitis, 303
Apprehension test, 115*f*
Appropriate health promotion, 7–8
Apraxia, 181
Aprosodia, 180, 181
Arcus senilis, 72
Argyll Robertson pupil, 72, 181
Arnold-Chiari malformation, 181
Arterioles, in eyes, 72
Arthritides, 209, 221*t*, 258*t*, 288–290, 289*t*
Arthritis
  enteropathy and, 264
  gouty, 264
  inflammatory, contraindications to joint manipulation in, 375
  psoriatic, 263
  spine pain and, 290
Arthritis profile, 204*t*
ASAP, as order note, 17
Ascites, 86
Asemia, 182
Asitia, 182
Assessment progress notes, POMR, 15
Astasia, 182
Astereognosis, 182
Asterixis, 171, 182
Asthenia, 182
Asthma
  in children, 42–43
  exercise-induced, 35
Astrocytomas, cerebral lesions and, 166*t*
Asynergia, 182
Ataxia, 169, 182
Athetosis, 167, 171
Atlantoaxial instability (AAI), 37
Atonia, 182
Atopic dermatitis, in children, 43
Atrial fibrillation, in elderly, 26
At-risk, definition of, 9
Atrophy, 167

Auditory disturbances, cervical spine trauma and, 350
Auscultation
of abdomen, 80
of extremities, 84
for heart examination, 78, 79*f*
of thorax/lungs, 76
Autonomy, patient, 331

B

Babinski response, 155–156, 157, 168
Back pain. *See* Cervical spine, trauma management; Low back pain
Backpacks
school, low back pain and, 41
weighted, for chronic low back pain, 364
Baker's cyst, 304
Bakody's sign, 97*f*
Ballismus, 167
Bamboo sign, 217*t*
Bankart lesion, 304
Basilar invagination, 165*t*, 290–291
Basophilic stippling, 189
Basophils, 189*t*, 190
Battle's sign, 84
Beatty's maneuver, 109*f*
Bechterew's test, 103*f*
Beer can test, 115*f*
Bell's palsy, 304
Belmont Report, 333
Beneficence, 330
Benign conditions
bone tumors, 218*t*, 280–284
definition of, 284
tumors and spinal pain, 292
Benign essential tremor, 305
Benign paroxysmal positional vertigo (BPPV), 325, 326*t*
Benign prostatic hyperplasia, 305
Berry aneurysm, 305
Bicarbonate, 194*t*, 197
Biceps tendinitis, 121*f*, 306
Biedermann, Heider, 38
Bilirubin, 192, 194*t*, 197
Bitemporal hemianopsia, 73, 172
Bladder cancer, 271, 275
Blade of grass sign, 217*t*
Blank spaces, in medical charts, 11–12
Blastic lesions, solitary or multiple, 212*t*
Blister of bone sign, 217*t*
Block vertebrae, 291
Blood. *See also* Serum chemistries
specimen tubes for, 246*t*
urinary, 192
Blood pressure, 64*t*
asymmetric, 67
in elderly, 26
normal pediatric ranges, 32, 33*t*
taking, 64
BMI (body mass index), 62, 63*t*
Bone cysts, 283
aneurysmal, contraindications to joint manipulation, 375
Bone destruction patterns, 220*t*
Bone islands, 280
Bone tumors
aggressive, 219*t*
benign, 218*t*, 280–284
contraindications to joint manipulation, 375, 376
common causes of, 221*t*
laboratory screening profile, 204*t*
malignant, 276–280
diagnostic imaging for, 275, 276*f*
examination for, 272
laboratory tests for, 274*t*
radiographic interpretation of, 208
Borchgrevink, G. E., 352
Boundary issues, 335
Boutonniere sign, 217*t*
Bowstring sign, 103*f*
BRACE (mnemonic), 341, 342*t*
Brachial neuropathy, shoulder depression test and, 101*f*
Brachial plexus lesions, 177
Bradycardia, in elderly, 26
Bradykinesia, 161
Bragard's test, 104*f*
Brain death, 177
Brain lesions, 159–162, 159*t*, 271, 293
Brain tumors, 179
Brainstem auditory evoked responses (BAER), 176–177
Brainstem lesions, 154, 165, 165*t*
Breast cancer, 270, 270*t*, 272, 274*t*
Broca's (expressive) aphasia, 181
Bronchitis, chronic, diagnosis of, 77
Brown-Sequard's syndrome, 160*t*, 163
Brudzinski's sign, 97*f*
Bulbar palsy, 182
BUN (blood urea nitrogen), 194*t*, 197
Burn's bench test, 95*f*
Burr cells, 188

Bursitis, 306
Button sequestrum, 217*t*

C

C1 fractures, differential diagnosis of, 214*t*
C2 fractures, differential diagnosis of, 214*t*
Cachexia, 167
Calcaneal apophysitis, 40–41
Calcaneocuboid joint mobilization, 410
Calcium, 194*t*, 197, 275
Calcium pyrophosphate crystal deposition disease, 264–265
Canadian law, material risks under, 332–333
Cancer. *See also* Neoplasms; Tumors
  diagnostic imaging for, 275–276
  introduction, 269
  laboratory investigation, 273–275
  physical examination, 271–273
  screening methods, 269–271, 270*t*
Candidiasis, oral, 75
Capsular patterns of joints, 407
Carcinoembyronic antigen, 274
Carcinoma, 284
Carcinoma *in situ*, 284
Cardiac ischemia profile, 204*t*
Cardiac risk profile, 204*t*
Cardiopulmonary resuscitation (CPR), 252–253
Carpal tunnel syndrome, 162, 306
  electromyography and, 178
  etiology of, 163*t*
  Phalen's test and, 124*f*
  prayer sign and, 125*f*
  Tinel's sign at the wrist and, 125*f*
Carpometacarpal (CMC) joint mobilization, 414
Case presentations, in hospitals/long-term care facilities, 48
Cauda equina syndrome, 160*t*, 165, 166, 182
Cauliflower ear, 73
Cellular inclusions, 189
Central cord syndrome, 160*t*
Central nervous system (CNS)
  lesion location and, 154
  malignancy
    diagnostic imaging, 275
    laboratory tests, 274*t*
    screening, 270*t*
Cerebellopontine angle tumors, 177
Cerebellum, lesions in, 154, 162, 169
Cerebral abscess, cerebral lesions and, 166*t*
Cerebral cortex, 154
  lesions in, 159, 161*t*
Cerebrovascular accidents, 307
  contraindications to joint manipulation, 376
  EEG for diagnosis of, 179
Cerumen, in ear canal, 74
Cervical collars, 348, 352
Cervical lateral glide mobilization, oscillatory, 385
Cervical spine
  compression test, 98*f*
  contraindications to joint manipulation, 376
  dislocations, differential diagnosis of, 214*t*
  distraction test, 98*f*
  fractures of
    differential diagnosis of, 214*t*
    Rust's sign and, 100*f*
  maximum compression test, 100*f*
  neurological lesions and, 166–167
  radiculopathy
    Bakody's sign and, 97*f*
    shoulder depression test and, 101*f*
    somatosensory evoked potentials and, 177
  referred spine pain and, 293
  tests, 97–102*f*
  trauma management
    ancillary diagnostic testing, 352
    ancillary therapies, 353–355, 354*t*
    examination, 348–350, 349*f*
    introduction, 347–348
    prognosis, 353
    radiography, 350–351, 351*t*
    side effects, 353, 354*t*
    treatment, 352–353
  visceral disease mimicry and dysfunction of, 296
Cervicogenic headache, 311
Cervicogenic vertigo, 325
Charts, medical
  hospitals' and long-term care facilities' procedures, 48
  state requirements for, 11
Chemotherapy, definition of, 284
Chest. *See also* Abdomen
  pain, 86–87
  radiograph interpretation, 237, 237*t*
  radiographic evaluation, 210–211
    consolidation, 223–224
    effusion (pleural), 224
    extrapleural sign, 224
    hilar enlargement, 224
    mediastinal masses, 224–225
    pulmonary nodules, 225

unresolving pneumonia, 225
Cheyne-Stokes respiration, 77, 78*f*
Chief complaint, 56–57
Children. *See also* Youth diseases
cardiopulmonary resuscitation for, 253
cervical spine, 36–38
common conditions of, 42–45
developmental red flags in, 35*t*
growth and development, 34
history and physical examination, 31–32
normal blood pressure, 33*t*
normal range and mean pulse for, 33*t*
orthopedic and sports injuries of, 38–42
pre-athletic physical examination, 34–36
Chloride, 194*t*, 198
Cholecystitis/cholelithiasis, 307
Cholesterol, 194*t*, 198
Chondroblastomas, 281
Chondrocalcinosis, differential diagnosis of, 212*t*
Chondromyxoid fibromas, 281–282
Chondrosarcoma, 278–279
Chordomas, 278, 292
Chorea, 167, 171
Chronic obstructive pulmonary disease, 307–308
Chronic pelvic pain syndrome (CPPS), 295–296
Chronic whiplash syndrome, 353–355
Chvostek's sign, 84
Circumlocution, 182
Clinical conditions. *See also specific conditions*
introduction to, 301
Clinical laboratory diagnosis, 187–204
for cancer, 273–275
complete blood count, 187–190
introduction, 187
serum chemistries, 193, 194–195*t*, 195–203
shorthand for, 188*f*
urinalysis, 190–193
Clonus, 154, 168
Closed-packed joint positions, 407
Clotting/bleeding disorders
contraindications to joint manipulation, 376
Clubbing (digital), 77, 84
Cluster headaches, 311–312
Cobb measurement method for scoliosis, 140*f*
Coccidioidomycosis, 291
Codman's sign, 116*f*
Cognitive impairment, cervical spine trauma and, 350
"Cogwheel" response, 154
Colic, 43–44
Colon cancer, 270, 270*t*, 272, 274*t*, 275
Colorectal cancer, 294
Community health, 4
Complete blood count (CBC), 187–190, 189*t*, 275
Comprehensive database, POMR, 13–14
Compression fractures, Soto-Hall test, 101*f*
Compressive neuropathy, electromyography and, 178
Computerized tomography (CT), 233–234, 234*t*, 351. *See also* Diagnostic imaging
Confabulation, 182
Congenital dysplasias, 291
Congenital lesions, 210, 221*t*
Congenital muscular torticollis (CMT), 38
Congenital/dysplastic spondylolisthesis, 144
Congestive heart failure, 77, 294
Conjunctiva, physical examination of, 69
"Connor" rating instrument, for ADHD, 44
Consolidation, of chest, radiographic interpretation of, 223–224
Constipation, 87
Continuous stretch mobilization (CSM), 408
Contract-relax (CR) therapy, 402, 404
Contrast baths, 395–396, 396*t*
Conus medullaris syndrome, 160*t*, 182
Corduroy vertebrae, 217*t*
Coronary artery disease (CAD), 293
Coronary disease, 294
Cortical lesions, 154, 161
Costoclavicular tests, 113*f*
Cotton wool sign, 217*t*
Cough, 87
Coupled motions, spinal, 288
Cozen's test, 122*f*
Cranial nerves, 154, 159, 167
Craniopharyngiomas, 176
Crank test, 116*f*
C-reactive protein (CRP), 203
Creatine phosphokinase (CPK), 194*t*, 198
Creatinine, 194*t*, 198
Crescent sign, 217*t*
Cruciate ligament tears, 308. *See also* Anterior cruciate ligament
Cryotherapy, 392–393
contraindications, 393*t*
effects, 392*t*
indications, 393*t*
for low back pain, 362
spray and stretch technique, 393–394
Cubital tunnel syndrome, 123*f*
Cullen's sign, 85

Cyanosis, 68, 77
Cysts, 284

D

Davis series radiographs, 351*t*
De Quervain's disease, 308. *See also* Stenosing tenosynovitis
Decerebrate posturing, 159–160
Decorticate posturing, 159–160
Deep tendon reflexes (DTRs), 154, 155*t*, 168
Degeneration, sub-acute combined, 325–326
Degenerative disc disease (DDD), 289
Degenerative joint disease, 265–266
Degenerative spondylolisthesis, 144
Dementia, 172, 182
Dental caries, 293
Dermatomes, 157, 158*f*
Diabetes mellitus
  chief complaint and, 59
  nerve conduction velocity for neuropathy in, 179
  oral candidiasis and, 75
  peripheral neuropathy and, 162, 163*t*
  retinopathy and, 72
  somatosensory evoked potentials and polyneuropathy in, 177
Diagnosis, as element in orders, 18
Diagnostic imaging. *See also* Radiology
  advanced, 233–236
    computerized tomography, 233–234, 234*t*
    magnetic resonance imaging, 234–235, 235*t*
    radionuclide bone scanning, 236, 236*t*
    ultrasound, 236, 236*t*
  introduction, 205
  plain film interpretation
    abdomen radiographs, 237, 238*t*
    chest radiographs, 237, 237*t*
    extremity radiographs, 238, 240*t*
    skull radiographs, 238, 241*t*
    spine radiographs, 238, 239*t*
Diarrhea, 87
Diastematomyelia, 182–183
Diastolic heart murmurs, 78
Diathermy, 394
Diffuse idiopathic skeletal hyperostosis (DISH), 266, 289
Digital rectal examination, 250–251
Digitalis effects in elderly, 26
Digits, clubbing of, 77, 84
Diplopia, 172, 183
Direct compression, 405
Disability, as element in orders, 18
Disc bulge, 292
Disc herniations
  central, 163
  chiropractic treatment of, 166
  compression and, 162–163
  nerve conduction velocity in, 179
  somatosensory evoked potentials and, 177
  whiplash and, 347
Disc lesions, 105*f*
Disc protrusion/extrusion/sequestration, 292, 308–309
Diskitis (aseptic), 290
Dislocation, spinal, 292
  contraindications to joint manipulation in, 375
Disp., as order in prescriptions, 19
Distal radioulnar joint mobilization, 413
Diuretics effects in elderly, 26
Diverticulitis, 309
Dizziness. *See also* Vertigo
  cervical spine trauma and, 350
  differential diagnosis of, 173
  EEG for diagnosis of, 179
"Double-Crush Syndrome," 179
Down syndrome, 37
Draping, during physical examination, 83
Dugas' test, 117*f*
Dysacusis, 183
Dysantigraphia, 183
Dysarthria, 167, 183
Dysbasia, 183
Dyscalculia, 167, 183
Dyschiria, 183
Dyschronation, 183
Dysdiadochokinesia, 183
Dysesthesia, 183
Dysgraphia, 180
Dyskinesia, 180
Dyslexia, 183
Dyslogia, 183
Dysmetria, 183
Dysmimia, 183
Dysmnesia, 181
Dysmorphophobia, 183
Dysnomia, 181
Dysphagia, 87, 183, 218–219, 349
Dysphasia, 181
Dysphonia, 181
Dysplasia, 284
Dyspnea, 87

Dyspraxia, 181
Dysreflexia, 183
Dyssynergia, 183
Dystonias, 171, 183
Dysuria, 87

E

Ears. *See also* Hearing loss
  physical examination of, 73–74
Echolalia, 183
Edema, peripheral, 88
Effective health promotion, 7–8
Ehlers-Danlos syndrome
  contraindications to joint manipulation, 376
Elbow
  dislocations, differential diagnosis of, 215*t*
  fractures, differential diagnosis of, 215*t*
  joint mobilization
    humeroradial, 413
    humeroulnar, 412
  tests of, 122–123*f*
Elbow fat pad sign, 217*t*
Electricity. *See* Galvanic current; Inferential current therapy; Microcurrent therapy; Sinusoidal current; Transcutaneous electrical nerve stimulation
Electrocardiogram (ECG), 249–250, 250*f*
Electroencephalogram (EEG), 179
Electromagnetic therapy, 353
Electromyography (EMG), 177–178
Ely's (heel-to-buttock) test, 104*f*
Emmetropia, 72
Emphysema, 76
Encephalitis, lumbar puncture and, 180
Enchondromas, 281
Endocrine lesions, 221*t*
Endometriosis, 294
Enostomas, 280
Enteropathic arthritis, 263, 290
Eosinophils, 189*t*, 190
Epistaxis, 74
Epley's maneuver, 326*t*
Erector spinae muscles, 106*f*
Ergogenic aids, athletes and, 36
Erythrocyte sedimentation rate, 204, 260
Escherichia coli, 291
Esophageal disease, 293
Ethics
  abandonment, 334–335
  advertising, 336
  boundary issues, 335
  caveat emptor *vs.* credat emptor, 329–330
  duties, 330–331
  fraud, 335–336
  "gaming the system," 335–336
  informed consent, 332–333
  Institutional Review Boards and, 334
  introduction, 329
  practice and research boundaries, 333–334
  research subjects, 333
  rights, 331
  self-regulation, 332
Evidence-based medicine (EBM)
  delivering individual health promotion with, 4–5
  principles of, 5–7
Evoked responses (EP), 176–177
Ewing's sarcoma, 279
Exercise(s)
  asthma and, 35
  cardiac abnormalities and, 35
  for cervical spine trauma management, 353
  chiropractic care of geriatric patients and, 27
  in elderly, 26
  as element in orders, 18
  for low back pain, 363
  spinal stabilization exercises, 405–407, 406*t*
Exostosis, 280–281
Expressive aphasia, 181
Extraocular muscles
  paralysis or palsy of, 72
  physical examination of, 70
Extrapleural signs, 224
Extrapyramidal system lesions, 161
Extras, as element in orders, 17
Extremities. *See also specific extremities*
  neurologic innervation of, 156*t*
  physical examination of, 84
  radiograph interpretation, 238, 240*t*
Eyelids, 69, 71, 72
Eyes
  abnormalities of, 71–72
  cardinal positions of gaze and ocular muscles, 71*t*
  normal retina of right, 69*f*
  physical examination of, 69–73
  pupil abnormalities, 70*t*

F

Face, physical examination of, 68–69
Facet disease, 98*f*, 105*f*
Facet planar motions, 288

Facet syndrome, 292, 309
Faintness, during exercise, 35
Fallen fragment sign, 217*t*
Family history
  adolescent athlete examination and, 36
  chief complaint and, 61
  of scoliosis, 138
  tree, 61*f*
Fasciculations, 155, 166, 171
Fat-blood interface, 217*t*
Fecal occult blood (FOB), 204
Female athlete triad, 36
Femoral epiphysis, slipped capital, 40
Festinating gait, 169
Fever, 309–310
  in elderly, 26
  neonatal, 44–45, 45*t*
  of unknown origin, 88
Fibrillations, 155, 178
Fibroids, 284
Fibromyalgia syndrome, 266–267
Fibrosarcoma, 279
Fibrous cortical defect with nonossifying fibroma, 283
Fibrous dysplasia, 283–284, 292
  contraindications to joint manipulation, 376
Fibroxanthomas, 283
Fidelity, 330
Fingers
  fractures of, differential diagnosis of, 215*t*
  joint mobilization, 414
Finkelstein's test, 124*f*
Fish vertebrae, 217*t*
Five I's (mnemonic), 21, 22*t*
Flaccid paralysis, 154
Fluorescent treponemal antibody absorbed (FTA-ABS), 198
Fluorimethane, 393
Foot
  fractures of, differential diagnosis of, 216*t*
  tests of ankle and, 133–135*f*
Foramen magnum, intracranial lesions and, 159
Foraminal encroachment
  cervical distraction test and, 98*f*
  neural, maximum cervical compression test and, 100*f*
Foraminal stenosis, intravertebral, joint manipulation and, 376
Forearm, fractures, differential diagnosis of, 215*t*
Fractures
  cervical spine, Rust's sign and, 100*f*
  compression, Soto-Hall test and, 101*f*
  contraindications to joint manipulation, 375, 376
  differential diagnosis of, 214–215*t*
  enchondromas and, 281
  metatarsal, Morton's test and, 133*f*
  scaphoid, snuff box palpation and, 125*f*
  spinal, 292
Fraud, 335–336
Freiberg test, 110*f*
Functional spinal units (FSU), 372
Fundoscopic examination, 71

G

Gaenslen's test, 110*f*
Gag reflex, 75
Gait, abnormal, 169, 171
Gallbladder disease, 294
Galvanic current, 392*t*, 398, 398*t*
"Gaming the system," 335–336
Gamma-glutamyl transpeptidase (GGT), 194*t*
Gardner's syndrome, 282
Gastroesophageal reflux disease, 310
Gastrointestinal malignancy, metastatic, 83
Gatterman, M. I., 371
Genital cancer, 270*t*, 271, 272
Gerber lift-off test, 117*f*
Gerber push-with-force test, 118*f*
Geriatrics/geriatric patients
  aging theories, 21, 23
  characteristic neuromusculoskeletal changes in, 24–25*t*
  chiropractic treatment of, 26–28
  clinical assessment, 23, 25
  Five I's for conditions in, 22*t*
  introduction, 21
  vital signs, 25–26
Giant cell tumor of bone, 279
  contraindications to joint manipulation, 375
Glaucoma, 72, 176
Glenohumeral joint mobilization, 411–412
Glioblastoma multiform, cerebral lesions and, 166*t*
Gliomas, 165, 165*t*, 166, 166*t*, 176, 284
Globulin, 194*t*, 198
"Glove and stocking" paresthesias, 162
Glucose, 191, 194*t*, 198–199, 261
Glutamic-oxoacetic transaminase, serum (SGOT), 195*t*, 197, 202

Glutamic-pyruvic transaminase, serum (SGPT), 193, 195*t*, 202
Glycosylated hemoglobin. *See* Hemoglobin A1C
Goldthwait's test, 104*f*
Gordon's Reflex, 157
Gout, chalky white deposits in pinna and, 73
Graded oscillatory mobilization (GOM), 381, 408
Green, L. W., 8
Grisel's syndrome, 37
Guillain-BarrÇ syndrome, 178, 179, 180, 310–311

H

'H' vertebrae, 217*t*
Hair-on-end sign, 217*t*
Hamartomas, definition of, 284
Hamstring spasm, 106*f*, 107*f*
Hand, tests of, 124–125*f*, 126*f*
Hay fever, 74
Head, physical examination of, 68–69
Headache, 173, 311
  cervicogenic, 311
  cluster, 311–312
  common causes for, 312*t*
  EEG for diagnosis of, 179
  evaluation of, 173*t*
  migraine, 313
  migraine-basilar artery, 313
  nervous system etiology, 314
HEADSS (mnemonic), 32
Health care, right to, 331
Health Insurance Portability and Accountability Act of 1996 (HIPAA), 19, 331
Health promotion, 3
  appropriate *versus* effective, 7–8
  delivering EBM for individuals, 4–5
  EBM principles in, 5–7
Hearing loss. *See also* Ears
  brain stem evoked response and, 177
  cerumen (wax) buildup in ear canal, 74
Heart
  adventitious sounds, 80*t*
  auscultation areas, 79*f*
  physical examination, 77–78
Heart failure, 78
Heart murmurs, 78
  common, 81*f*
  grading system, 82*t*
Heart rate, in elderly, 26
Heartburn, 88
Heat therapy, 394
  contraindications, 395*t*
  effects, 392*t*
  indications, 395*t*
  for low back pain, 363
Heel pad sign, 217*t*
Heel-to-buttock test, 104*f*
Hemangiomas, 280
  contraindications to joint manipulation, 376
Hematemesis, 88, 222
Hematochezia, 222
Hematocrit (Hct), 187, 189*t*, 190
Hematomas
  contraindications to joint manipulation with, 375
Hematopoiesis, extramedullary, 188
Hematuria, 88
Hemiballismus, 171
Hemiparesis, 169
Hemiplegia, 183
Hemoccult, 273
Hemoglobin (Hgb), 187, 189*t*, 190
  glycosylated, 194*t*
Hemoglobin A1C, 194*t*, 199
Hemoptysis, 88
Hemorrhage, poikilocytosis and, 188
Hepatic profile, 204*t*
Hepatitis, electromyography and, 178
Hepatomegaly, 88, 222
Herpes zoster (shingles), 163, 294, 314
Hiatal hernia, 294
Hibb's test, 126*f*
High velocity low amplitude (HVLA) manipulation, 371
High-density lipoprotein (HDL) cholesterol, 199
Hilar enlargement, 224
Hip, 126–129*f*, 216*t*, 409
Hip disease, 126*f*, 128*f*, 294
Hip flexion contracture, 128*f*
Hippocrates, 19
  oath of, 330
H.I.S.T.O.R.Y. (mnemonic), 57, 59, 59*t*
History and physical examination (H&P)
  for adolescents, 34–36
  for children, 31–32
History of present illness (HPI)
  allergies, 57
  chief complaint, 56–57
  events of, 61

History of present illness (HPI) (*continued*)
  family history, 61, 61*f*
  general history, 57
  last menstrual period/last meal, 61
  medications, 57
  mnemonics, 59*t*
  past medical history, 57, 58*t*, 59, 60*t*
  psychosocial history, 61
  tips in taking, 55–56
HIV (human immunodeficiency virus), 178, 199
HLA-B27 test, 260
HLA-DR4 test, 261
Hodgkin's lymphoma, 314–315
Hoffman's Reflex, 156, 168
Homan's sign, 85
Hoover's sign, 95*f*
Hospitals/long-term care facilities
  case presentations, 48
  charting procedures, 48
  chiropractor roles in, 50–51, 50*t*
  clinics and ward rounds, 48
  general institutional protocols, 47–50
  institutional committees, 48–49
  introduction, 47
  surgical procedures, 49–50
Howell-Jolly bodies, 189
Human chorionic gonadotropin (HCG), 194*t*, 199, 275
Human T-lymphocyte virus (HTLV), 199
Humeral epiphysitis, proximal, 39
Humeroradial joint mobilization, 413
Humeroulnar joint mobilization, 412
Hydrocollator packs, 394
Hydroxyapatite deposition disease, 265
Hyperchromic anemia, 189
Hyperglycemia, 162
Hyperhomocystinemia, 378
Hypermobility, intervertebral, 290
Hyperopia, 72
Hyperparathyroidism, 291
Hyperpathia, 183
Hyperplasia, 284
  benign prostatic, 305
Hyperreflexia, 154, 174
Hypertension, 67, 315
Hypertensive retinopathy, 72
Hypertonicity, 154
Hypertrophy, 284
Hyperventilation, EEG and, 179
Hypoacusis, 184
Hypochromic anemia, 188, 189
Hypomobility, intervertebral, 290
Hypoplasia, 37
Hyporeflexia, 154, 174
Hypotension, orthostatic, 67
Hypothyroid patients, 69
Hypotonicity, 154

I

Ice, 392
Ice massage, 393
Iliac artery aneurysms, 83
Iliac compression, 111*f*
Illness, definition of, 9
Individual health behaviors, 8–10
Infants
  brain stem evoked response and hearing loss in, 177
  cardiopulmonary resuscitation for, 253
  nerve conduction velocity in, 178
Infection
  contraindications to joint manipulation with, 375
  radiographic interpretation of, 210
Inferential current (IFC) therapy, 399–400, 400*t*, 401*t*
Informed consent, 332–333
Infranuclear lesions, 159
Infrared therapy, 394
Infraspinatus disease, 121*f*
Infraspinatus isolation test, 118*f*
Infratentorial lesions, 160–161, 161*t*
Initial plans, POMR, 13, 13*t*, 14–15
Injuries, chief complaint and, 59
Instability
  contraindications to joint manipulation with, 375
Institutional Review Boards, 334
Internuclear ophthalmoplegia, 184
Interphalangeal joint mobilization, 411, 414
Intervertebral foramen, 163
Intervertebral hypermobility, 290
Intervertebral hypomobility, 290
Intracranial lesions, 154, 177
Intracranial pressure, lumbar puncture and, 180
Intradiscal vacuum cleft, 217*t*
Intravertebral foraminal stenosis
  contraindications to joint manipulation, 376
Intravertebral vacuum cleft, 217*t*
Involuntary movements, abnormal, 171–172
Iris, examination of, 70

Iron, 194*t*, 199
Iron binding capacity, total (TIBC), 194*t*, 199
Irritable Infant Syndrome of Musculoskeletal Origin (IISMO), 44
Ivory phalanx, 217*t*
Ivory vertebra, 213*t*, 217*t*

J

Jaundice, 68, 71, 88
Jobe test, 119*f*
Joint disease, degenerative, 265–266
Joint manipulation
  adverse reactions to, 377–380
  under anesthesia/conscious sedation, 380
  benefits of, 374*t*
  contraindications, 374–377
    absolute, 375–376
    relative, 376–377
  evidence for, 372*t*
  indications, 373–374, 373*t*
  introduction, 371
  rationale for spinal, 372
Joint mobilization, 407–414
  acromioclavicular, 412
  ankle mortise, 410
  elbow, 412–413
  glenohumeral, 411–412
  hip, 409
  interphalangeal, 411
  knee
    femoral-tibial, 409
    tibiofibular, 410
  metatarsophalangeal, 411
  with movement, 380–381
    clinical examples of, 383–386
    grades, 381
    principles of, 381
    types, 381–383
  scapulothoracic, 412
  spinal, 408–409
  sternoclavicular, 412
  subtalar joint, 410
  tarsometatarsal, 411
  wrist, 413–414
Jumper's knee, 40
Justice, 330–331
Juvenile kyphosis, 39

K

Kemp's test, 105*f*
Kernig's sign, 105*f*
Ketones, 192
Kidney, calcification in, 223
Kidney cancer, 273, 274*t*
Kidney disease, 294
Kidney profile, 204*t*
Kinematic imbalances caused by suboccipital strain (KISS), 38
KISS syndrome, 38
Kleist's Hooking Sign, 156–157
Klippel-Feil Syndrome, 37–38
Knees
  anterior drawer sign of, 129*f*
  femoral-tibial joint mobilization, 409
  fractures of, differential diagnosis of, 216*t*
  jumper's, 40
  meniscus tears, 316–317
  tests of, 129–132*f*
  tibiofibular joint mobilization, 410
Kohler's disease, 40
Koplik's spots, 85
Kreuter, M. W., 8
Kyphosis, juvenile, 39

L

Laboratory
  diagnosis (*See* Clinical laboratory diagnosis)
  as element in orders, 17
Labral disease, anterior, 120*f*
Labral lesions, 116*f*
Lachman's test, 131*f*
Lacrimal apparatus, examination of, 69
Lactate dehydrogenase (LDH), 194*t*, 200
Laryngeal disease, 293
Larynx, whiplash and lacerations of, 347–348
LATER DUDES (mnemonic), 17
Lateral decubitus traction/extension, 384–385
Lateral epicondylitis, 122*f*, 315
Lateral recess stenosis, 184
  contraindications to joint manipulation, 376
Lateral spine, 157
Legg-Calve-Perthes (LCP) disease, 39–40
Legs
  apparent length, 102*f*
  seated straight raise test, 96*f*
  straight raise test, 108*f*
Leiomyomas, 284
Leukemias, 273, 275, 316
Leukoplakia, 75
Levine's sign, 85
Lewin's test, 106*f*

Lhermitte's sign, 99*f*
Liability claims, medical recordkeeping and, 11–12
Libman's test, 94*f*
Ligament tears, whiplash and, 347
Linder's sign, 99*f*
Lipase, 194*t*, 200
Lipomas, 284
Little League elbow, 39
Little League shoulder, 39
Liver cancer, 272–273, 275
Liver disease, 188
Low back pain (LBP)
  Burn's bench test for, 95*t*
  in children, 41–42
  Milgram's test and, 106*f*
  tripod sign and, 109*f*
Low back pain (LBP) management
  diagnostic evaluation, 360–361, 361*f*
  introduction, 359–360
  prognosis, 365
  treatment, 361
    acute, 362–364, 362*t*
    chronic, 364–365
    evidence for manual techniques in, 372*t*
    prognosis for success with manipulative, 365
Low-density lipoprotein (LDL) cholesterol, 194*t*, 200
Lower body screening examination, 147–148, 149*t*
Lower motor neuron lesions (LMNLs), 154, 155*t*, 157, 157*t*
Lucent lesions, 212*t*, 213*t*
Lumbar puncture (LP), 179–180
Lumbar rotation stretching mobilization, progressive or continuous, 385
Lumbar shear stability, 106*f*
Lumbar spinal canal stenosis, 364
Lumbar spine
  contraindications to joint manipulation, 375
  disease, straight leg raise and, 108*f*
  fractures of, differential diagnosis of, 214*t*
  referred spine pain and, 294–295
  tests, 102–109*f*
  visceral disease mimicry and dysfunction of, 297
Lumbosacral transitional segments, 291
Lungs
  adventitious sounds, 77*t*
  cancer, 269, 270*t*, 272, 275, 277*f*
  chronic disease, clubbing of digits and, 77
  chronic obstructive pulmonary disease, 307–308
  multiple or solitary nodules, 225
  physical examination of, 75–77
  referred spine pain and, 294
Lupus erythematosus cell preparation (LE prep), 200, 260
Lyme disease, 316
Lymph nodes, 83
Lymphadenopathy, 89, 293
Lymphocytes, 189*t*, 190
Lymphomas, 83
  of bone, 280
  diagnostic imaging for, 275
  examination for, 273
  Hodgkin's, 314–315

M

Maffucci's syndrome, 280
Magnetic resonance imaging (MRI), 234–235
  appropriate use of, 206–207
  cervical spine trauma, 351
  common indications and contraindications, 235*t*
  evoked potentials and, 176
Malignant conditions. *See also* Bone tumors, malignant; Neoplasms
  contraindications to joint manipulation with, 375
  definition of, 285
  tumors and spinal pain, 292–293
Malingering tests, 95–96*f*
Mankopf's test, 96*f*
Manual force mechanically-assisted procedures, 371
Marfan's syndrome
  contraindications to joint manipulation, 376
Massage, 401–402, 403*t*
McBurney's sign, 85
McMurray's test, 132*f*
Mean cellular volume (MCV), 187, 188
Mean corpuscular hemoglobin, 187, 189
Mean corpuscular hemoglobin concentration, 187
Mechanical force manually-assisted (MeFMA) procedures, 371
Mechanical supports, 407, 407*t*
Medial epicondylar apophysitis, 39
Medial-lateral grind test, 131*f*
Mediastinal masses, 224–225

Medical recordkeeping
introduction, 11–12
orders in, 16–18
patient confidentiality, 19
prescription writing, 18–19
problem-oriented, 12–16
specialized notes, 16
Medications
chief complaint and, 57
effects in elderly, 26
MEDLINE, 5
Melena, 89, 222
Meniere's disease, 74
Meningeal irritation, 97*f*, 99*f*
Meningeal tumors
contraindications to joint manipulation with, 375
Meningiomas, 165, 165*t*, 176
Meningitis, 99*f*, 105*f*, 166, 166*t*
Meniscal damage
Apley's compression test and, 130*f*
knee, 316–317
McMurray's test and, 132*f*
medial-lateral grind test and, 131*f*
Menstrual distress, female athlete triad and, 36
Mental status examination, 167
Metabolic lesions, 221*t*
Metacarpophalangeal (MCP) joint mobilization, 414
Metaplasia, 285
Metastasis
definition of, 285
spinal cord lesions and, 165
spine pain and, 293
Metatarsal fracture, 133*f*
Metatarsophalangeal joint mobilization, 411
Microcurrent therapy (MCT), 363, 364, 400–401
Migraine headaches, 313
Migraine-basilar artery headaches, 313
Milgram's test, 106*f*
Miller, Joyce, 44
Mill's test, 122*f*
Mimicry syndromes, 295–298, 404
Minor's sign, 107*f*
Mnemonics
AMPLE, 59*t*
BRACE, 341, 342*t*
Five I's, 21, 22*t*
HEADSS, 32
history, 59*t*
H.I.S.T.O.R.Y., 57, 59, 59*t*
LATER DUDES, 17
OPPQRST, 56, 59*t*
SOAP, 15–16
Mobilization with movements (MWMs), 380–382, 408. *See also* Joint mobilization, with movement
Monocytes, 189*t*, 190
Mononucleosis, recurrent, 35
Monospot, 200
Morton's test, 133*f*
Motor evoked potentials (MEP), 177
Motor examination, 169
Multiple myeloma, 276–278, 293
Multiple sclerosis, 317
brain stem evoked response and, 177
Lhermitte's sign and, 99*f*
lumbar puncture and, 180
motor evoked potentials and, 177
optic neuritis and, 72
visual evoked potentials and, 176
Murphy's punch test, 85
Murphy's sign, 85
Muscle energy techniques, 402–404
Muscle rigidity, 154
Muscle strength grading, 168*t*, 169
Muscle tears, whiplash and, 347
Muscle tone, 154
Myasthenia gravis, 178, 179, 317
Mydriasis, 72
Myelopathy, 184
contraindications to joint manipulation with, 375
spondylotic, 185
Myoclonus, 171
Myofascial conditions, spine pain and, 295
Myofascitis, 290
Myopia, 72, 73
Myxedema, 85

N

Nail pitting, 85
National Library of Medicine, MEDLINE, 5
Natural apophyseal glides (NAGs), 381, 382–383
Neck pain, cervical spine trauma and, 348–349
Neer impingement test, 119*f*
Nelson, C. F., 8
Neonatal fever, 44–45, 45*t*
Neoplasms. *See also* Cancer; Malignant conditions
brainstem lesions and, 165, 165*t*
Neri's bowing test, 107*f*

Nerve conduction velocity (NCV), 178–179
Nerve root compression or adhesions, 108*f*
Nerve root lesions, 157, 157*t*, 162–163, 164*t*
Nerve root tension, 99*f*, 102*f*, 103*f*, 106*f*, 107*f*
Neural mobilization, 414–415
Neuritis, optic, 72
Neurogenic claudication, 322. *See also* Spinal canal stenosis
Neurologic sequelae, in cervical spine trauma, 350*t*
Neurology
- abnormal gait, 169, 171
- abnormal involuntary movements, 171–172
- differential diagnosis of, 172–175
  - anisocoria, 172
  - bitemporal hemianopsia, 172
  - dementia, 172
  - diplopia, 172
  - dizziness, 173
  - headache, 173, 173*t*
  - hyperreflexia, 174
  - hyporeflexia, 174
  - muscular weakness, 175
  - ophthalmoplegia, 174
  - polyneuropathy, 174
  - syncope, 174–175, 175*t*
  - tremors, 175
  - vertigo, 175
- etiology of lesion, 162–166
  - nerve root lesions, 162–163
  - peripheral, 162
  - spinal cord, 163, 165
- examination, 167–169
  - cerebellum, 169
  - cranial nerve, 167
  - mental status, 167
  - motor, 169
  - reflexes, 168
  - sensory, 168–169
  - visual inspection, 167
- introduction, 153
- location of lesion, 153–162
  - deep tendon reflexes, 154, 155*t*
  - fasciculations or fibrillations, 155
  - paralysis/paresis/muscle tone, 154, 155*t*, 156*t*
  - pathologic reflexes, 155–157
  - peripheral neuropathy, 162
  - radiculopathy, 162
  - spinal cord, 157, 159, 159*t*
- peripheral neuropathy, 169
- specialized testing, 176–180
  - electroencephalogram, 179
  - electromyography, 177–178
  - evoked responses, 176–177
  - lumbar puncture, 179–180
  - motor evoked potentials, 177
  - nerve conduction velocity, 178–179
- treatment or treatment contraindications, 166–167

Neuromas
- acoustic, 74, 165, 165*t*
- Morton's test and, 133*f*

Neutrophils, 189*t*, 190
Nitrites, urinary, 192
Noises, loud, hearing loss and, 74
Nonmaleficence, 330
Nose, examination of, 74
Nosebleeds, 74
Nuremberg Code, 333

O

Ober's test, 127*f*
Objective progress notes, POMR, 15
O'Brien's test
- supinated position, 120*f*
- thumbs down position, 120*f*

Obturator sign, 85
Occipitocervical transitional segments, 291
Ochronosis, 73
Ocular pressure examination, 71
Oculocephalogyric reflex (OCGR), 402, 404
Odontoid aplasia, atlantoaxial instability and, 37
Oliguria, 89
Ollier's disease, 281
Oncogenes, 285
Oncology, clinical. *See* Cancer
Onset, of complaints, 56
Open-packed joint positions, 407
Operations. *See also* Surgery
- chief complaint and history of, 59

Ophthalmoplegia, 174, 184, 185
Oppenheim's Sign, 157
OPPQRST (mnemonic), 56, 59*t*
Optic neuropathy, 176
Orders
- types of, 17–18
- writing, 16–17

Orthopedics. *See also* Physical examination
- angular deformities of, 149*t*
- ankle/foot tests, 133–135*f*

elbow tests, 122–123*f*
hand tests, 126*f*
hip tests, 126–129*f*
introduction, 93
knee tests, 129–132*f*
malingering tests, 95–96*f*
pelvic tests, 109–112*f*
range of motion, 135, 136–137*t*
scoliosis evaluation, 135, 137–141, 138*t*, 140*f*, 141*f*, 142*t*, 143
screening examinations
lower body, 147–148, 149*t*
upper body, 146–147, 147*t*
shoulder tests, 114–122*f*
spine tests
cervical, 97–102*f*
general, 94*f*
lumbar, 102–109*f*
thoracic, 102*f*
spondylolisthesis, 143–146, 145*t*
thoracic outlet tests, 112–113*f*
useful tests/signs, 93
wrist/hand tests, 124–125*f*
Orthoses, 407, 407*t*
Os odontoideum, atlantoaxial instability and, 37
Oscillatory cervical lateral glide mobilization, 385
Osgood Schlatter's disease, 40
Osteoarthritis of the facet articulations, 290
Osteoblastomas, 282
contraindications to joint manipulation, 375
Osteochondritis dissecans, 317–318
Osteochondromas, 280–281
Osteogenesis imperfecta, 71
contraindications to joint manipulation with, 375
Osteoid osteomas, 282
contraindications to joint manipulation, 375
Osteomas, 282
Osteopenia, in males, 213*t*
Osteopoikilosis, 280
Osteoporosis, 291, 318
contraindications to joint manipulation, 376
Osteosarcoma, 278
Otitis externa, 73
Otitis media (OM), 42, 74
Otoscopic examination, 73
Ovarian disease, 294

P

Pace test, 111*f*
Paget's disease, 292
Pain. *See also* Spine pain
abdominal, 86
chest, 86–87
inferential current for management of, 400
lateral spinal cord and, 157
Libman's test for, 94*t*
movement in pinna and, 73
neurological root lesions and, 157
whiplash-induced, 347
Pain medications, effects in elderly, 26
Palliative factors, of complaints, 56
Palpation
of abdomen, 81, 83
for abdominal aortic aneurysms, 84
of extremities, 84
for heart examination, 77–78
snuff box, 125*f*
of thorax/lungs, 75
Pancoast's tumor, 293, 318
Pancreatic calcification, 222
Pancreatic cancer, 273, 275
Pancreatic disease, 294
Pancreatic profile, 204*t*
Papilledema, 72
Papillomas, 285
Paragraphia, 184
Paralysis, 154
ascending, 310–311 (*See also* Guillain-Barré syndrome)
neurosurgical referrals for, 166
Paraphasia, 184
Paraplegia, 184
Parapnasia, 184
Parathyroid hormone (PTH), 195*t*, 200
Paresis, 154, 184
Paresthesias, 349
Past medical history, 57, 58*t*, 59
Pathologic spondylolisthesis, 144
Patient confidentiality, 19
Patrick-FABER test, 112*f*
figure four test, 127*f*
Patte test, 121*f*
Pediatrics. *See* Children
Pedicles, missing, 212*t*
Pelvic disease, 111*f*
Pelvic floor strengthening exercise, 27
Pelvic fractures, 214*t*
Pelvic inflammatory disease, 294

Pelvic pain syndrome, chronic (CPPS), 295–296
Pelvic tests, 109–112*f*
Peptic ulcer disease, 294, 318–319
Percussion
  of abdomen, 80, 83*t*
  of extremities, 84
  for heart examination, 78
  spinous, 94*f*
  of thorax/lungs, 75
Periodontal abscess, 293
Peripheral mobilization with movements (MWMs), 383, 384
Peripheral nerve compression syndromes, 162
Peripheral nerve lesions, 157, 157*t*
Peripheral nervous system, 154
Peripheral neuropathy, 162, 169
  common causes, 170*t*
  of cranial nerves, 154
  Lewin's test and, 106*f*
  Neri's bowing test and, 107*f*
  nerve conduction velocity in, 179
  straight leg raise and, 108*f*
Peritonitis, 83
Personal health, definition of, 4
pH, urinary, 191
Phalen's test, 124*f*
Phantom limb, 184
Pharyngeal disease, 293
Pharynx, whiplash and lacerations of, 347–348
Phlebitis, 319
Phlebotomy, 245–247, 248*f*
Phonophoresis, 398
Phosphorus, 195*t*, 200
Photic stimulation, 179
Physical examination, 61. *See also* Orthopedics
  abdomen, 79–81, 82*f*, 83–84, 83*t*
  abnormal pulses, 65*t*
  body mass index, 63*t*
  for cancer, 271–273
  cervical spine trauma, 348–350, 349*f*
  Cheyne-Stokes respiration, 78*f*
  draping during, 83
  ears, 73–74
  extremities, 84
  eyes, 69–73, 69*f*, 70*t*, 71*t*
  general signs, 61–62, 61–62*t*
  head/face, 68–69
  heart and great vessels, 77–78, 79*f*, 80*t*, 81*f*
  nose, 74
  pulse pressure abnormalities, 67*t*
  respiratory abnormalities, 66*t*
  skin, 68
  special tests/signs in, 84–86
  thorax/lungs, 75–77
  throat, 74–75
  vital signs, 63–64, 64*t*, 67
Physical medicine
  effects, 391, 392*t*
  introduction, 391
  specific types, 391
    contrast baths, 395–396, 396*t*
    cryotherapy, 392–393, 393*t*
    galvanic current, 398, 398*t*
    heat therapy, 394, 395*t*
    inferential current therapy, 399–400, 400*t*, 401*t*
    joint mobilization, 407–414
    massage, 401–402, 403*t*
    neural mobilization, 414–415
    orthoses, 407, 407*t*
    sinusoidal current, 398–399, 399*t*
    spinal stabilization exercises, 405–407
    spray and stretch technique, 393–394
    traction, 401, 402*t*
    trigger point/tender point therapy, 404–405
Physician-patient relationship, boundaries and, 335
Piriformis syndrome, 109*f*, 110*f*, 111*f*, 184, 319–320
Pituitary tumors, 176
Pivot shift test, 132*f*
Plagiocephaly, 38
Plans in POMR progress notes, 15–16
Plantar fascitis, 41, 320
Platelet count, 187, 189*t*, 190
Platybasia, 165*t*
Plegia, 167
Pleural effusion, 224
Pneumonia, unresolving, 225
Pneumoperitoneum, 223
Poikilocytosis, 188
Polycythemias, 188
Polyneuropathy, 174
POMR. *See* Problem-oriented medical recordkeeping
Posterior cord syndrome, 160*t*
Posterior joint pathology, 100*f*, 102*f*
Posterior spine, 157
Post-facilitation stretch therapy, 402, 404
Post-isometric relaxation (PIR), 402, 403–404

Postures
intracranial lesions and, 159–160
spine pain and, 295
Potassium, 195*t*, 201
Prayer sign (reverse Phalen's test), 125*f*
Pregnancy, 295
contraindications to joint manipulation, 377
Pre-hypertension, 67
Pre-participation physical examination (PPE) for athletes, 34–36
Presbycusis, 73
Presbyopia, 72
Prescription writing, 18–19
Preventive health, definition of, 8
Privacy Rule, HIPAA, 19
Problem list, POMR, 13, 13*t*, 14
Problem-oriented medical recordkeeping (POMR), 12–16
complete problem list components, 13*t*
comprehensive database, 13–14
initial plans, 13*t*, 14–15
progress notes, 14*t*, 15–16
Progress notes, POMR, 13, 14*t*, 15–16
Progressive stretch mobilization (PSM), 381, 408
Pronator drift, 169
Pronator teres syndrome, 320
Proprioception function, 157
Proprioceptive neuromuscular facilitation (PNF), 402
Prosopagnosia, 184
Prostate, benign hyperplasia of, 305
Prostate cancer, 270*t*, 271, 274*t*
Prostate specific antigen, 275
Protein electrophoresis, serum (SPE), 201, 201*f*, 275
Protein, serum, 195*t*, 202
Provocative factors, of complaints, 56
Pseudobulbar palsy, 184
Pseudomonas, 291
Psoas sign, 85
Psoriasis, ear canal and, 74
Psoriatic arthritis, 263, 290
Psychosocial history, chief complaint and, 61
Pulse (resting), 32, 33*t*, 63, 64*t*, 65*t*, 78
Pulse pressure, 67, 67*t*
Pupils, 70, 70*t*, 72
Pyrosis, 88

Q

Quadriplegia, 184
Quality, of complaints, 56

R

Raccoon eyes, 85
Radial artery insufficiency, 113*f*
Radial ligaments, 123*f*
Radiation, of chief complaint, 56
Radiculoneuropathy, 105*f*
Radiculopathy, 162
bowstring sign and, 103*f*
cervical
Bakody's sign and, 97*f*
shoulder depression test and, 101*f*
somatosensory evoked potentials and, 177
cervical compression test and, 98*f*
contraindications to joint manipulation with, 375
definition of, 184
electromyography and, 178
signs and symptoms of, 164*t*
symptoms of, 162–163
Radiocarpal joint mobilization, 413–414
Radiography, cervical spine trauma, 350–351, 351*t*
Radiohumeral bursitis, 122*f*
Radiology
abdomen and chest evaluation, 211, 216, 218–219, 222–225
basic interpretation rules, 207–211
arthritides, 209
bone tumors, 208
congenital lesions, 210
general bone studies, 208
infection, 210
soft tissues, 210–211
trauma, 209
basic physics
procedures, 226, 228–229, 228*t*
rules, 225–226
common causes of common lesions, 211, 221*t*
common indications for musculoskeletal, 206*t*
differential diagnosis and follow-up imaging, 211, 212–216*t*, 217–218*t*, 219*t*, 220*t*
as element in orders, 18
reports, 229, 231–232
selected techniques, 230*t*
lower extremity, 232*t*
upper extremity, 231*t*
standard kVp for different body regions, 227*f*
standard views, 229, 233*t*
ten rules of, 205–207

Radionuclide bone scanning, 236, 236*t*
Range of motion, 135, 136–137*t*
Raynaud's disease, 321
Raynaud's phenomenon, 85
Receptive aphasia, 181
Reciprocal inhibition, 402, 404
Rectal examination, digital, 250–251
Red blood cell (RBC) count, 187, 188, 189*t*
Refills, as order in prescriptions, 19
Reflexes, examination of, 168
Rehabilitation. *See also* Physical medicine
  introduction, 391
Reiter's syndrome, 263–264, 290
Remission, definition of, 285
Renal calcification, 223. *See also under* Kidney
Research subjects, 333
  practice boundaries and, 333–334
Respiration, Cheyne-Stokes, 77, 78*f*
Respiratory rate, 26, 64, 64*t*, 66*t*
Reticuloendothelial cancer tests, 274*t*
Retinitis pigmentosa, 72
Retinopathy, 72
Retrobulbar neuritis, 176
Review of systems (ROS), 59, 60*t*
Rheumatoid arthritis, 261–262, 290
Rheumatoid factor (RA latex), 195*t*, 202, 260
Rheumatology. *See also* Arthritides
  disease classification, 257
    history, 257, 259
    laboratory investigation, 260–261
    physical examination, 259–260
    radiographic investigation, 261
  disease types, 261–267
    ankylosing spondylitis, 262
    calcium pyrophosphate crystal deposition disease, 264–265
    degenerative joint disease, 265–266
    diffuse idiopathic skeletal hyperostosis, 266
    enteropathic arthritis, 264
    fibromyalgia syndrome, 266–267
    gouty arthritis, 264
    hydroxyapatite deposition disease, 265
    psoriatic arthritis, 263
    Reiter's syndrome, 263–264
    rheumatoid arthritis, 261–262
  introduction, 257
Rhinitis, allergic, 74
Rib lesions, 294
Right to health care, 331
Rigidity, abdominal, 83
Rinne's test, 73
Risser-Ferguson measurement method for scoliosis, 141*f*
Risser's sign of skeletal maturation, 141*f*
Romberg test, 169
Rotator cuff disease, 121*f*, 321
Rotator cuff tear/rupture, 116*f*
Rothwell, D. M., 378
Rust's sign, 85, 100*f*
Rx, use in prescriptions, 18–19

S

Sacroiliac disease, 111*f*, 112*f*, 126*f*, 127*f*
Sacroiliac joint disease, 129*f*
Sacroiliac joint dysfunction, 297, 321–322
Sacroiliac lesion, 104*f*, 110*f*
Sacroiliitis, 213*t*
Sail sign, 217*t*
Sarcoma, definition of, 285
Sausage digit, 217*t*
Scaphoid fracture, 125*f*
Scapulothoracic joint mobilization, 412
Scheuermann's disease, 39
Schilling's test, 202
School backpacks, 41
Sciatica, neural mobilization and, 415
Scissor gait, 171
Sclera, 69, 71
Sclerotic vertebra, 213*t*
Scoliosis, 135
  Adam's position and, 102*f*
  benign bone tumors and, 282
  Cobb measurement method for, 140*f*
  curvature progression, 143
  epidemiology, 138*t*
  etiology, 137
  family history of, 138
  painful, differential diagnosis of, 213*t*
  physical examination, 138–139
  radiographic examination, 139
  Risser-Ferguson measurement method for, 141*f*
  Risser's sign of skeletal maturation and, 141*f*
  treatment, 139–141, 142*t*, 143
Scotty dog sign, 217*t*
Seatbelts, whiplash injuries and, 348
Seated straight leg raise test, 96*f*
Secondary tumors, definition of, 285
Sedation, conscious, joint manipulation under, 380
Seizures, 172
  aquatic sports and, 36
  contraindications to joint manipulation, 377

EEG for diagnosis of, 179
photic stimulation and, 179
Self care, definition of, 9
Sensory examination, 168–169
Serum chemistries, 193, 195–203
acid phosphatase, 193
albumin, 193, 195
albumin/globulin ratio, 195
alkaline phosphatase, 195–196
alpha-fetoprotein (AFP), 196
amylase, 196
anti-double stranded DNA antibody, 196
antinuclear antibody, 196
antistreptolysin-o titre, 196
bicarbonate, 197
bilirubin, 197
calcium, 197
chloride, 198
cholesterol, 198
common values, 194–195*t*
creatine phosphokinase (CPK), 198
creatinine, 198
fluorescent treponemal antibody absorbed, 198
gamma-glutamyl transpeptidase, 198
globulin, 198
glucose, 198–199
glutamic-oxoacetic transaminase, 197, 202
glutamic-pyruvic transaminase, 193, 202
hemoglobin A1C, 199
high-density lipoprotein cholesterol, 199
human chorionic gonadotropin, 199
human T-lymphocyte virus, 199
iron, 199
iron binding capacity, total, 199
lactate dehydrogenase, 200
lipase, 200
low-density lipoprotein cholesterol, 200
lupus erythematosus cell preparation, 200
monospot, 200
parathyroid hormone (PTH), 200
phosphorus, 200
potassium, 201
protein, 202
protein electrophoresis, 201, 201*f*
rheumatoid factor, 202
sodium, 202
special studies, 203–204
specific panels, 204, 204*t*
thyroid stimulating hormone, 202
thyroxine, 203
triglycerides, 203
triiodothyronine, 203
troponin I, 203
uric acid, 203
venereal disease research laboratory, 203
vitamin B12, 202
Serum glutamic-oxoacetic transaminase (SGOT), 195*t*, 197, 202
Serum glutamic-pyruvic transaminase (SGPT), 193, 195*t*, 202
Setting, of chief complaint, 56
Sever's disease, 40–41
Shekelle, P. G., 377
Shingles. *See* Herpes zoster
Short leg syndrome, 295
Shoulder depression test, 101*f*
Shoulder dislocation, 117*f*, 215*t*
Shoulder fractures, 215*t*
Shoulder, tests of, 114–121*f*
Shuffling gait, 171
SI joint dysfunction, 297. *See also under* Sacroiliac
Sick role, definition of, 9
Sickle cell anemia, 188
Sig., use in prescriptions, 19
Simple bone cysts, 283
Sinding Larsen-Johansson disease, 40
Sinusoidal current, 392*t*, 398–399, 399*t*
Sitting slump test, 108*f*
Skeletal malignancy. *See* Bone tumors, malignant
Skin, examination of, 68
Skull radiograph interpretation, 238, 241*t*
Slipped capital femoral epiphysis (SCFE), 40
Snuff box palpation, 125*f*
SOAP (mnemonic), 15–16
Sodium, 195*t*, 202
Soft tissues, radiographic interpretation of, 210–211
Somatosensory evoked potentials (SSEP), 176, 177
Soto-Hall test, 101*f*
Space-occupying lesions, 100*f*
Spastic gait, 171
Spastic paralysis, 154
Specialized notes, 16
Specific gravity, of urine, 191
Spinal canal stenosis, 184, 322, 364
contraindications to joint manipulation, 376
Spinal cord compression, 99*f*
Spinal cord injuries, 177
Spinal cord lesions, 157, 159, 159*t*, 163, 165
common, 165*t*
examination for, 271

Spinal cord syndromes, 160*t*
Spinal cord transection, 165
Spinal cord tumors, 294, 295
  contraindications to joint manipulation in, 375
Spinal joint dysfunction, 290
Spinal lesions
  differential diagnosis of, 214*t*
  unstable, 220*t*
Spinal manipulative therapy, 365, 372
Spinal stabilization exercises, 405–407, 406*t*
Spinal tap, 179–180
Spinal tumors, lumbar puncture and, 180
Spine
  biomechanics, 288
  contraindications to joint manipulation, 375
  joint mobilization, 408–409
  radiograph interpretation, 238, 239*t*
  structural landmarks, 287
Spine pain
  introduction, 287
  mimicry syndromes, 295–298
  referred, 293–295
  vertebrogenic
    arthritides, 288–290
    biomechanical, 290
    common causes of, 289*t*
    developmental, 290–291
    infectious, 291
    metabolic, 291
    miscellaneous, 292
    trauma, 292
    tumors, 292–293
Spine tests
  cervical, 97–102*f*
  general, 94*f*
  lumbar, 102–109*f*
  thoracic, 102*f*
Spleen, calcification in, 223
Splenomegaly, 88, 223
Splinter hemorrhages, 85
Spondylitis, ankylosing, 262, 288–289
Spondylolisthesis, 143, 292
  clinical findings, 143–144
  contraindications to joint manipulation, 377
  diagnosis, 144–145
  grades, 145*t*
  pathogenesis, 144
  treatment, 145–146
Spondylolytic spondylolisthesis, 144
Spondylosis, 177
Spondylotic myelopathy, 185
Sprains. *See also* Sprain/strain management
  cervical compression test and, 98*f*
  differential diagnosis, 340*t*
  grading system, 340*t*
  management, 342–343
  signs and symptoms, 341*t*
  spinal, 292
Sprain/strain management, 340–341. *See also* Sprains; Strains
  introduction, 339–340
  prognosis, 344
Spray and stretch technique, 393–394
Spurling's maneuver, 102*f*
Standing orders (SO), 16
STAT, as order note, 17
State laws
  common reportable patient care circumstances under, 12*t*
  on medical recordkeeping, 11–12
  on prescriptions, 18
Stenosing tenosynovitis, 124*f*, 308
Stenosis. *See also* Spinal canal stenosis
  lateral recess, 184
Steppage gait, 171
Sternoclavicular joint mobilization, 412
Stomach cancer, 273, 275
Straight Back Syndrome, 295
Strains. *See also* Sprain/strain management
  differential diagnosis of, 340*t*
  grading system, 340*t*
  management of, 343–344
  signs and symptoms of, 341*t*
  spinal, 292
Strawberry tongue, 86
Stroke, manipulation-related, 378
Subarachnoid hemorrhage, lumbar puncture and, 180
Subcortical lesions, 154, 161*t*
Subjective progress notes, POMR, 15
Subluxation, 121*f*
Subscapularis dysfunction, 117*f*
Subscapularis tendinitis, 118*f*
Subtalar joint mobilization, 410
Supplements/nutraceuticals, 18
Supranuclear ophthalmoplegia, 185
Supraspinatus impingement, 119*f*
Supraspinatus musculotendinous disease, 115*f*
Supraspinatus tendinitis, 119*f*
Supratentorial lesions, 160–161, 161*t*
Surgery, in hospitals/long-term care facilities, 49–50
Sustained natural apophyseal glides (SNAGs), 381, 383
Swan neck deformity, 217*t*

Swimmer's ear, 73
Symbols (abbreviations chart), 417–429
Syncope, 35, 174–175, 175*t*, 179
Synesthesia, 185
Synovitis, 292
Syphilis, 72
Syringomyelia, 165, 177, 185
  contraindications to joint manipulation, 377
Systems, review of
  chief complaint and history, 59
  elements in, 60*t*
Systolic heart murmurs, 78

T

Tabes dorsalis (neurosyphilis), 163
Talonavicular joint mobilization, 410
Target cells, 188
Tarsal tunnel syndrome, 163*t*
Tarsometatarsal joint mobilization, 411
Telephone orders, 17
Temperature, 64*t*, 157
Temporomandibular joint disease, 293
Tender points, 404–405
Tensor fascia lata contraction, 127*f*
Tentorium cerebelli, 160–161
Teres minor, 121*f*
Terry Thomas sign, 217*t*
Third-party payers, medical recordkeeping for, 11–12
Thomas test, 128*f*
Thompson's test, 134*f*
Thoracic extension, progressive or continuous, 385
Thoracic outlet neurovascular compression syndrome, 112*f*, 113*f*
Thoracic outlet syndrome, 113*f*, 162, 163*t*, 179, 322–323
Thoracic spine
  contraindications to joint manipulation, 376
  fractures of, differential diagnosis of, 214*t*
  referred spine pain and, 293–294
  tests, 102*f*
  visceral disease mimicry and dysfunction of, 296–297
Thoracolumbar back pain, 349
Thorax, 75–77, 76*t*
Throat, examination of, 74–75
Thrombophlebitis, 319
Thumb, 124*f*, 414
Thyroid cancer, 274*t*
Thyroid stimulating hormone (TSH), 195*t*, 202
Thyroxine (T4 total), 195*t*, 203
Tibial tubercle apophysitis, 40
Tic Douloureux, 323–324
Tics, 167, 172
Timing, of chief complaint, 56
Tinel's sign
  at the elbow, 123*f*
  at the wrist, 125*f*
Tinnitus, 185
Tongue
  cranial nerve lesions and, 75
  strawberry, 86
Topagnosis, 185
Traction, 401
  contraindications, 402*t*
Transcutaneous electrical nerve stimulation (TENS), 399–400
Transient ischemic attack, 323
Transitional segment, lumbosacral, 323
Transverse friction massage (TFM), 402
Transverse tarsal joint mobilization, 410
Trauma, 209, 214*t*, 221*t*, 292
Traumatic spondylolisthesis, 144
Treatment, as element in orders, 17
Tremors, 167, 175
Trendelenburg's test, 128*f*
Triano, J. J., 372
Trigeminal neuralgia, 323–324
Trigger points (TrPs), 295, 297–298, 404–405
Triglycerides, 195*t*, 203
Triiodothyronine (T3 RIA), 195*t*, 203
Tripod sign, 109*f*
Trolley-track sign, 217*t*
Troponin I, 195*t*, 203
Tuberculosis, 291
Tumors, 59, 69, 285, 292–293

U

Ulnar artery insufficiency, 113*f*
Ulnar ligaments, 123*f*
Ultrasound
  diagnostic, 236, 236*t*
  therapeutic, 392*t*, 396, 398
    contraindications, 397*t*
    indications, 397*t*
Unicameral bone cysts, 283
Unilateral organs, exercise and, 36
Unstable injuries, definition of, 348
Updates, as element in orders, 18
Upper body screening examination, 146–147, 147*t*
Upper motor neuron lesions (UMNLs), 154, 155*t*

Uric acid, 195*t*, 203
Urinalysis, 190–193
  bilirubin, 192
  blood, 192
  glucose, 191
  ketones, 192
  nitrites, 192
  normal values, 191*t*
  pH, 191
  specific gravity, 191
  urobilinogen, 193
Urine casts, 192*t*
Urine specimen collection, 247–248
Urobilinogen, urinary, 193
Uterine cancer, 295
Uvula, cranial nerve lesions and, 75

V

Vacuum phenomenon, 217*t*
Valgus stress
  of the ankle/foot, 135*f*
  of the hand, 126*f*
  ligamentous stability in fingers, 126*f*
  of the radial (lateral) collateral ligament, 123*f*
  of the ulnar (medial) collateral ligament, 123*f*
Varus stress
  of the ankle/foot, 135*f*
  of the hand, 126*f*
  ligamentous stability in fingers, 126*f*
Vas deferens calcification, 223
Vascular claudication, 324
Vascular diseases
  brainstem lesions and, 165, 165*t*
  cerebral lesions and, 166*t*
  common causes of, 221*t*
  George's tests for, 378
Veins, right antecubital fossa, 247*f*
Venereal disease research laboratory (VDRL) tests, 203
Venipuncture, 245–247, 248*f*
Venules, in eyes, 72
Veracity, 331
Verbal dysdecorum, 185
Verbal orders, 16–17
Vertebrae. *See under* Spinal; Spine
Vertebral anomalies, 291
Vertebral artery dissection, 324–325
Vertebrobasilar artery damage, manipulation and, 378, 379
Vertebrobasilar ischemia/dissection, 379*t*
Vertigo. *See also* Dizziness
  benign paroxysmal positional, 325, 326*t*
  cervical spine trauma and, 350
  cervicogenic, 325
  differential diagnosis of, 175
Virchow's node, 83
Vision examination, 70
Visual evoked potentials (VEP), 176
Visual fields
  examination of, 71
  loss of, 72
Vital signs, 63
  for adults, 64*t*
  for children, 32
  clinical pearls, 63–64, 67
  for elderly patients, 25–26
Vitamin B-12
  deficiency, 177, 325–326
  Schilling's test for, 202

W

Weakness
  muscular, 175, 178
  subjective, 35
Weber's test, 73
Weed, Larry, 12–13
Weight loss, unexplained, 89
Wellness, 8–9
Wernicke's (receptive) aphasia, 181
Wheezing, 35, 89
Whiplash, 347
Whiplash syndrome, chronic, 353–355
Whirlpool baths, 394
White blood cell (WBC) count, 187–188, 189, 189*t*, 275
White blood cell (WBC) differential, 190
World Health Organization, 21
Wright's hyperabduction test, 113*f*
Wrist
  dislocations, differential diagnosis of, 215*t*
  fractures, differential diagnosis of, 215*t*
  joint mobilization, 413–414
  tests of, 124–125*f*
Written orders, 16

Y

Yeoman's test, 129*f*
Yergason's test, 121*f*
Youth diseases. *See also* Children
  chief complaint and, 59